# PRIMARY CARE in the HOME

# PRIMARY CARE in the HOME

**LAWRENCE H. BERNSTEIN,** M.D.
*Mansfield Family Practice*
*Storrs, Connecticut*
*Assistant Clinical Professor in Medicine*
*University of Connecticut School of Medicine*
*Farmington, Connecticut*

**ANTHONY J. GRIECO,** M.D.
*Professor of Clinical Medicine*
*New York University School of Medicine*
*Medical Director, Cooperative Care Center*
*New York University Medical Center*
*New York, New York*

**MARY K. DETE,** R.N., B.S.N., P.H.N.
*Vice President, Patient Services*
*Hospital Home Health Care Agency of California*
*Torrance, California*

 **J. B. Lippincott Company**
Philadelphia
*London*
*Mexico City*
*New York*
*St. Louis*
*São Paulo*
*Sydney*

Acquisitions Editor: Patricia Cleary
Sponsoring Editor: Joyce Mkitarian
Manuscript Editor: Judith Ebbert
Indexer: Maria Coughlin
Art Director: Tracy Baldwin

Designer: Susan Hess
Production Supervisor: Carol Florence
Production Assistant: Barney Fernandes
Compositor: Circle Graphics
Printer/Binder: RRD

6 5 4 2

**Library of Congress Cataloging-in-Publication Data**

Primary care in the home.

Includes bibliographies and index.
1. Home nursing. I. Bernstein, Lawrence H.
II. Grieco, Anthony J. III. Dete, Mary K.
[DNLM: 1. Home Care Services. 2. Primary Health
Care. WY 115 P952]
RT120.H65P75 1987 649'.8 86-20857

The authors and publisher have exerted every effort to ensure that drug
selection and dosage set forth in this text are in accord with current
recommendations and practice at the time of publication. However, in
view of ongoing research, changes in government regulations, and the
constant flow of information relating to drug therapy and drug reactions, the reader is urged to check the package insert for each drug for
any change in indications and dosage and for added warnings and
precautions. This is particularly important when the recommended
agent is a new or infrequently employed drug.

To our patients and to their families
and care partners, who make home
care work so well

# Contributors

**Steven Abramson, M.D.**
Associate Professor of Medicine
New York University School of Medicine
New York, New York

**Joseph Agris, M.D.**
Plastic and Reconstructive Surgery
Texas Medical Center
Houston, Texas

**Lisa E. Babitz, M.D.**
Teaching Assistant in Medicine
New York University School of Medicine
Fellow in Geriatrics
New York University Medical Center
New York, New York

**Barbara Z. Berk, M.D.**
Teaching Assistant in Medicine
Fellow in Geriatrics
New York University School of Medicine
New York University Medical Center
New York, New York

**Lawrence H. Bernstein, M.D.**
Mansfield Family Practice
Storrs, Connecticut
Assistant Clinical Professor in Medicine
University of Connecticut School of Medicine
Farmington, Connecticut

**Diane S. Blum, M.S.W.**
Director of Social Work
National Cancer Care Foundation
New York, New York

**Ronald H. Blum, M.D.**
Professor of Medicine
New York University School of Medicine
Associate Director, Rita and Stanley H. Kaplan
  Cancer Center
New York University Medical Center
New York, New York

**Mitchell H. Charap, M.D.**
Assistant Professor of Medicine
New York University School of Medicine
New York, New York

**Richard Conviser, Ph.D.**
Project Specialist
Empire Blue Cross and Blue Shield
New York, New York

**Dianna M. D'Amico, R.N., B.S.N., C.R.R.N.**
Independent Living Experience Coordinator
Rusk Institute of Rehabilitation Medicine
New York, New York

**Mary K. Dete, R.N., B.S.N., P.H.N.**
Vice President, Patient Services
Hospital Home Health Care Agency
  of California
Torrance, California

**Eduardo M. Farcon, M.D.**
Clinical Associate Professor of Urology
New York University Medical Center
New York, New York

**Michael L. Freedman, M.D.**
Professor of Medicine
New York University School of Medicine
Director, Division of Geriatrics
New York University Medical Center
New York, New York

**Stuart M. Garay, M.D.**
Assistant Professor of Clinical Medicine
New York University School of Medicine
New York, New York

**Shirley Garnett, R.N., M.S.**
Manager, Education Center
Cooperative Care Center
New York University Medical Center
New York, New York

**Eli Ginzberg, Ph.D.**
Professor of Economics
Director, Conservation of Human Resources
Columbia University
New York, New York

**Thomas H. Gouge, M.D.**
Associate Professor of Clinical Surgery
New York University School of Medicine
New York, New York

**Jeffrey Greene, M.D.**
Clinical Associate Professor of Medicine
New York University School of Medicine
New York, New York

**Robert M. Greenstein, M.D.**
Professor of Pediatrics
University of Connecticut School of Medicine
Director, Research and Training Center for
    Pediatric Rehabilitation
Farmington, Connecticut

**Anthony J. Grieco, M.D.**
Professor of Clinical Medicine
New York University School of Medicine
Medical Director, Cooperative Care Center
New York University Medical Center
New York, New York

**Suzanne Stefanowski Hudd, M.P.H.**
Director of Information and Resource
    Development
Research and Training Center for Pediatric
    Rehabilitation
University of Connecticut School of Medicine
Farmington, Connecticut

**Martin L. Kahn, M.D.**
Professor of Clinical Medicine
New York University School of Medicine
New York, New York

**Owen P. Kieran, M.D.**
Clinical Instructor of Rehabilitation Medicine
New York University Medical Center
New York, New York

**Wanda Kowalski, R.N., M.A.**
Clinical Assistant Director of Nursing
Cooperative Care Center
New York University Medical Center
New York, New York

**Paul S. Kurtin, M.D.**
Assistant Professor of Pediatrics and Medicine
Tufts University School of Medicine
Chief, Division of Pediatric Nephrology
New England Medical Center
Boston, Massachusetts

**Abraham N. Lieberman, M.D.**
Professor of Neurology
New York University School of Medicine
New York, New York

**Mack Lipkin, Jr., M.D.**
Adjunct Associate Professor of Medicine
New York University School of Medicine
Director, Primary Care Program
New York University Medical Center
New York, New York

**Michael R. McGarvey, M.D.**
Corporate Vice President, Health Affairs
Empire Blue Cross and Blue Shield
New York, New York

**Patricia Minuchin, Ph.D.**
Research Professor
Department of Psychiatry
New York University School of Medicine
New York, New York

**Salvador Minuchin, M.D.**
Research Professor
Department of Psychiatry
New York University School of Medicine
New York, New York

**Pablo A. Morales, M.D.**
Professor and Chairman
Department of Urology
New York University School of Medicine
Director of Urology
Bellevue Hospital Center and New York
    University Medical Center
New York, New York

**Grace Phelan, R.N., M.S.N.**
Supervisor, Education Center
Cooperative Care Center
New York University Medical Center
New York, New York

**Laurie R. Stuhl Prowler, O.T.R.**
Specialist in Barrier Free Design
Rusk Institute of Rehabilitation Medicine
New York, New York

**Elizabeth A. Purcell, R.N., B.S., E.T.**
Clinical Nurse Specialist, Enterostomal
    Therapist
New York University Medical Center
New York, New York

**Alex Rosen, Ph.D.**
Formerly Dean, School of Social Work
New York University
New York, New York

**Howard G. Thistle, M.D.**
Associate Professor of Clinical Rehabilitation
    Medicine
New York University School of Medicine
New York, New York

**Mary Ellen Wadsworth, R.N., M.P.H.**
Coordinator of Outpatient Education
Cooperative Care Center
New York University Medical Center
New York, New York

**John Whelan, R.N., B.S.N.**
Urology Department Head
Rusk Institute of Rehabilitation Medicine
New York University Medical Center
New York, New York

**Sarah Williams, M.D.**
Clinical Instructor in Medicine
New York University School of Medicine
New York, New York

**Michael D. Witt, Pharm.D., J.D.**
Attorney, Health Care Department
Warner and Stackpole
Boston, Massachusetts

# Preface

We have written this book on home care to share our excitement about the changing style of medicine. Home care is an entity composed of many facets—people, supplies, technology, and programs; therapists, commodes, parenteral nutrition, and care plans. But the whole, the end result, is greater than the sum of its parts. It is this end result, the impact on the patient, that we have tried to articulate through the individual chapters, hoping to convey the flavor of the process. An understanding of this process will embody the concept of "team"—the glue that holds all of this together.

If we are to define home care as, in large part, a process, we should be able to define the proceedings better. For that purpose, we have included a fair amount of didactic material in the book, but there also is a component of style. Certainly, we cannot provide home care without the requisite knowledge; it is equally difficult without adapting our style. Some of the chapters focus on knowledge, others on style; it is the combination that results in successful home care. If, with this book, we are able to spread our enthusiasm for both these components, we will be gratified.

*Lawrence H. Bernstein, M.D.*

*Anthony J. Grieco, M.D.*

*Mary K. Dete, R.N., B.S.N., P.H.N.*

# Contents

# Introduction

## ELI GINZBERG

Some years ago I was called out of a business meeting at noon to answer a telephone call from our long-term family physician, Dr. K., a distinguished internist with 30 years' experience. My wife had not been feeling well for some time, and under pressure from both of us the doctor had arranged to have her x-rayed that morning by one of the city's leading radiologists. He had just gotten the report: my wife had tuberculosis. Admission to the hospital (a prominent teaching institution) was urgent, and the doctor would try to arrange for a consultation late that afternoon. Had I not been rattled, I would have questioned the diagnosis since my wife had been gaining, not losing, weight. Later in the day it took the consultant no more than three questions to settle the matter: the correct diagnosis was a lung abscess; the proper therapy, an 8-day cycle of antibiotic treatment to be administered twice daily.

After two or three days, my wife suggested that Dr. K. send her home and she would arrange with the Visiting Nurse Service for her daily injections. The doctor said that was impossible because my wife would need the antibiotic injections over the weekend. She explained that the VNS made weekend calls, but Dr. K. remained unconvinced. My wife was discharged from the hospital against advice, and, Dr. K.'s skepticism notwithstanding, she made a normal recovery at home.

This condensed tale helps to highlight several aspects of "home care," each of which warrants brief attention. The first and most important is that physicians in the post–World War II era have become hospital-fixated for good and bad reasons: it is often easier to diagnose and treat a patient in a hospital setting; it is more convenient (and also more profitable) for the physician to have a number of patients congregated in the hospital where he can draw upon an elaborate support staff, from residents to consultants; and until recently most insurance policies provided coverage only for patients who were hospitalized.

How different the situation was in my youth. Both my sister and I were born at home (1914 and 1911, respectively), and my sister had her tonsils removed at home (on the kitchen table) by a surgeon who was assisted by our family doctor.

Shortly after the end of World War II, Dr. E.M. Bluestone, the then head of Montefiore Hospital, developed a "home health care program" with the aim of speeding the discharge of his predominantly chronic patient load. Although the program caught the attention of many hospital planners and administrators, it was not broadly replicated and with time it stagnated even at Montefiore as the hospital became increasingly a tertiary-care institution.

Now, a third of a century later, the subject of "home care" is once again on the nation's health agenda, and for a variety of reasons it is likely that this time it will become an institutionalized modality of care. Since the explicit purpose of this text is to assist the "primary care physician and nurse to provide better patient care in the home," it highlights the differences that confront the medical team in providing treatment in the home rather than in the office or in the hospital. Several chapters emphasize various aspects of the physician's "management" of such care through intermediaries, principally family members and ancillary professional and paraprofessional personnel, the home-care nurse being the most prominent.

A look at the chapter titles in Part 3, Providing Care at Home, reveals that this volume is heavily focused on patients with serious chronic conditions that require ongoing medical attention. This sensible and desirable emphasis requires that the full reach of home health care be described briefly, if only to provide an overview of the entire terrain and to distinguish among the major patient groups.

The first differentiation relates to the large numbers of "frail elderly" who, because of reduced physical vigor (often associated with some loss of mental acuity), can no longer be solely responsible for their own maintenance and functioning. They require varying degrees of assistance, from continuous (in the case of the bedridden) to periodic help with shopping, housekeeping, and other activities such as taking a walk, going to church, keeping a doctor's appointment, and so on. The key to their continued ability to live at home is the presence of one or more persons, usually family members, who are able and willing to provide the range of support services required, often supplemented by assistance from paid health-care and personal-care workers and from volunteers.

Many of the frail elderly have no specific health condition that requires continuing observation and treatment, but this does not mean that such a condition will not develop. The odds are that sooner or later one or more—acute or chronic—will. The greater the number of the frail elderly who are encouraged and assisted to live at home, the more important it becomes that they have ongoing access to medical care: for the mobile, in a physician's office or nearby clinic; for the immobile, through a house call and nursing visits.

At the opposite end of the spectrum of patients requiring home health care are those who have been discharged from the hospital because their physician believes that their convalescence can proceed satisfactorily at home, often with some continuing professional attention, be it medical, nursing, or physiotherapy. Whether and to what extent the hospitalized patient can be discharged earlier than in the past depends on the presence of support personnel in the home and the availability of qualified professional personnel (*i.e.,* physicians and others) who will provide essential services, when needed, in the home during the remaining period of the patient's convalescence. In a visit some months ago to a leading academic health center in the Midwest I was startled to hear the comment, "Our patients are now being discharged in a sicker condition than when they entered the hospital." Clearly such patients need to be monitored, assessed, and often treated at home.

In addition to the frail elderly and the convalescent discharged from an acute-care hospital—two large groups of individuals who under varying conditions will need health services in their homes—this book is focused on a third group—the many children, adults, and older persons who suffer from a serious ailment that requires ongoing medical management. Among these are young people with genetic illnesses; patients suffering from neurologic disease; patients requiring parenteral therapy; cancer victims; terminal patients; and still others who must be under a physician's care even if much of the actual service will be rendered by nurses and paraprofessionals.

One more observation about the categorization of home-care patients. There is nothing stable or static about the medical status of most individuals and about their need for medical attention and treatment. The convalescent cardiac patient, recently discharged from the hospital, can acquire an upper respiratory disease that must be diagnosed and treated. The homebound, chronically ill individual may develop an acute condition totally unrelated to his principal disability that requires attention. Alternatively, many persons with chronic illness reach a stage at which their condition stabilizes and they are better able to cope with it. Some bedridden patients regain mobility and others who were ambulatory become bedridden. A major challenge to effective home health care is to ensure that the physician and the other members of the treatment and support team do not assume that their initial assessment and therapeutic plan will continue unaltered. Periodic reassessment is critically important if homebound patients are to receive adequate care, with the nurse playing an integral role.

It may be illuminating to review, at least briefly, the congeries of mutually reinforcing factors that have effected a resurgence of home health care after decades of decline, almost to the point of disappearance. Without attaching any special significance to their order, the following factors help to explain the new thrust to home care.

The determination of the payers for health care (particularly government and insurance, which together provide almost 7 out of every 10 dollars) to contain their outlays is a major element in the new equation. With acute hospital care accounting for roughly $160 billion out of $400 billion total health-care expenditures in 1985, payers are looking for alternatives to costly hospitalization. They believe that they have found a good alternative in discharging patients more quickly than in the past. The rapid decline in average length of hospital stay of the elderly from mid-1983 and continuing into the first half of 1985, amounting to around 15%, is strongly supportive of this approach.

But the trend toward earlier discharge has not gone unchallenged. There is considerable anecdotal evidence to the effect that many patients are being discharged prematurely and, to make matters worse, adequate home health-care services are not available to provide the professional and social supports that they require. Admittedly, a great many new home health-care programs are being put in place by acute-care hospitals and nonprofit and for-profit providers, and many older, established programs are being expanded. But patients, their families, and their physicians are only slowly becoming aware of the potential of the new, expanded capacity and how best to make use of it.

A second force that is giving a boost to home health care is the growing awareness of many laymen and physicians that hospitals represent an environment that is not free of risk to the patient. The less time a patient is in a hospital, the less likely that he will be exposed to the dangers of infection, errors in medication, or other dysfunctional experiences. If one needs hospitalization, the risks are worth it, but once one can convalesce at home, there is no point to continuing to tempt fate.

One of the principal reasons for the stagnation of the Montefiore home health-care program of the late 1940s was the general shortage of physicians, which encouraged doctors to allocate their time with the aim of treating an optimal number of patients. Requiring the patient to come to the physician's office or retaining him in the hospital was a way of conserving the physician's time. The last decades have seen a substantial increase in the number of physicians per 100,000 population, from around 140 after World War II to about 220 per 100,000 population in 1985. This represents an increase of more than 50% even if one disregards the fact that the typical physician today is better prepared, having undergone seven or more years of formal training compared to five years of training in the earlier period. Moreover, the "pipeline" is full of new physicians, and each year will see many more physicians entering than retiring from practice. To put the matter starkly, up to the early to mid 1970s, patients encountered difficulties in getting appointments with physicians; in recent years, more and more physicians have been experiencing gaps in their appointment books. A secondary reason for the return of home health care is the growing scramble of physicians for patients and the opportunities that some of them are finding to establish or expand their practices by treating patients at home.

Still another factor that is operating to expand home health care is patient demand. In the early years of Medicaid, nursing homes expanded rapidly and many families, especially those in the lower income brackets, welcomed the opportunity to transfer to them difficult members of their households who could use institutional supervision and care. But governments, finding their outlays for nursing-home care growing out of control, have erected barriers to their continued expansion and, more important, many of the elderly have evinced strong preferences for avoiding institutionalization as long as possible. These combined forces are helping to ensure that more of the elderly, both frail and sick, remain at home where many of them require medical attention.

Also leading to the expansion of home health care are recent developments on the entrepreneurial and delivery fronts. Upjohn, a leading for-profit pharmaceutical company, has long been an important provider of home health-care services. In the past few years several other for-profit and nonprofit organizations have entered the field. In the face of a declining inpatient census, many hospitals have established home health-care departments; also, there are old and new community agencies that have expanded or started such programs. The recent rapid expansion in HMO enrollments is also encouraging some of the plans to explore and undertake these activities. The inclusion of another low-cost setting in their panoply of treatment sites is a way of improving the range of their services within a total price that remains competitive.

There is no need to extend this list. Clearly a great many potent forces—economic, professional, entrepreneurial, and consumer preference—are reinforcing each other to speed the growth of home health-care programs. It would be an error, however, to conclude from the foregoing that home health care is the wave of the future and that its indefinite growth is ensured. Consider the following: A major determinant of the feasibility of caring for a sick person at home, especially one with a serious chronic condition, is the presence of one or more able-bodied members of the household who will assist in the care of the invalid. We know that only a minority of aged parents still live in the same household with one of their children or in close proximity. We know further that fewer than 25% of all persons aged 75 and above are living with a spouse. Moreover, even among those who do, the spouse may be too feeble to provide the care that the sick member requires and there may not be sufficient income to hire full-time or even part-time help.

Put another way, home health care has much to commend it if there are capable, nonemployed members of the household available to care for a sick child, adult, or elderly parent or spouse. But the key is the presence of the able-bodied, nonemployed household member. The demographic trends are, however, clearly moving in the opposite direction. More and more women are more or less regularly attached to the labor force, and increasing numbers of the frail and sick elderly are over 75 years of age and likely to be living alone. Even if they are fortunate enough to have a spouse, the elderly may lack the physical strength to provide the necessary support.

Money is always a key determinant of the type and range of health-care services to which different groups in a community have access. With respect to money, the outlook for expanded home health care is not unfavorable although it cannot be assessed as good or excellent. The last decades have seen a marked improvement in the financial status of the elderly so that half of them are at least reasonably well off. They should have relatively little difficulty in buying as much as 20 hours of personal care a week for a period of years. With Medicare B coverage, most or all of their physician visits would be covered. Admittedly they could be under financial pressure if they had to purchase expensive drugs for an indefinite period. Many would also find it burdensome or impossible to hire full-time around-the-clock support personnel. As noted above, 20 hours would be reasonably easy; 168 hours would be beyond the means of most.

As for the many—about half of all the elderly—who live in poverty or with incomes less than double the poverty line, the financial drain of maintaining a chronically ill person at home could prove much more difficult if not impossible. With the exception of New York City, which has a liberal home health-care benefit for the Medicaid population (its beneficiaries utilize on average over 50 hours of paid external help), there are only limited public funds available to assist low-income, chronically ill persons to remain in their homes.

Some experimental programs, federal and state, are aimed at exploring the potential of redirecting some of the present flows of Medicare and Medicaid funds from institutional (hospital and nursing home) to home health care. There is no evidence, however, that such a redirection can be accomplished without increasing substantially the total amount of funding, for the reason that the number of people opting for governmentally supported home health services will increase once they become reimbursable. The difficulty lies in the fact that neither Medicare nor Medicaid was initially designed to provide the eligible groups with broad access to home health-care services and, as a result, up to now these services have been covered for the most part by consumers' out-of-pocket expenditures. Short of fundamental reforms in Social Security, Medicare, and Medicaid coverage and payment systems, together with the inclusion of significant home health-care benefits by private insurance, the financial base will be inadequate to encourage any substantial increase in home health-care services for the low-income population. However, this caveat does not extend to the more affluent among the elderly who are currently able to draw on private resources to supplement their Medicare B coverage.

Major financial reforms are a necessary precondition for the full flowering of home health-care programs, but they are not the only precondition. The other major factor relates to the pace of innovation in therapeutic and rehabilitative procedures and devices. There are rumors afloat that the hospital and medical supply companies are far advanced in development efforts aimed at the introduction of new products that will make it easier, less expensive, and more efficient and effective to care at home for patients who in the past have been routinely treated in a hospital or a nursing home. The odds are that some of the heralded breakthroughs may never materialize or at least not in the near term. It is likely, however, that much of what is in the wings will be available by the end of this decade or the beginning of the next and will effectively expand the demand for home health care.

There is one more major theme that relates to the primary-care physician who will inevitably have to carry most of the responsibility for turning the potential of more and better home health care into reality. This key concept is that of "linkage" between the physician and his patient, the patient's family, the hospital discharge staff, the community agencies that provide home health-care services (from the VNS to old and new nonprofit and for-profit companies), medical supply houses and their range of products, and public and volunteer agencies that provide a variety of services (from visitors to special transportation) for the homebound.

This list should suffice to make perhaps the most important point: the physician who wants to provide quality home health services for his patients must take the time and trouble not only to become well informed about the relevant medical infrastructure, in-hospital and in the community, but he must also enlarge his knowledge of the social agencies that, in turn, are providers of critical adjunct services. In addition, the primary-care physician must budget his time to talk at length both with his patient and with the responsible members of the patient's household who will be important members of the enlarged therapeutic team. In fact, these responsible relations will make or break whatever plan the physician works out for his patient.

In small and medium-sized communities it may prove relatively easy for the interested physician to become acquainted with the infrastructures on which he will need to draw in planning and implementing a desirable home health-care program for his patient. The challenge is more formidable in a large urban environment where the web of medical and social welfare agencies is far more complicated.

There is no question that the present fee schedule is a disincentive to the primary-care physician to take the time both to acquire the basic information he needs and to engage in appropriate consultation and discussion before formulating a home health-care program for his patient. There is a minimal prospect, not much more, that the years ahead will see some reforms in the structure of physician payment that will reward more liberally than in the past those primary-care physicians who engage in the important task of patient management, including the management of home health care. We will also see the expansion of many more prepayment arrangements, which will provide incentives to corporate and group practices to be guided in the selection of treatment sites and modalities of treatment by criteria of efficiency and effectiveness, and these should encourage greater reliance on home health care.

There are those who believe that the HMO will be the delivery system of the future. I expect it to grow, probably to a point where it will encompass up to one third of the population, but not more. In the event that my more cautionary estimate proves correct, the fact that so many people will remain outside of prepayment plans will make for organizational difficulties in developing home health care as rapidly or as universally as would be possible under a more structured payment and delivery system.

As one who has observed at close quarters the changing health-care delivery system in the United States during the last six decades, I have learned that one must always be attuned to the new and not underestimate its potential for growth. At the same time, one must continue to give proper weight to the institutional, financial, and value systems in place that will militate against the rapid advance of the new. Home health care is definitely an important innovation, making a strong reappearance for the first time in this century. I have every reason to believe that there is a sufficient number of powerful forces at work to encourage its growth so that before too long it will become a major setting for the provision of health care for the homebound elderly and chronically ill.

As noted above, however, there are a number of factors that will hobble its full development, factors that span a wide area, from the complexity of the infrastructure to the payment systems for physicians. In his choices whether to play a larger or a smaller role in the expansion of home health care, the primary-care physician will in large measure determine how quickly and how effectively the potential of home health care is realized. If he fails to take the lead, it will advance, but slowly. If he is out front, it may prove to be an exciting new frontier.

# PART I

# Preparing for Care at Home

# 1
# The Role of the Physician

LAWRENCE H. BERNSTEIN

## A NEW ORIENTATION

Home care is rapidly entering the mainstream of medical practice in this country, a change that is being fueled by dramatic economic and social mandates. For many reasons, physicians have not fully and enthusiastically embraced the idea of home care. Patients, on the other hand, have always preferred home care, or care in the home. As physicians, we have all been asked questions such as "Why can't I go home sooner?"; "Can this be done in one day?"; "Why does grandma have to go into a nursing home—isn't there another choice?" Even when faced with these and other such questions we generally fail to consider home care as a viable option. Although home care is not a panacea, it is an option offered too infrequently by the physician. But why don't we think of home care more often, especially if it is the best response to some specific and direct requests from patients? Why is the physician still wedded to the idea of caring for patients in the hospital or office but not in the home?

The answer to the first question is that the current generation of physicians has had little training or exposure to home care either in theory or in practice. Most medical students and hospital staff spend the formative, impressionable years of their careers in the urban tertiary-care referral centers. The training process all too often focuses on disease rather than on people—not that the two are mutually exclusive. Home care is more people oriented, requiring a shift in focus from disease alone to the complete context of disease, patient, family, and environment. Life goes on beyond the walls of the hospital. When the problems are finally resolved for the hospital staff, they are just beginning for the people at home. For the physician concerned exclusively with inpatient care, there is an element of "out of sight, out of mind" when a patient is discharged from the hospital. The discharge process and the patient's continuing convalescence at home are not nearly as important to the young physician in training as are the more exciting and immediate demands of acute care. This is particularly true when all contact with the patient is lost after discharge. Advancement in the teaching setting is usually tied to such activities as acquiring grants, publishing, and research, and not to direct patient care. It is therefore not surprising that a doctor who makes house calls is a rare species in the medical center—a role model the student is unlikely to encounter and emulate. In this setting, little opportunity exists to put forth the values inherent in home care.

Because the current generation of practitioners is not experienced in home care there is a general lack of familiarity with the jargon, techniques, and equipment used in home care.

Home care requires a different approach to the patient. The current underutilization of home care is as much a manifestation of an unfamiliarity with this approach to the patient as it is a lack of knowledge *per se*. Home care is a way of dealing with a person that is strongly biased by our interpretation of that person's capacity to function independently, our willingness to extend ourselves, and our propensity to look at illness in its full social and cultural context. It is our perceptions of the particular individual (and the elderly in general) that largely determine whether or not we will care for this person in the home. How we view this individual and his family outside the context of his illness has a major bearing on whether or not we will practice home care. This is in distinction to our, of necessity, being less selective in deciding whether we will care for most other patients presenting to our office or hospital.

There is little opportunity to learn about home care, even for the physician who is so motivated. There are few articles in the medical literature on this topic. Similarly, continuing medical education courses have ignored this area. The nursing literature (books and periodicals) is an excellent source for articles dealing with the clinical, psychological, and socioeconomic issues of home care, but most physicians consider it beneath their dignity to read a nursing journal. As a result, most physicians have not been trained in this mode of health-care delivery and have insufficient opportunity to learn about it or gain experience in it. Are there other reasons physicians have been slow to adapt to the changing trend in home care?

Although home care may lack the glamour of the high-tech cutting edge of medicine, we must begin to integrate its concepts into the mainstream of medical education. Only then will we see physicians broadly and openly accepting home care as a valid part of primary-care medicine. This does not mean we need a separate academic department, but rather an acceptance of an approach that is different from what we are doing now.

## BECOMING MORE INVOLVED: WHAT DOES HOME CARE OFFER THE PHYSICIAN?

What arguments can be put forth to encourage the physician to become more involved? The strongest case is that to discharge a patient to the home and not remain actively involved in that patient's care is a form of abandonment—not abandonment in the strictly legal sense, but rather an abdication and moral abandonment of our responsibility for the continuing care of the patient. We have deferred to the nursing profession, which has responded with dedication, compassion, and skill—and with all too little support from us. If we are intimately and intensely involved with the patient in the office and hospital, why such an abrupt change in the level of participation when the patient becomes a home patient? The patient and family certainly don't view hospital discharge as a divorce but rather as part of a continuum. In the following discussion, we will present the positives of adopting such an attitude.

What specifically does home care have to offer the physician in addition to an enhancement of patient care? In an era of cost containment, home care offers the opportunity to choose a less costly method of care for many patients; not all, but many. Home care is an integral component of an expeditious discharge process. Chapter 2 presents an elegant approach to this problem and carries the concept of continuity of care to a high level of refinement. If discharge planning is done well it should mean less trouble for the physician as well as being advantageous for the patient. A carefully thought out and orchestrated plan anticipates potential problems the patient may have at home and provides a structure not only for preventing difficulties but also for resolving many issues that may arise. By forging a strong working relationship with the nurses who will be helping in the home, the physician will be better able to respond to any number of acute problems.

As the care partner begins to experience increasing stress and fatigue, as so often happens, an attentive nurse can identify this and begin to deal with the issues long before the problem becomes a major difficulty. Dealing with the impacted patient is far easier if you learn about the problem early rather than late. If your patient's mobility is gradually diminishing, it will probably be the nurse who will first notice this and inform you of it. When an acute illness intervenes, the people working in the home will be able to suggest the best ways of dealing with the patient and family if they are familiar with your style and the particular problems this patient has been having all along. But all of this requires your working in concert with the home care nurses. This is an asset for both physician and patient.

If the physician has forged a good working relationship with the discharge planner and community providers, the process will be considerably less time consuming and onerous than imagined. Although it takes time and experience to get to know these people and for them to feel comfortable with you, it is time well invested.

One of the hallmarks of medicine in the 1980s is competition. As much as home care may not be discussed in the literature and at meetings, competition among physicians is. Responding to a patient's medical, social, psychological, and financial needs in the setting most desirable for the patient certainly enhances the physician–patient relationship. The physician who is viewed by the community as someone who takes care of people at home, even if this is primarily by telephone with occasional house calls, has an advantage over his colleagues. As patients (sometimes referred to as *consumers*) become more sophisticated in their use of health services they are beginning to expect this kind of physician response.

## HOME CARE: A MATTER OF STYLE

Given a choice between institutionalization and staying at home, most patients opt for home. We as physicians are too quick to choose institutionalization for them because it is a quicker, neater, and cleaner solution to the problem—for us. But is this really what the patient wants and needs? How much extra effort are we willing to expend to try and keep that patient at home? The answers to these questions are really at the heart of quality primary care—at least as much as astute diagnosis and treatment. Some of the most grateful patients are the patients who, through the efforts of their physician, have been able to stay at home. A firm commitment has been made to care for these people at home and they are appreciative. Do not underestimate the positive public relations from "doing good." At a time when the high-tech end of medicine is booming and the physician image is suffering, home care can benefit both doctor and patient.

None of us likes to lose contact or control of a patient, but when we abdicate our responsibility to the home care nurse this is exactly what we do, and apparently willingly. This is not an all or none process or even a power struggle over control. (The nurses would welcome our input!) It is an issue of a participatory role versus a perfunctory distant role where our most notable activity involves signing forms. Our involvement also demonstrates a sense of responsibility and fairness to the nurses who are on the front lines taking care of our patients. They are functioning as our hands, eyes, and ears in the home, for which we owe them a large debt of gratitude. That debt can easily be repaid by increasing our involvement.

If we are asking for an increase in the level of involvement from physicians, what sort of introspection and soul searching are going to be necessary first? If home care is viewed as, in large measure, a matter of style as well as substance, perhaps a fitting place to start is to look at some of our preconceived ideas about the elderly. What notions do we bring with us when we are confronted with an elderly patient whose faculties are dwindling and who is unable to continue functioning in the fashion to which he has become accustomed over the years? This is the person who needs help with washing, cooking, and shopping. Perhaps his hygiene isn't as good as it could be. Carrying laundry up and down the stairs is a treacherous effort at best. Although the family is around, everyone works and can only contribute minimal amounts of time. Anyway, the grown children think it may be time to consider the nursing home. The arthritis is acting up and the heart failure isn't under very good control, partly because of the inability to stay on a sodium-restricted diet. You, as the physician, are constantly getting phone calls from the family and the patient and are starting to feel uncomfortable with both the situation and the process.

This is a time of reckoning for everyone involved, but let's focus on the physician. In a very fundamental sense how are you going to view this person? Is he capable and able to function independently, or do you feel he is in need of institutionalization? Do you think of this person as being sick because he is sick or because he is old? Do you have a fatalistic attitude toward aging? Do you view age as a disease or do you tend to look at a person with heart failure as an old person with heart failure or a person with heart failure who also happens to be old? It is a matter of emphasis—disease or age. If our inclination is to perceive the age dimension as the major determinant in the process, our approach to the patient will be more fatalistic than if we focus on the disease. By focusing on age, the patient sees himself in a more passive role because, after all, you can attempt to alter a disease process, but age is inexorable. Remember, old people are sick because they are sick, not just because they are old. This is not to deny the intangible aspects of aging nor is it meant to imply that all disease can be or even should be treated. We do not need to exhaustively work up all symptoms, but rather exercise judgment.

There is a tendency to foster learned helplessness where perhaps learning independence might be more appropriate. Certainly the reimbursement system fosters our doing things *to* our patients instead of structuring a program of independence for them. I do not have the answer for changing that, but we should not allow the reimbursement patterns to dictate our practices completely.

Do we, as very individual, idiosyncratic practitioners, have our own propensity to foster needless dependence? How much of this is fulfilling our needs to be in control? Are the patients themselves striving for independence, while we are (perhaps unwittingly) working counter to this goal? Is there a conflict between the patient's wishes and what the family thinks is best? You may have an entirely different set of ideas about what you think is best. How do you resolve these issues? Whose "side" do you take? For whom are you serving in an advocacy role? The resolution of these dilemmas involves questions of liability, allegiance to the patient, and a response to the concerns of the family—not an easy task. But these are important questions to answer for yourself. Your attitude will largely determine your response to this and other analogous scenarios.

On a broader scale we should briefly mention the role of government and third-party reimbursement. Almost all the forces that are brought to bear encourage institutionalization and discourage the physician from aggressively being the ombudsman for his patient. This statement is not meant to be interpreted with a sense of oblivion to the financial issues. There is a gray area between allowing this to rule our decision making and forcing the patient into financial ruin. Part of the answer is to better educate ourselves about the particular reimbursement patterns in our state, particularly Medicare. Having the knowledge of what is and is not reimbursable puts you in a better position to discuss these issues with your patient. When you are not conversant with the ground rules of the game you may be inclined to avoid the topic entirely. This does not imply that you will only discuss options that are fully reimbursed, but the more informed you are, the more actively you will participate in the process.

## THE DEMANDS OF HOME CARE: HOW IS THE HOME DIFFERENT?

What additional demands are placed on the physician as he accepts a fuller responsibility for these patients? Remember, we are stepping out of our high-tech hospital and office settings and entering an environment that is foreign to many of us. Isn't it a bit odd that we all were raised in homes, live in homes, and care for patients who have homes, but we don't usually think of the home as a place to deliver care? Specifically, how is the home setting different from any other place in which we care for patients? What is different about the process, our interactions with the patient, and our behavior? As we discuss home care, it seems appropriate to spend some time discussing the home itself as a component of the care. We have always viewed the hospital setting as an integral part of our inpatient care. There is an entire literature dealing with the impact of the physical environment of the hospital on patient care—noise levels, arrangement of rooms, accessibility by nurses, lighting, ambience, and so on. The home environment deserves no less attention.

In what specific ways is the home a different place to care for people? The most striking difference is that the home contains the patient's familiar surroundings; his family, cultural milieu, personal objects, comfortable bed, and, most important of all, the schedule and routine that have been maintained for several decades. Let us not underestimate the dehumanizing aspects of strange surroundings, a new shift of nurses every eight hours, a schedule finely tuned to the needs of an institution, not a home, and the enormous sense of loss of control that occurs as an inpatient. Most patients feel like captives in the hospital or, at best, a guest in the physician's office. Now think of the physician's position as he enters the patient's home. The shoe is on the other foot. The physician is a guest in the patient's house where the patient writes the rules and has expectations of the physician's behavior and where the physician feels a bit out of place. The patient now has the greater sense of control, which is probably as it should be.

How has this impacted on the physician–patient relationship? As the physician entering a patient's home, especially for the first time, I find myself thinking much more about the patient's cultural differences and physical surroundings than I do when I am in my office or hospital. I begin to think about what the patient and his family are expecting of my behavior and what my behavior should be. Here are some simple common examples. In the home I ask if I can use the telephone to call the pharmacy; in the hospital, I do it without really giving it much thought. In the home I ask where I can wash my hands and have a clean towel; in the hospital I know exactly where all these items are located. When I enter the home I ask where to put my coat and at least think a bit about where I am going to sit to write notes and so on; in the patient's hospital room, I am perhaps a bit more brazen about where I throw my coat and where I sit down to write. All of these nuances of behavior have an impact on how the physician–patient interaction is going to take place. If the patient is feeling more secure and confident, his ability and willingness to partake in the discussion and specifics of a care plan will be enhanced. The same applies to the family's participation. By meeting them, to a greater extent than previously, on their terms, I have begun to remove barriers to their accepting me and my suggestions. I, on the other hand, have fewer barriers to overcome in accepting the patient and family within the context of all that is so terribly important to their life in many fundamental ways.

I now at least know what my patient's home looks like. Think about that for a moment. Think what it means when you discharge a stroke patient home from the hospital with all sorts of new problems such as poor mobility and difficulty bathing and eating, as well as inadequate bowel and bladder function. What does it tell the patient when you talk about "getting around the home" when you don't have the slightest idea what the home is like? Compliance, which is a major problem for so many of our patients, is improved when the patient feels that he both understands and controls the process. In the home it is considerably easier to set the stage for that to happen.

An essential part of home care is the expanded role of the family as both care partners and just plain family with all of the connotations of the concept of kinship. There is no better place to begin to appreciate and understand the dynamics of the family than in the home. Each home has its own unique environment; as a physical place with poor lighting and steep stairs; as a cultural background with its unique ambience, sense of the past, taboos, and so forth; as a place "that I built by the sweat of my brow." You first start to get a sense of what the home really means to your patient when you go inside. But you have to *allow* yourself the time to taste, feel, and touch these nuances before you begin to ask the patient's spouse to do things he or she has never dreamt of doing before. At the same time, your own biases and cultural background will permeate the way you present options to the patient and family and how you expect them to participate in the care process.

Everything we have said about the patient's culture, history, and family lore applies equally well to the past history the physician brings to the relationship. This becomes particularly poignant in the home setting. We need to constantly look in the mirror and ask questions of and about ourselves. In the office it is easier to insulate ourselves and view ourselves as only a physician and not a total person. When you open the patient's front door you become a more complete person in the eyes of your patient. Through this process I become more human to the patient and treat him more humanely.

In what ways is the process in the home different? The basics of medicine still hold. We take a history, make our observations, do an examination, come to a diagnosis, and initiate treatment. In the home setting we essentially go through the same steps but with a somewhat different emphasis and even a subtly different goal. The goal of treating disease, be it physical or emotional and in the hospital, office, or home, is the amelioration of pain or discomfort and the resolution of the presenting complaint. This doesn't change in different settings, but the process and sequence of events do.

The sequence of the diagnostic and therapeutic process in the home is sometimes different from what we conventionally do in the office or hospital. In the home there are times when we need to treat a problem before we have made a diagnosis. This is heresy in the teaching setting, except for life-threatening problems. Let's take a specific example and expand on this a bit. You are caring for an elderly patient who is essentially living a bed-to-chair existence. One of his problems is urinary incontinence, although his bowel patterns are not troublesome. His wife is arthritic and the washing machine is in the basement. Changing the bed linen is a major chore for her and this factor alone is beginning to impact on her ability to continue to care for her husband at home much longer. For the sake of simplicity, let's pretend that there is no alternative available for extra help in the home. This is rarely the case, but it will allow us to focus on the problem more easily.

What are your goals when you first learn about the problem? The first concern is to keep the bed sheets dry. Initially the patient and his wife aren't too concerned with prostatic hypertrophy, an intravenous pyelogram, or prostatectomy or a differential diagnosis of urinary incontinence. They both want to keep the patient dry so that a nursing home doesn't become a possibility. Before you do much in the way of diagnostic maneuvers, you need to come up with a mechanism to keep this fellow dry. The solution may be nothing more than a simple adult diaper or one of the newer, more sophisticated urine collection devices. A urinal or bedside commode may be appropriate. The point is, you are on the spot and need to be familiar enough with these options to comfortably and confidently make the recommendation. In addition to resolving the immediate issue (drenched bed linen) you have also earned some credibility with your patient.

If this patient were in the hospital we would have the luxury of having the sheets changed every several hours as we proceed down the diagnostic pathway. Depending on the size and sophistication of the hospital and availability of consulting staff, a very high degree of diagnostic certainty can be achieved. How is it different in the home? Often in the home we will try a therapeutic or palliative maneuver and then take some diagnostic steps followed by another therapeutic attempt. If that fails we may need to do more testing. This can be done in a stepwise fashion, whereas in the hospital the diagnostic process is more likely to be a straight line.

This strategy requires the cooperation of the family and patient. It also requires a physician who is able to tolerate a degree of uncertainty as the process evolves. Remember, we and the patient may be more or less tolerant of uncertainty to different degrees and at different junctures. It is essential that this be shared openly. We need to ask ourselves occasionally whether our anxiety is fueling the diagnostic steps or does the patient really want to proceed at the same pace as we are moving? If the alternative is hospitalization, a nursing home, or invasive testing, the patient is often willing to be a bit more tentative in the approach. We already are accustomed to different levels of uncertainty in different settings. The diagnosis of the etiology of chest pain in a 60-year-old is far less certain on the telephone than if that same person were in the emergency room, and that is less certain compared to injecting dye into the person's left anterior descending coronary artery. But we have learned what problems need to be treated in what settings and how aggressive to be at the moment. The home is part of that spectrum and not an entirely foreign land; it's just that we have not gotten used to it yet.

Back to our patient. A diaper and bed pad at night coupled with a commode during the day may achieve the results you want. Is it essential to go ahead with a full diagnostic work-up? That is a medical decision that can only be answered knowing all the facts about the individual patient. But, and this is an important point, you have resolved the immediate problem before doing any testing, and for some patients that may be sufficient provided they are then informed of the potential reversible problems, complications, and so on. In the home you still need to be concerned about liability issues. This is an appropriate time to add that this sort of process will probably decrease, not increase, your liability risks. If you can keep that patient dry and avoid nursing home placement, the patient and family will be grateful indeed—and that gratitude is the single greatest factor in avoiding a law suit. We need to keep the patient's perspective in mind constantly, and that is easier to do in the home setting far removed from the subtle pressures we all feel in the hospital. The patient and his problem become the primary focus. Perhaps removing the specter of multiple third parties peering over our shoulder allows us to relate more directly to our patient without interposing "the chart" between us.

## WORKING WITH NURSES

Another way in which the process is different at home has to do with how we work with nurses. Most of our experience in working with nurses comes either from our office or the floor nurse in the hospital. Let's look at the role of the doctor and nurse within the context of the process at home. We need to share care with the nurse and relinquish some of the control we are accustomed to exerting. There is all too often an element of intimidation in the way we deal with nurses in the hospital. This benefits no one and creates an even greater problem in the home. Home care nurses are more knowledgeable and more experienced than we are in a whole host of areas. We need to allow the nurse to make decisions based on her expertise and more intimate involvement with the patient. This nurse may be seeing the patient on a daily basis for weeks or months. Doesn't it seem that there should be some sharing of information and management based on that? We as physicians may be made to feel less knowledgeable about the patient's condition when we speak with the nurse but that's the reality of the situation. By analogy, the same holds true with a coronary care unit nurse reporting the vital signs on an acutely ill patient: at the moment she knows the most about that patient and we have learned how to use that information for the benefit of the patient. It's really quite similar at home. If we allow ourselves, we can learn a great deal about home care from an experienced nurse.

The telephone can be the bane of our existence but a source of enormous comfort and security to our home patients. It is also our main link with the nurse at home. When the nurse calls on the telephone, we can learn a great deal more in a two- or three-minute conversation than we will ever learn from a standardized form we are required to sign every 60 days. By listening to the nurse we will be better informed when we speak to the patient or family, and they will have more of a sense of our involvement in their care.

This raises the issue of availability. A large part of the success of a home care program is the physician's availability, both by telephone and in person. Most patients will be quite tolerant of their disease at home if they know they can reach the physician when needed, and these patients are rarely abusive of the privilege. "Just knowing you were there got us through" is a common form of "thank you."

What about house calls? If you are going to be involved in home care—involved heart and soul—you will occasionally need to venture beyond your familiar office or hospital. Yes, it will take time and may be inconvenient, and it may not pay well, but it will make all the difference in keeping the patient at home. Your mere presence in the patient's home makes an eloquent statement about your concern for that patient. There is a special bonding that develops, with very positive ramifications for all aspects of the care of that patient. Yes, house calls are burdensome but they are not without their gratifications.

## A BROADER APPLICATION OF HOME CARE CONCEPTS

Thus far we have been discussing patients with generally clearly identifiable problems who are then designated as recipients of home care. I will not attempt to define either the concept of home care or the characteristics of the home care patient population rigidly. For most of our practices home care patients are a small segment of our total patient population. If this is the case, is there a more broadly useful application of the material regarding home care? Is the information we categorize as pertaining to home care relevant only for our "home care" patients? I would like to state the thesis that there are many patients for whom information relevant to home care is indeed important material, but we do not always recognize their problems when we see these patients outside the context of "home care." Or, to look at it from another angle, our propensity to look for a given problem is largely determined by our awareness of possible solutions. We don't think of the solutions so we are less likely to be attuned to the problem. This is more an issue of a sensitivity to a problem than it is a perplexing diagnostic and therapeutic dilemma.

Let's take another hypothetical patient and elaborate on this idea. You are doing a physical examination on a 75-year-old man with some minor well-controlled hypertension and chronic lung disease. He is rather independent in most of his daily comings and goings and only minimally confused at times. At home he and his wife are doing well together, with some help from family and helpful neighbors. During the examination you notice some dampness and yellow staining of his underpants. There are several approaches to the problem. First, you can ignore it entirely and assume that the patient would mention the incontinence if he thought it were important enough. Or, you do what we were all taught to do so diligently in medical school, and that is a careful review of systems. For the male genitourinary system the review goes something like this: we run through a litany of symptoms including pyuria, dysuria, hematuria, hesitancy, urgency, strength of the stream, and so on. You may well draw all negative responses because you are looking for a specific disease for which you are well prepared to go down a specific diagnostic and therapeutic path. How about asking the patient "How do you pee?" It doesn't sound very scientific, but it gets to the point for the patient. His answer might then be "Well, to tell you the truth, Doc, at night I sometimes lose control because, well, I get a little confused at night. A few nights ago I started to get up and felt a little dizzy. And with that long dark hallway I'm sort of afraid of falling. I don't like to wake the wife because then she has trouble falling back to sleep and with her bad arthritic legs that's a real problem. I know my daughter was concerned about my wife carrying all that laundry down the stairs and isn't too crazy about the smell of urine when she comes over on Sunday afternoon."

Now you are first starting to get a sense of what "a little incontinence" means to this patient and his family. Remember, this is a patient with no specific "home care" needs as we have conventionally defined them. But we can certainly begin to apply some of the things we have learned about durable medical equipment and consumable supplies to this situation. The subsequent diagnostic process will be a matter of judgment not to be touched on here. The point is that we need to have solutions in mind if we are going to think of asking the right questions. As was mentioned earlier, this is as much a matter of style as it is an issue of didactic learning. Perhaps our review of systems for the elderly should be modified to look for some of the problems that are so troublesome for them but mundane for us.

The same approach can be taken in inquiring about a patient's bathing habits. "How do you bathe? What's it like when you climb in and out of the tub? Do you take a bath less often because of a fear of falling? Tell me a bit about the layout of your bathroom." By asking these sorts of questions, you will begin to uncover another set of problems you would have missed if you had confined your review of systems to "joint pain, swelling, redness, morning stiffness, response to aspirin," and so on. As a result of asking pertinent questions you are more likely to suggest grab bars or a transfer bench.

The patient is worried about breaking her hip in the shower. The family is worried about inadequate hygiene. And you are most concerned with making an accurate diagnosis of the precise type of arthritis she has—or at least that is the message you give. Our elderly gent is dreadfully afraid of soiling the bed linen. His daughter is unhappy about his urinating in bed as well as dribbling during the day. The family thinks the doctor needs to order all sorts of tests before he can solve any aspect of the problem. More importantly, they think you are really missing the boat in terms of their real problems. We need to at least partially look at this situation from the vantage point of what is most acutely painful for the patient at the moment.

Likewise, mobility issues can be addressed by asking about how the house is arranged. "Are stairs becoming more difficult? If you could walk better how would things be different for you? Do you need to make some simple changes such as additional railings or re-arranging furniture? What kind of floor coverings do you have and what sort of shoes do you wear in the house?" Yes, these are questions usually asked by our physical and occupational therapy colleagues but can be easily incorporated into our questions as well. Only by assessing the physical environment by direct questions (or, better still, by a home visit by you or the nurse) can you begin to understand how your patient functions. By asking the questions with a functional emphasis, the solutions (such as commodes, walkers, and canes) are more likely to become apparent.

There are many other questions to be asked of both our homebound and ambulatory patients. Dental care can be provided for house-confined patients through special programs and devices designed by the American Dental Association. Some of the basic screening and preventive procedures we do so readily in the rest of our population sometimes get forgotten with our homebound patients. These people need to have their teeth cleaned, have Pap smears if appropriate, and receive periodic complete examinations and laboratory work as you would order for any other patient, except that we need to work a bit harder to get it all done. But that does not diminish the necessity.

We often assume that the national associations for the deaf, blind, or handicapped are only for the people who are totally deaf or severely handicapped or legally blind. This is not the case. The associations have a great deal to offer people with only modest deficits. But the physician is usually the only medical contact for these patients. If we don't ask the right questions and come up with the appropriate answers it is unlikely that anyone else will. Part of our job in caring for these people involves our playing the roles of physician, teacher, and ombudsman—in equal parts. Omitting any facet of this markedly diminishes our effectiveness in dealing with the elderly and the homebound in particular.

My plea is that when we do our review of systems with our patients we keep in mind the activities of daily living in a functional sense and from the patient's perspective. We need to ask about bathing, eating, dressing, bowels, and mobility. These are the basic activities of daily living (ADL) and appropriately get at the essential facets of one's well-being. But we need to go one step further and take a closer look at some of the more cerebral functions. In addition to the usual query about orientation and alertness, we should look more closely at the functional implications. "Can you balance your checkbook, maintain your home as you would like it, enjoy reading or social functions?"

The answers to these questions and others like them will give you a much better sense of the patient's functioning and any potential deficits. The process is less structured than what we were taught and may seem less goal oriented than the detailed neurologic reports we are accustomed to receiving. But, keeping these ideas in mind, as we take our history and speak with our patients we will more appropriately identify the patient's necessities and be prepared to respond. Much of that response is the substance of home care. A bedside commode, a urinal, or a diaper is just as applicable for our ambulatory as for our homebound patients. We need not make such a sharp distinction between the two patient groups.

Home care is taking care of people in the home; that is, taking care of all their multiple needs from the patient's, the family's and physician's perspective, yet integrating all of this in such a fashion that you are able to deliver high-quality medical care. The future of medical care is going to be partially shaped by our ability to do this and by our ability and willingness to respond to the economic and social changes occurring in health care.

# 2
# Preparing for Home While in the Hospital

ANTHONY J. GRIECO

What does it mean to be a patient in a hospital? Hospitals are designed as the best physical environment in which to treat acute medical problems. Hospitals consolidate sophisticated medical resources, providing patients with intensive, continuous monitoring. All resources, technical or human, are available in the immediate environment. Yet, hospitals may adversely influence the way patients respond to illness and consequently to the course of their recovery. We know that the very fact of being hospitalized engenders extraordinary stress—a stress imposed on an already sick person. Furthermore, the hospital experience may also limit the patient's ability to adapt to a change in life-style that illness may necessitate.[1]

One of the greatest pitfalls in the treatment of patients is the acute-care hospital setting itself. The traditional hospital is frightening and dehumanizing. In part, this is caused by the notorious lack of privacy, which is the accepted means of ensuring adequate observation by the professional staff in order to provide safety for clinically unstable patients. Bedrest is encouraged from the moment of admission, as the patient is stripped of clothing, dons pajamas, and is placed into a bed. It is from the recumbent position that the patient views the nurses, aides, interns, residents, attending physicians, technicians, and staff.

Dependency is not merely encouraged, but is demanded, as medications used prior to admission are confiscated, even if the identical drugs are to be continued during the hospital stay. The patient, who until the time of admission had been in control of his or her medications and environment, is now considered totally incapable of being entrusted with any active role in care. Control is forcefully shifted to the hospital staff. At home, the physician's words were recommendations and advice. In the hospital, the physician writes "orders."

To ensure that proper treatment is provided, hospital nurses are trained to administer each medication and to observe the patient swallow every tablet or capsule. How can the patient be expected to understand the complexities and nuances of changes in drug dosage and timing? How can the hospital keep track of narcotics, sedatives, and other controlled drugs if the patient were responsible for self-administration of medications? How can charting be accurate under such conditions? The major question asked is "How can patients be trusted?"

Since the locus of control is the hospital staff rather than the patient, it is not an urgent consideration to provide detailed information to the patient about the treatment regimen. Everything is expected to happen automatically, without any thought being required on the patient's part. The family, likewise, has no responsibility other than to visit and provide

**19**

support. The family is expected to encourage the patient to submit passively to uncomfortable invasive testing, procedures, and treatments. The promise is that, after discharge, further solace will be provided in a more personal fashion at home.

In an acute-care hospital emphasis is maintained on cure of disease rather than on care of the patient. Certainly care is provided abundantly, but the highest stated goal is treatment and cure. To underscore that philosophy, how often does someone convey the impression that "nothing more can be done" when a disease is considered incurable. That does not imply that care is not needed. On the contrary, the patient in that situation often requires the greatest efforts of true devoted care and attention to comfort. "Nothing more can be done" are terrible words, even more terrifying if used as parting words on discharge. Then, they mean nothing more of the glory-laden treatments, but everything more of affectionate care to be provided at home by the family.

> Modern hospitals, which require a complicated administrative and professional service, often weigh heavily on the budgets of states, municipalities, or private charity and are presenting an increasingly grave and difficult economic problem.[2]

Those words, originally written in Italian by Professor Castiglioni in Italy in 1936, sound as though they had been written in the United States today. They support early discharge as an economic necessity. As the pace of financial life has quickened, the pressures for earlier discharge have heightened in intensity. Discharge planning now begins even before admission, and is refined during the hospital course.

From the time of Hippocrates, the skill of making an accurate prognosis was considered of greatest importance.[3] His words, "I hold that it is an excellent thing for a physician to practice forecasting,"[4] perhaps represent historical support of the idea of prognosticating as the first step of discharge planning.

Published nationwide norms for length of stay by diagnosis-related group (DRG) aid in the process of predicting the day of discharge. DRG labeling has dramatically affected both the hospitals' and physicians' thinking about the duration of hospitalization needed. The economic incentives and fiscal penalties have driven down the length of stay, which at this time is still falling, throughout the country.

Earlier discharge makes "anticipation" the key word. It is necessary to anticipate not only the date of discharge, but also the needs for durable medical equipment and supplies; the needs for concrete services; the needs for home care nursing, home health aides, and home physiotherapy; transportation requirements; and the needs for the entire home contingent, including the family.

How can the hospital stay itself be used to prepare the patient more fully for home? The answer is: by openly sharing information.

Preparing the patient for home starts by openly sharing thoughts and information about the diagnosis being considered. No diagnosis is too sensitive to be disclosed to the patient. The family's fears of the patient's possible anguish in learning of a serious diagnosis must be recognized and handled with compassion. Treatment plans, including the various options being considered, should be discussed as they are being proposed and evaluated by the professionals, not merely after a decision has been reached. Possible side-effects of the work-up and treatment are faced with less trepidation if understood and anticipated by the patient and family.

Medications in the hospital are the purview of the professionals. At home, prior to hospital admission, the patient and family were totally responsible for purchasing, storing, and administering all medications. They had to juggle timing to coordinate with the other activities of each day, such as traveling to work, eating meals, shopping, and sleeping. It was necessary for the patient to keep track of inventory, knowing when to refill prescriptions, as well as remembering to take the various drugs on the predetermined schedule.

On admission to the hospital, all this changes. It starts with the patient describing the medications in use prior to hospitalization. At times there may be a discrepancy between the attending physician's recollection or records and the description of medications as related by the patient. Either could be in error. The physician is generally more likely to be correct in naming the drugs and their dosages, but at times the physician will truly know only that a certain class of drug was prescribed (*e.g.,* a beta-blocker) rather than remembering which agent in that class had been prescribed. The patient, however, is always more reliable than the physician in reporting the frequency and timing of administration of medications, since only the patient really knows what the compliance has been to the physician's prescription.[5]

While the medications are being reviewed, they are often inspected by the nurses and house staff. This is excellent practice to verify accuracy. However, it is frequently accompanied by confiscation of the drugs. In some hospitals this step is a deliberate policy. In others, it is often a failure to remember, on the part of busy staff, that the medications are to be returned, and they may remain on the nursing desk or in the house officer's pocket to be reviewed again later with the other members of the team.

Patients accept being relieved of their home medications, since they understand that the acute hospitalization may necessitate changes in the drug regimen. That interactions could occur between the prior medications and those to be ordered in the hospital is well understood by the general public. It takes a compulsive patient to say, "Where are my eyedrops for glaucoma? I need to use them right now!" or "I need my regular 2:00 PM pills right now." The hospital takes charge. The message to the patient by nursing and medical staffs is the same: "Don't worry." "You are in good hands." "Leave it to us." "We will handle everything." "It is our responsibility, not yours."

At the time of discharge, the roles shift again dramatically. Up until the moment of departure, the hospital must control every dose of medication. From the next moment on, the patient and family are totally responsible. With unit dose dispensing, remaining pills are not given to the patient on discharge, but rather are returned to the hospital pharmacy so they can be administered to another inpatient. Therefore, the first medication crisis the patient faces is that the medication prescriptions must be filled promptly on the way home from the hospital or doses will be missed.

At home, the patient and family face the task of deciphering drug names and instructions. The names used by the hospital doctor and nurse may differ from the names on the pharmacist's label, since generic and brand names are quite dissimilar. The pills, capsules, and tablets used in the hospital may differ in appearance from those dispensed by the pharmacist for home use, since different brands may be encountered. The superficial instructions given at discharge, in the flurry of excitement about being released from the hospital, may prove inadequate for correct and confident medication administration at home.

The information needed by the patient and family to become fully capable of accurate medicating following the transition home includes understanding the indications for which each drug was started, the situations in which changes in dosage would be considered, and the interactions between the multiple drugs prescribed, as well as potential interactions with foods, alcohol, and common over-the-counter agents. Both the patient and family need to become familiar with the expected side-effects and other less common adverse reactions that are possible, as well as the desired therapeutic effects. They must know whether it is important to be rigidly accurate in timing of dosage or whether they have some latitude. They should have a procedure to follow in the event that a dose is inadvertently missed. All this is too much education to accomplish at the time of discharge. However, it is easily accomplished if planned as a goal early in the hospitalization.

Sharing information about diagnostic tests and procedures is considered obligatory in order to obtain informed consent. It also helps to prepare the patient for home. An invasive diagnostic or therapeutic procedure can serve as a focus for educating the patient and family about the disease condition and diagnoses being considered. Knowing what to do in anticipation of the test, what sensations will be experienced during the test, and what the patient should do following completion of the test to minimize complications are easily met educational objectives. The information that is expected to be gleaned from having the test performed should be discussed beforehand. The actual results and their implications must be shared with patient and family promptly afterward.

By having the thought processes of the medical and nursing team openly discussed with the patient and family prospectively, rather than retrospectively, they can see and become part of the process of formulation of these ideas into conclusions. They can become involved in planning management as they help to make decisions, with their knowledge developing in this seminar-like manner.

Do patients want to make medical decisions regarding their care? One study[6] found that 54% of community hospital patients wanted to help make decisions. This figure is probably low. The passive patient role, fitting with medicine's traditional power and its mystique of omniscience, is changing. More decisions are being challenged. Second opinions are mandated before surgery by many third-party payers. Many decisions are being challenged after the fact by malpractice suits. The obvious benefit of having the patient and family participate from the early data-gathering stage through the formative diagnostic stage to the therapeutic decision-making stage is therefore much greater than just preparation for discharge.

Many other opportunities exist for enhancing preparation for the transition to home while the patient is still in the hospital. Unnecessary bedrest must be discouraged. Physical activity should be demanded, not merely encouraged, so that the appropriate limits of tolerance will be reached. A simple technique is to walk the patient around the hospital unit while discussing symptoms, findings, management, or plans.

## COOPERATIVE CARE DURING HOSPITALIZATION

Is it really feasible to have full patient and family involvement in care during an acute hospitalization? "Cooperative care" is a working model that accomplishes that goal, thereby comprehensively laying the groundwork for management at home.

The first cooperative care unit in the United States opened in 1979 at the New York University Medical Center in New York City. The unit, a 104-patient wing of the 735-bed university hospital, is an integral part of that acute-care hospital. The same clinical criteria are used for deciding on admission to the cooperative care unit, and for continuing the stay, as are used for admission to or continued stay in the traditional part of the hospital. Utilization review procedures are identical in the two parts of the institution. Days that patients spend in the cooperative care unit replace days that otherwise would have been spent in the traditional part of the university hospital, not additional days, so that the overall duration of hospitalization is not prolonged.

The cooperative care unit, although providing acute care, does so in a setting that appears dramatically unlike that of a traditional hospital unit. The major difference is that, throughout the hospitalization, the patient is accompanied by a family member or close friend, who lives in the room with the patient. That individual, who is selected by the patient, is called a "care partner." The care partner's role is very similar to what would be expected of a family member at home. Providing one-on-one personal attention to the patient, the care partner brings home-style emotional support and gives physical assistance. The care partner is responsible for helping with transferring from bed to chair and to toilet, and for all other activities of daily living. Together, the twosome should achieve independence in the room.

The patient rooms in the cooperative care unit are designed to be home-like. Each room has two beds—one for the patient, one for the care partner. Privacy is ensured, since the room can be locked. Access to the room is controlled by the patient and care partner, as it would be at home.

The floors that house the patient rooms have no nursing stations, and no nurses or nurse-aides are regularly present on these floors. Observations that need to be made while the patient is in the room are the full responsibility of the care partner. Clinically important observations are made and recorded by the care partner and become the foundation on which management is built. An intelligent family member who knows the patient intimately can, with the addition of instruction by the professional staff, easily detect subtle changes in the patient's appearance. Those important discoveries, as well as a myriad of details to which the care partner's attention is directed, become part of the report given to the nurses and physicians responsible for managing the patient's illness. Overall, though, supervision is maintained by the professional staff.

Administration of medication in the room becomes a responsibility of the patient–care partner team. Many treatments are performed in the room by the care partner, rather than by the hospital staff. Unlike a traditional hospital unit, in which all the services come to the bedside, in cooperative care the patient, with the assistance of the care partner, comes to the centralized services. If the patient is not fully ambulatory, it is the care partner who pushes the wheelchair. They go together to the site of clinical nursing care at the "therapeutic center," to the site of instruction at the "education center," and to meals in the dining room.

How can an acute-care hospital function with the active presence of so many family members? Don't they produce too much interference? Don't they slow down the effectiveness and efficiency of the facility? A study of hospital care in a foreign culture noted the following:

> Visitors may sometimes become a strain for both patient and staff merely because there are too many of them or because they tend to disregard hospital rules and regulations. A particular problem is posed by visitors who expect to stay with the patient throughout his hospitalization, whether or not there are special facilities for them to do so, and this is common practice in many countries. In Malawi, for instance, a patient has "guardians" who accompany him from his village into hospital, look after him while he is there, and accompany him back to his village on discharge. In the Philippines these people are known as "watchers," and they are very common among all classes in rural as well as urban areas. Though their presence is accepted in both private and government hospitals, the watchers often cause a great deal of trouble with their many belongings, sharing the patient's bed, occupying a vacant bed in the ward, or simply spreading themselves out on the floor. In the vast majority of cases they are given no instructions. . . . [7]

That is the problem. When no instruction is given, the visitors become obstructionists. Given instruction, knowledge, and direction, visitors become extenders of the hospital staff, capable of assisting in many important tasks. The net result is diminished need for the professional staff to perform simple but time-consuming tasks so they can instead care more effectively for a greater number of patients. The cost saving can be startling.

How are patients selected for entry into the cooperative care unit? The attending physician makes the decision to admit his or her patient to the unit by initially determining that acute-care hospitalization is required by the severity of illness or the need to perform an inpatient invasive procedure. Three additional factors must then be taken into consideration to decide that admission to cooperative care, rather than to the traditional part of the hospital, is possible. First, the medical condition must be judged by the physician to be stable enough so that for periods of time the patient can be maintained out of view of the professional nursing staff. Second, the patient must be mobile enough, with the assistance of the care partner, so that together they will be able to manage in the room and be able to come to the centralized clinical, educational, and dining facilities. Third, an adequate care partner must be available.

The care partner need not be just one person. The role of care partner could be a shared responsibility among several family members or friends. For example, one person could serve as a care partner during daytime hours, while another who is employed days could come at night. In some instances, it may be more convenient for one individual to serve as a care partner one day, with a different family member or friend serving the next day. The advantage of sharing the responsibility in this way is that more family members can become trained, confident, and competent. That benefit more than outweighs the loss of continuity and the added burden of training the additional people to become care partners.

Patients enter cooperative care by one of two routes: by being directly admitted from home, or by being transferred to cooperative care from the traditional part of the hospital. Examples of the types of situations that would lead to direct admission are the need for cardiac catheterization, myelography, chemotherapy, intravenous antibiotics, management of congestive heart failure, brittle diabetes, and intractable angina. Examples of the transfers from the traditional part of the hospital include postoperative care of patients who have undergone major surgery, such as coronary artery bypass grafting, cardiac valve replacement, colon resection, resection of lung cancer, neurosurgery, and urologic surgery. Following stabilization, patients with myocardial infarction and other major medical disorders are likely to be transferred to cooperative care until they are ready for discharge.

## PLAN OF CARE

The first stop on arrival in the cooperative care unit, after the usual paperwork formalities at the admitting office, is the education center. It is so extremely important for the successful functioning of the cooperative care program to have a fully informed patient and care partner, that an educational assessment is performed before a clinical assessment is made.

The education center is a large area containing smaller conference rooms, for individual and group instruction, and carrels at which the patient and care partner can view videotape and slide presentations. After providing a videotape introduction and orientation to cooperative care, a nurse-educator meets with the patient and care partner and determines their educational needs. Some needs will be addressed immediately, but others will be met by instruction sessions scheduled for later in the hospital course. Teaching will be provided during the stay by members of the multidisciplinary education team. The team consists of a nutritionist, pharmacist, social worker, and recreation therapist, in addition to the nurse-educator.

The nurse-educator is primarily responsible for teaching regarding the diagnosis, the scheduled diagnostic procedures, the treatments, and the observations that are to be made during the hospitalization by the care partner. None of the clinical care responsibilities usually associated with nursing are assigned to the nurse-educator. Thus, the educational objectives remain the nurse-educator's top priority and are not relegated to second-level importance when pressures are imposed by urgent clinical demands. Written materials are given to the patient and care partner in conjunction with the nurse-educator's teaching, and are useful for reinforcement and review. The folder provided for these materials will be added to repeatedly throughout the stay in cooperative care as the other members of the education center team step in along predetermined stages.

The nutritionist meets with the patient and care partner to assess nutritional status and the diet that the patient had followed at home prior to admission, and to then discuss the prescribed diet to be followed while in cooperative care. This is necessary at the beginning of the hospitalization, rather than at the end, in order to prepare the patient for selecting foods from the cafeteria-style service in the dining room. Later, at mealtimes, the nutritionist will have repeated opportunities to reinforce the teaching while observing whether the patient's food choices have been made correctly.

The social worker may be needed at the time of admission to intercede, particularly if a care partner problem is present. The problems that would trigger immediate intervention on arrival include the absence of a care partner, a care partner who is not fully adequate for the expected responsibilities, and excessive anxiety or worry on the part of either the patient or care partner, so that counseling and support are needed to a greater extent than ordinarily provided by the nursing staff.

The pharmacist enters the picture later, as does the recreation therapist.

Following the screening, evaluation, and initial teaching performed in the education center, the second stop for the patient on admission to cooperative care is the therapeutic center. This is the area in which the nurse-clinicians are located and to which the patients come at appointed times for clinical assessment, treatment, and care. Patients are seen in examining rooms, quite like those of physicians' offices.

Nurse-clinicians are required to have three to five years of prior medical–surgical acute-care hospital nursing experience, in addition to a minimum of a bachelor's degree and supplemental education and training, before being considered eligible for a position in cooperative care. Maturity, experience, and competence are all needed attributes for the nurse-clinician to deal effectively with the patient who is out of the professional's sight and to confidently marshal the services of the care partner as an intermediary. Most difficult, for the hospital-based nurse, is the absence of complete control, since the responsibilities progressively follow an evolutionary process, passing from the professionals to the care partner and patient.

Other than performing the physical assessment of the patient at the time of admission, which is done much as it would be in a traditional hospital setting, the nurse-clinician must also, at that time, prepare the patient and care partner for their roles in observing, recording, reporting, and treating. A schedule will be created, which will incorporate the later planned visits to the therapeutic center, diagnostic tests, and x-ray examinations.

The physical plant of the New York University Medical Center Cooperative Care Unit is housed on the seven upper floors of the 15-story Arnold and Marie Schwartz Health Care Center. The top floor holds the dining room, lounge, and recreation therapy area. The fourteenth floor is the location of the reception desk, admission department, pharmacy, education center, and therapeutic center. Patient rooms are on the remaining five floors (the ninth through the thirteenth). With 20 to 21 rooms on each of those floors, the capacity of the unit is 104 patients and, in addition, 104 care partners.

When the elevator doors open and the patient and care partner step out to go toward their room, they first appreciate that no nurses at all are on the floor. It is quiet, despite full occupancy, since it is lacking the clatter and clutter of a traditional nursing unit. That is left behind on the fourteenth floor, with its centralized services having a slight flavor of chaos at times.

Using the key to enter their room, the patient and care partner find it to be home-like. It is simply furnished, and missing are the accouterments of the technology-intensive traditional hospital room. For example, the beds are low, without siderails or electrical controls. One bed is for the patient, one for the live-in care partner. A sitting area, with chairs, small table, dresser, and television, gives the room the appearance of a small studio apartment. Each room has a private bathroom, some with bathtub, others with wheelchair-accessible shower stall.

The rooms lack in-wall oxygen outlets and in-wall suction apparatus. If oxygen is required, and if oxygen will be needed also after discharge, such as for a patient with chronic pulmonary disease, the patient and family will be better prepared for home if they learn how to use the home oxygen devices while still in the hospital. In that instance, a portable tank or oxygen concentrator will be used in the room. The educational session will then have obvious immediate relevance. The practical hands-on experience will reinforce the teaching and make it more effective and memorable. The philosophy is that, while in cooperative care, the patient and care partner should deal with the realities they are to expect at home.

Cardiac monitors are not used in the patient rooms. This avoids the situation of increased anxiety created by suddenly removing the telemetry device upon discharge. Having looked upon the monitoring as a needed safety measure, perhaps even after it was truly needed, the sudden loss of its "protection" is felt by patient and family as additional reason for fear of going home. If monitoring is required in cooperative care, the patient will be brought to the six-bed observation unit, which is part of the fourteenth floor therapeutic center. Although the care partner is present and plays a supplementary and supporting role in the observation unit, here the professional nurse is constantly present and has full responsibility. The care partner is a trainee in that environment.

Patients are not assigned to the observation unit as if they were being transferred to a traditional hospital intensive care unit. Rather than having the room assignment changed, they remain in the observation unit only a few hours, similar to the pattern of a recovery room. They then return to their original patient room floor, where the care partner again becomes the primary observer.

What if a medical emergency occurs while the patient is in the home-like room and only the care partner is present? How is safety ensured? In a traditional hospital, safety is maintained by keeping the room door open, permitting nurses, aides, and others to witness obvious crises. Very little additional medical security results from the "buddy system" of two patients assigned to a semiprivate room. If one patient becomes somewhat pale, has some discomfort, or acts a bit strangely, the other patient in the room is not likely to intercede unless the change is quite dramatic. Certainly, if one patient has a grand mal seizure, the other patient will call for help. More subtle but substantial and important clues to changes in the clinical condition will not be recognized or acted on by the uninvolved, uninterested roommate who is, after all, a patient, too.

By contrast, in cooperative care, the care partner is a nonpatient who knows the patient well and has a vested interest in his or her well-being. The care partner, having been given instruction and direction by the education center and therapeutic center, is knowledgeable and feels responsible, as though "on duty." As in any acute-care hospital, emergencies do arise unexpectedly. In cooperative care, the premonitory symptoms and signs are usually noticed earlier by the care partner than they would be noted by professional staff in the traditional setting. Attuned to the need to observe and record changes in condition and appearance, the care partner becomes a reliable early warning detection mechanism. This human alarm triggers an immediate response from the nurse-clinicians. It cannot be ignored the way an imperfect electrical or mechanical device may be.

Faced with what appears to be an emergency, the care partner calls the therapeutic center on the "hot line." Literally in seconds, as in any acute-care hospital, nurse-clinicians arrive at the room. Additional emergency equipment and personnel are summoned as necessary. After initial stabilizing in the room, the patient is brought to the observation unit. Since the observation unit provides a high level of care, if emergent transfer to the traditional wing of the hospital is appropriate, it would most likely be to the intensive care unit.

Maintaining the distinction from the usual hospital procedures, in cooperative care, meals are provided in the top-floor dining room for both the patient and the accompanying care partner. Food is not served on a prearranged tray. Instead, each meal is considered an educational opportunity. Cafeteria-style, the patient must select each food according to the principles taught by the nutritionist on admission. With supervision and repeated reinforcement, by the time of discharge it is quite clear that even restaurant menu selection will pose no difficulty.

What if the patient on a low-salt diet selects food that is high in sodium content while in cooperative care? Won't that interfere with the plan of treatment? On the contrary, having the patient totally responsible for determining what is to be selected makes it more likely that the diet in the hospital will bear a strong resemblance to that which will be accepted and followed at home.

If a patient with congestive heart failure is hospitalized, three therapeutic interventions of significance must be recognized. First, physical activity is minimized. Second, the diet is severely restricted in sodium content. Third, a medication regimen is instituted. Not all the improvement is due to the prescribed drugs; some is the result of the reduction in activity and salt. At home, it is impractical to assume that the patient will continue to follow stringent sodium restriction and remain at bedrest. The diuretic dosage that was effective in the hospital may no longer be adequate when the activity level is increased and the salt content becomes that of a more palatable diet. With the patient at home, after discharge, the physician must retitrate the diuretics in order to maintain the therapeutic effect that was achieved in the hospital.

In cooperative care, the patient retains the right to eat with or without regard to the severity of the restrictions prescribed. Therefore, with the diet more akin to the post-discharge menu, the physician will be able to titrate the diuretic dosage in the hospital more accurately for home. The patient who is poorly compliant with the prescribed diet will be able to select food without regard to the ordered restriction. The resulting diet will be high in salt and, although it may be imperfect, it is more realistically like that which will be followed at home. Since activity and diet have already been restored to home-like levels, no further diuretic titration is likely to be required after discharge.

Coordinating management and expediting referrals between the therapeutic center and education center staffs are accomplished by a daily conference on the patient plan of care. Each nurse-clinician briefly presents his or her case load, with the nurse-educator, nutritionist, social worker, pharmacist, and recreation therapist present. If additional formal instruction or counseling is needed, it can be arranged at this time. The interdisciplinary exchange detects problems from differing viewpoints and stimulates creation of innovative solutions. The recreation therapist, for example, may be the first to appreciate the overprotectiveness of a spouse dissuading the patient from enjoying moderately vigorous leisure activities. Bringing that problem into the open here permits intervention, such as simply demonstrating the safety of a graded increase in energy expenditure.

The plan-of-care conference may identify the pharmacist as a needed referral. Most patients in cooperative care self-administer medications. This procedure, familiarly called "SAM" by the staff, is a four-step process. It starts with educating the patient and care partner about the drug regimen to be used, followed by evaluating their knowledge and understanding of each item, proceeds to dispensing the medications for self-administration, followed by auditing frequently for accuracy of timing and of recording.

In teaching about the prescribed medications, the pharmacist will cover the generic and brand names of each agent; reasons for use of the medication; its actions, expected side-effects, potential hazards, and interactions with other drugs and with foods; and proper timing and dosage. Written summaries are used for review. The nurse-clinician later independently verifies that the patient and care partner have retained the information prior to starting them on SAM. The medications are packaged and labeled as they would be for outpatient use and the patient–care partner team then becomes responsible for each dose, as they would be at home. They record each medication administered on sheets similar to traditional hospital medication records. At each subsequent nursing visit at the therapeutic center, the records are reviewed and discussed to confirm that the timing and dosage have been as prescribed.

## OUTCOME OF COOPERATIVE CARE

By its comprehensive educational program of education of the patient and education of the family, the cooperative care stay provides better preparation for home care after discharge than does a traditional hospitalization. Because of their active involvement in care and treatment decisions during the acute illness, the patient and family become better managers of chronic disease at home. Having had first-hand experience and working as a team, the patient and care partner can more confidently handle minor crises at home, avoiding their magnification and evolution into major crises. More appropriate utilization of health-care resources should follow. There should be a reduction of emergency room visits and rehospitalizations, with a concomitant increase in telephone contacts with the physician and of elective office visits.

Greater accuracy in following the prescribed treatment regimen is an outgrowth of the fuller understanding developed during the stay in cooperative care. Fewer medication errors are committed. The diet is followed to the same degree as that for which the medications were adjusted. The disease process and diagnosis are known in detail. Risk factors can be recognized and possibly avoided. Patient satisfaction and family satisfaction are enhanced. Anxiety is reduced.

Despite the need for additional food and space for the care partners, cooperative care is cost-effective. Two people—the patient and care partner—cost approximately one-third less than one patient in a traditional semiprivate acute-care hospital room. The savings result from the reduced staff required, as well as the centralization of services.

## FOLLOW-UP AFTER DISCHARGE

The average length of stay in cooperative care is four days. It is not permissible to extend the duration of hospitalization beyond that needed for clinical care, even if the educational objectives have not yet been fully met. Therefore, follow-up education is part of the outpatient program. All the disease-specific programs available for inpatients are available, in separate sessions, to outpatients. Group courses in risk factor intervention, particularly weight reduction and smoking cessation, are provided.

Linkage with home care services, as from conventional hospitals, is provided for those patients requiring such care. Home care nurses, aides, durable medical equipment, and supplies need to be arranged. Verbal and written reports are exchanged. Feedback from the home care service is incorporated into subsequent treatment plans.

After discharge, physician office visits become extensions of the educational process.

The physician–patient interaction gives patients an opportunity to increase their understanding of the medical process, particularly the logic of treatment and follow-up. Patients who do not use this opportunity effectively may not acquire the knowledge, skill and, more importantly, the confidence and sense of control they need in the daily management of chronic disease.[8]

Having been in cooperative care, with its emphasis on sharing of control and information, patients are well equipped to take full advantage of the physician follow-up.

## ADAPTING COOPERATIVE CARE TO SMALL HOSPITALS

Can a large program, such as that of the cooperative care unit at the New York University Medical Center, be translated into a form that would be suitable for preparing patients for home while in a small community hospital? What are the essential ingredients to be incorporated into such a plan? Is expensive capital construction necessary? How can all the teaching staff be supported?

Many small hospitals already contain cooperative care-like units. Pediatric services are, in essence, cooperative care units for children. It is openly acknowledged that children must have education about their condition and that their parents are indispensable ingredients in helping to provide inpatient care. Cooperative care extends the benefits of family participation and education, widely available for children, to the adult hospitalized patient. Thus, the groundwork has already been laid for implementing such programs. Live-in maternity units likewise have much of the structure of cooperative care in place. This background experience of many hospitals can be expanded upon easily.

Step one is to keep the patient as active as possible, commensurate with good clinical judgment. Step two is to get the family involved from the start. Step three is to develop a formal education protocol for each major category of illness or type of patient, involving personnel already on the hospital staff. Step four is to look carefully at the other models in existence at the hospital, such as the maternity and pediatric units mentioned above. The fifth step, not previously possible but now a potentially available avenue of approach, is to take advantage of the decreased hospital inpatient occupancy spreading across the country in conjunction with DRGs. As empty beds become available, consider using two-bed rooms for one patient plus one care partner.

The philosophy is important, not the structure. Hospitals should be looked upon as high-technology home-extensions, not as castles of treatment guarded by protectionist policies that safeguard all control into the hands of the professionals. Preparing the patient for home while in the hospital begins by preparing the hospital for home-like involvement of patient and family. That is the modern advance made by cooperative care. It has brought hospital care full cycle, from the ancient hospital in which care-givers were helped by family, past the traditional hospital in which the care givers are watched by the family, to the futuristic hospital in which care givers and family are merged. Preparation for home care is then ideally accomplished.

## REFERENCES

1. Bedell SE, Cleary PD, Delbanco TL: The kindly stress of hospitalization. Am J Med 77:592–596, 1984
2. Castiglioni A (translated by Krumbhaar EB): A History of Medicine, 2nd ed, p 1130. New York, Alfred A Knopf, 1947
3. Ibid, pp 167–168
4. Lyons AS, Petrucelli RJ II: Medicine: An Illustrated History, p 216. New York, Harry N Abrams, 1978
5. Price D, Cooke J, Singleton S, Feely M: Doctors' unawareness of the drugs their patients are taking: A major cause of overprescribing? Br Med J 292:99–100, 1986
6. Strull WM, Lo B, Charles G: Do patients want to participate in medical decision making? JAMA 252:2990–2994, 1984
7. Eldar R, Eldar E: A place for the family in hospital life. Int Nurs Rev 31:40–42, 1984
8. Greenfield S, Kaplan S, Ware JE Jr: Expanding patient involvement in care: Effects on patient outcomes. Ann Int Med 102:520–528, 1985

# 3
# Preparing the Physical Environment

HOWARD G. THISTLE
DIANNA M. D'AMICO
LAURIE R. STUHL PROWLER

The rehabilitation medicine practitioner will find it relatively easy to identify and assess a variety of potential or existing patient disabilities and, likewise, that particular patient's home care needs. However, many medical practitioners find it difficult to do so. Not only are they unable to identify which patients need home care, but they are often unaware of the kind of home care needed or how to provide necessary environmental modifications, equipment, and services. The patient may be discharged home with no arrangement having been made for home care. Increasingly, however, as hospital stays are shortened and patients are managed more at home, it is incumbent upon the physician to identify a patient's home care needs and understand how to utilize appropriate resources to meet those needs. Only then can the patient hope to function optimally. Home care needs may range from providing a simple self-help device to something more complex such as modifying the home for accessibility. Safety, of course, must always be a major consideration.

To identify the nature and degree of disability, there are a variety of assessment tools available to the practitioner and he or she may, rather quickly, identify the patient's limitations that need to be addressed. Once identified, and with the knowledge of appropriate resources, the physician can direct the patient to avenues for self-help, home modification, equipment, or community services. Often, information gathered from evaluation devices may have therapeutic implications that could not be derived from a knowledge of clinical diagnoses or laboratory test results alone.

The available assessment devices include the PULSES profile, Bartel and Katz Index, and Kenny Self-Care Evaluation, as well as the rehabilitation indicators. Some are cumbersome and time consuming and, therefore, impractical as a simple, concise method for identifying patients with disabilities requiring modifications in the home. The PULSES profile is one of the least cumbersome and can provide the practitioner with a fast, easy method for assessing functional abilities and disabilities. Although it was originally devised by Drs. Moscowitz and McCann for working with chronically ill and aging persons, it can be applied to all age groups, impairments, and disabilities.

## PULSES PROFILE*

A patient may have impairments in one or more of six areas and may range from no impairment to mild, moderate, or severe impairment. The patient is rated on a scale of 1 to 4 in each of the following six areas:

P—physical condition: basic health/illness status

U—upper limb functions: self-care activities (drinking, eating, dressing upper/lower body, donning brace or prosthesis, washing/bathing, perineal care)

L—lower limb functions: mobility (transferring) chair/toilet/tub or shower, walking, climbing stairs, propelling wheelchair)

S—sensory components: sight, communications (verbal/hearing)

E—excretory functions: control of sphincters (bladder/bowel)

S—support factors: psychological/emotional, family/social/financial supports

In addition to the above, some of the common broad categories of physical limitations to consider are whether the patient is independent or dependent, bedridden, wheelchair-bound or ambulatory, hearing or visually impaired. While your patient may not fall into any of these categories directly, they may serve as a guide in your evaluation phase.

Preparing the patient for return home is multifaceted. The planning must include an assessment and *then* preparation of both patient and home environment so as to facilitate the safest and smoothest transition.

## ASSESSMENT OF THE PATIENT'S NEEDS

Table 3-1 is an aid to planning and recommending equipment for your patient to facilitate independence and safety at home. We have chosen to divide the chart into broad categories of limitations with specific equipment suggestions.

Examples of disabilities in each category are the following:

*One-sided impairment*
   Hemiplegia
   Amputation

*Lower extremity impairment*
   Paraplegia
   Multiple sclerosis
   Cerebral palsy
   Spina bifida
   Amputation

*All extremities impaired*
   Quadriplegia
   Arthritis
   Cerebral palsy

*Low endurance*
   Cardiac disease
   Chronic obstructive pulmonary disease
   Cancer

*Visual impairment*
   Low vision problems
   Blindness

*Auditory impairment*
   Deafness

When assessing the home environment, both the exterior and interior of the house or apartment must be considered. You should be most concerned about accessibility, obstacles, and safety. The following home evaluation will determine what modifications are

(*Text continues on page 38*)

* Granger CV, Albrecht GL, Hamilton BB: Outcomes of comprehensive medical rehabilitation; measurement by PULSES profile and the Bartel Index. Arch Phys Med Rehabil 60:145, 1979

**TABLE 3-1. ASSESSMENT OF EQUIPMENT NEEDS FOR THE DISABLED PATIENT**

| Activity | Problem | Equipment | Comments |
|---|---|---|---|
| *Transfers* | One-sided impairment | Sliding board | A smooth-surfaced wooden board with a center hole placed between patient and transfer object. The board is placed under patient's upper thigh. |
| | Lower extremity impairment | Sliding board, trapeze | |
| | All extremities impaired | Sliding board with one-person assist | |
| | | Hoyer lift | The Hoyer lift is a hydraulic lift using a sling to hold patient. It may also be useful with an overweight dependent patient. |
| | Low endurance | Sliding board | |
| | Visual impairment | Not applicable* | Orientation to environment |
| | Auditory impairment | Not applicable | |
| *Mobility* | One-sided impairment | Manual wheelchair with one-hand drive, ambulatory with walker, cane (straight, narrow-base or wide-base quad), or crutches | |
| | Lower extremity impairment | Manual wheelchair (standard or sports model), ambulatory with braces and assistive devices | |
| | All extremities impaired | Manual wheelchair with lugs | Lugs allow patient with limited grasp to propel a wheelchair. Lugs are protrusions from the rim of the wheelchair. Gloves are recommended to provide better traction. |
| | | Motorized wheelchair with specific drive control (hand, breath, chin) | The various drive controls are specific to patient's functional ability. Breath and chin controls are used for patients who have no function in upper extremities, but who have good head and neck control. The hand control can be adapted with differently shaped devices. |
| | Low endurance | Manual wheelchair, motorized wheelchair, motorized scooter | Patient must have good balance to operate motorized scooter. |
| | Visual impairment | Seeing eye dog; cane | Orientation to environment. If a person leads the patient, patient must hold onto the person's upper arm and be given verbal cues. |
| | Auditory impairment | Not applicable | |

| Activity | Impairment | Equipment | Comments |
|---|---|---|---|
| **Toileting** | One-sided impairment | Toilet bars, raised toilet seat, bedpan, bedside commode, shower commode chair, toileting stick | The shower commode chair can be placed directly over toilet. The toileting stick is used by patients who have limited reach. It holds toilet paper and assists with cleaning. |
| | Lower extremity impairment | Toilet bars, bedside commode, shower commode chair, suppository insertor, digital stimulator | These are used to assist patient with limited mobility/grasp. |
| | All extremities impaired | Bedside commode, toileting stick, shower commode chair, suppository insertor, digital stimulator | |
| | Low endurance | Bedside commode | |
| | Visual impairment | Not applicable | Orientation to environment; consistency maintained with placement of objects |
| | Auditory impairment | Not applicable | |
| | Bedridden | Bedpan or urinal, absorbent pads | |
| **Feeding** | One-sided impairment | Dycem pad | Dycem pad is a nonskid rubber pad that prevents an object from skidding. It is placed beneath the object. |
| | | Rocker knife | Rocker knife is a curved-blade knife that allows patient to cut food with one hand by using a rocking motion. |
| | | Scoop dish, plate guard | Both devices have high sides so patient can push food against the sides, preventing food from sliding off plate. |
| | Lower extremity impairment | Not applicable | |
| | All extremities impaired | Electric self-feeder | Electrically brings utensil to patient's mouth |
| | | Utensils with built-up handles ADL/universal cuff, C-clip holder | Used for patients with decreased grasp. Both devices wrap around palm of hand to hold utensils. They are used by patients who have limited or no grasp. |
| | Low endurance | Long straw, mug | Pace activity level. |
| | Visual impairment | Not applicable | Consistency in organization; verbal cuing; exploration of dish; memory training. When cuing the individual, you must describe position of food, utensils, and beverage by associating the positions with the numbers on a clock. |
| | Auditory impairment | Not applicable | |

*(continued)*

**TABLE 3-1. Continued**

| Activity | Problem | Equipment | Comments |
|---|---|---|---|
| ***Hygiene*** | | | |
| Brushing hair/combing hair | One-sided impairment | Not applicable | |
| | Lower extremity impairment | Not applicable | |
| | All extremities impaired | Long-handled brush or comb, built-up handle, C-clip holder | |
| | Low endurance | Not applicable | Pace activity level. |
| | Visual impairment | Not applicable | |
| | Auditory impairment | Not applicable | |
| Brushing teeth | One-sided impairment | Suction denture brush | Patient needs to place toothbrush on counter to stabilize. Open toothpaste tube with one hand and squeeze onto toothbrush. |
| | Lower extremity impairment | Not applicable | |
| | All extremities impaired | Suction denture brush, built-up handle, C-clip holder, electric toothbrush | |
| | Low endurance | Electric toothbrush | |
| | Visual impairment | Use braille labels on items | |
| | Auditory impairment | Not applicable | |
| Bathing | One-sided impairment | Long-handled sponge, suction nail brush, soap on a rope, wash mitt | |
| | Lower extremity impairment | Long-handled sponge | |
| | All extremities impaired | Long-handled sponge, suction nail brush, wash mitt, soap on a rope, digital read-out temperature faucets | Water temperature must be checked on *full* sensation areas. Nonskid surface is recommended in tub. |
| | Low endurance | Long-handled sponge | |
| | Visual impairment | Raised letters on faucets | Consistency in organization of supplies is helpful. |
| Shaving | Auditory impairment | Not applicable | |
| | One-sided impairment | Electric shaver | |
| | Lower extremity impairment | Not applicable | |
| | All extremities impaired | Electric razor, C-clip holder for razor (manual or electric), shaving cream dispenser handle | The shaving cream dispenser handle is a lever apparatus attached to spray nozzle to assist in pressing down. This is for patients with limited hand control. |

| Activity | Impairment | Adaptive device | Comments |
|---|---|---|---|
| | Low endurance | Built-up handle for manual razor | Decreases chance of cutting oneself |
| | Visual impairment | Electric razor | |
| | Auditory impairment | Electric razor | |
| | | Not applicable | |
| **Dressing** | | | |
| Putting on lower extremity clothing | One-sided impairment | Dressing stick | Wooden stick with hook on the end to aid in reaching and hooking clothing |
| | | Stocking aid | Oval-shaped plastic device with loops on top. Stocking is fitted over plastic, foot is placed into stocking, and loops are pulled upward. |
| | Lower extremity impairment | Reacher | |
| | | Dressing stick, reacher, trouser and sock pulls | The pulls are loops that are attached to clothing. Patient places hand or wrist through loop. The wrist is used for pulling by patients who lack grasp. |
| | | Leg lifter | The leg lifter may be either webbing or a strap to assist patient in lifting leg for positioning to dress. |
| | All extremities impaired | Dressing stick, reacher, trouser pull, stocking aid, zipper pull | The zipper pull is a small loop or ring attached to the zipper for a patient with limited hand control. |
| | Low endurance | Reacher | Patient sets up own system for identifying colors and styles, for example, by using a different knot on the label to distinguish clothing of different colors (e.g., red = 2 knots). |
| | Visual impairment | Not applicable | |
| Putting on upper extremity clothing | Auditory impairment | Not applicable | |
| | One-sided impairment | Velcro closure for bras or shirts, front closing bra, button hook | |
| | Lower extremity impairment | Not applicable | |
| | All extremities impaired | Velcro closure for bras, button hook, dressing stick | |
| | Low endurance | Not applicable | |
| | Visual impairment | Not applicable | Pace activity level. |
| | Auditory impairment | Not applicable | |

*(continued)*

**TABLE 3-1. Continued**

| Activity | Problem | Equipment | Comments |
|---|---|---|---|
| ***Dressing*** | | | |
| Putting on shoes | One-sided impairment | Elastic laces, Velcro closure, long shoe horn, slip-on shoes | |
| | Lower extremity impairment | Not applicable | |
| | All extremities impaired | Elastic laces, Velcro closure, long shoe horn, slip-on shoes | |
| | Low endurance | Long shoe horn, Velcro closure, slip-on shoes | |
| | Visual impairment | Not applicable | |
| | Auditory impairment | Not applicable | |
| ***Communication*** | One-sided impairment | Low mounted telephone, portable telephones, shoulder rest for telephone, intercom systems, personal alarm systems | |
| | Lower extremity impairment | Low mounted telephone, portable telephone | |
| | All extremities impaired | Dialing stick | Stick is placed in a hand splint or in the mouth to assist with dialing telephone. |
| | | Push-button telephone, automatic dialer, speaker telephone, alternate telephone devices: MED Micro-dec, Prentke Romich, Du-it Mecca | The alternate telephone devices are used to gain access to telephone. The specific type of control depends on patient's upper extremity function. |
| | Low endurance | Portable telephone | Place within easy access. |
| | Visual impairment | Large number outlays for telephone with raised numbers or braille: automatic dialer | |
| | Auditory impairment | Telecommunicator (teletype or telecommunication device) | This provides a visual display or printout of incoming messages when attached to the telephone. Telephone may also be installed with a light system to indicate incoming calls. |
| | | Volume control on hand set | |

## Meal Preparation

| Impairment | Equipment | Notes |
|---|---|---|
| One-sided impairment | Rocker knife; rehabilitation cutting board | The rehabilitation cutting board is a wooden board with two stainless steel nails projecting to secure food for cutting. |
| | Dycem pad | |
| | Cart | To transport food |
| | Cane holder | Holder clips onto cane to balance on the countertop. |
| All extremities impaired | Adapted utensils | Joint protection techniques for arthritics. Utensils are adapted with built-up handles or clips to secure onto hand if patient has poor control. |
| | Dycem pad | |
| | Rehabilitation cutting board | |
| | Zim jar opener | |
| | Electric can opener | |
| | Lapboard | |
| | Reacher | To transport items |
| | Bag attached to wheelchair | |
| | Lower countertops | Modification for the wheelchair-bound patient |
| Lower extremity impairment | Reacher, lapboard, bag attached to walker, lower countertops | |
| Low endurance | High stool | Pace activity level. A high stool enables patient to sit while working, thereby decreasing energy expenditure. |
| Visual impairment | Not applicable | Consistent organization, labeling, using touch, verbal cuing, marking dials, long oven mitts, memory training, orient to environment |
| Auditory impairment | Not applicable | |

* No specific equipment recommendations are required.
† For specific showering equipment recommendations, see the section on the bathroom under Preparation of the Physical Environment, later in this chapter.

needed. The modifications may be as simple as widening a doorway or as complex as making major renovations within the house. The following questions may be helpful:

With whom does the patient live?

Type of house
   Apartment?
   Privately owned or rented?
   Number of stories?
   Garage—attached (street level or under house)? Detached? How many cars can be accommodated?

Entrances
   How many and where?
   Number of steps outside and inside the entrance door?
   Location of handrails at steps?

Elevators (where applicable)
   Is the elevator big enough to accommodate the person with the wheelchair?
   Is the door wide enough?
   Can the person reach and operate the elevator controls?
   Are the controls audibly and tactily suitable for the patient?
   Does the door close automatically?
   Does the elevator level off at landings?

First floor
   List the rooms.
   What are the floor coverings?

Stairway
   Is it straight?
   Does it have one or more turns?
   Are these turns wedge-shaped steps or landings and more steps?
   Location of handrails?
   Floor coverings?

Other floors and stairways
   Repeat the same questions.

Kitchen
   What is the general layout?
   Who prepares the food?
   Will the patient be involved?

Laundry
   Location?
   Who does the laundry?

Bathrooms
   Where are the bathrooms located that the patient will use?
   Get the following information about all pertinent bathrooms:
      Floor location in house
      Width of doorway
      Direction of door swing
      Presence of threshold and its height
      Layout of bathroom—have the patient draw it or describe it as you draw it.
   Ask one by one about the following fixtures:
      Lavatory—wall hung or in a vanity?
      Toilet—tank or flush valve?
      Combined tub with shower curtains or sliding doors?
      Separate shower stall—height of lip, size of stall, curtain or shower door opening
      Separate bathtub—curtain or sliding doors?
      Does patient have a hand-held shower spray, grab bar(s), or shower seat of any kind?

Bedroom
  Doorway size?
  Hallway width just outside the bedroom door?
  Size and type of bed?
  Amount of space around bed?
  Are stored clothes accessible?

Doorways
  Width of doors?
  Direction of door swing?
  Presence of threshold and its height?

Upon completion of the evaluation, list all of the areas that appear to present a problem. Modifications of the specific interior and exterior areas of the house are discussed under Preparation of the Physical Environment, below.

## PREPARATION OF THE PATIENT

### SUPPORT SYSTEM

Once a clear and thorough assessment of the patient's realistic abilities and needs for equipment and home modifications has been made, you then need to identify the patient's support system upon discharge.

If the patient is planning to return home alone, is that a feasible plan? Can a family member adequately provide assistance, or does it need to be supplemented by a nurse, aide, or homemaker?

The patient's insurance benefits to cover assistance at home will need to be checked by the social service department or through direct contact with the insurance carrier.

Whoever has been chosen as the care partner for the patient should be involved with the rehabilitation team for the preparation for home. The care partner should be made aware of the patient's needs, such as assistive devices, home modifications, and the implications regarding the patient's safety.

### SAFETY

Maintaining the patient's safety at home is a major component of discharge planning. All individuals involved with the patient need to be aware of safety precautions and management concerning such areas as falls, fires, and minor and major emergencies.

The following are some basic considerations that need to be discussed to ensure one's safety at home:

1. What are possible safety hazards in the patient's home, such as insufficient lighting, clutter in walkways?
2. How will the patient's limitations, such as sensory, judgment, physical, or communicative impairments, interfere with his safety?
3. How would assistance be obtained, if needed, for the patient once he is home? Would a personal alarm system or intercom system be feasible? Personal alarm systems are very appropriate for patients who will be home alone for extended periods of time. They allow the patient constant communication with assistance at the tip of his finger. Listed in the Appendix are several manufacturers to contact for information relevant to your patient's specific needs.
4. Has a fire plan been prepared and practiced, taking into consideration the limitations of the patient?
5. How should emergencies be managed at home?

The preparation of the patient and his care partner is only the first step in discharge planning. The second consideration is the preparation of the patient's physical environment as he returns home with different capabilities.

## PREPARATION OF THE PHYSICAL ENVIRONMENT

### BEDROOM

**Size.** The bedroom must be large enough to accommodate a bed, clothing storage, and any necessary medical equipment, and still be large enough for the patient's mobility. If a patient is ambulatory, make sure there are no objects blocking paths leading to furniture. If a patient is in a wheelchair, there should be aisle spaces of 3 to 4 feet between pieces of furniture and room next to the bed for transfers. The bed should be at a height that is level with the wheelchair and high enough for an ambulatory patient to stand up easily from the side of the bed.

**Storage.** Storage spaces should be arranged so that clothing is within reach. Clothing in a bureau or in dressers should be arranged so that drawers can be opened easily. Clothing in closets can be made accessible by adding an additional rod at a lower level. For wheelchair-bound patients, appropriate height of objects is no higher than 48 inches from a front approach and 54 inches from a side approach.

**Electrical Outlets.** Electrical outlets should be grounded to accommodate medical equipment such as an electrical hospital bed, or respiratory or heart monitors. In addition, there should be a sufficient number of outlets for environmental control units. The number of outlets needed will be determined by the number of pieces of equipment the patient needs.

### BATHROOM

**Tub.** The following equipment may be recommended for the patient's use, depending on the level of independence:

1. Tub shower chair—a chair without arms placed in the tub to sit on while bathing, especially if endurance is low. The patient must be ambulatory and safe in making a transfer into the tub.
2. Tub bench—a bench extending over the edge of the tub to sit on while bathing. It is recommended for patients with poor or unsafe transfer skills and low endurance, as well as for patients with lower extremity weakness or paralysis.
3. Grab bars—these may be installed to improve mobility within the bathtub.
4. Hand-held shower spray—this can be used to direct and bring the water source closer.

There should be adequate space adjacent to the tub to bring the commode/wheelchair close to promote safe transfers. Shower doors should be removed when using the tub bench. If the shower doors remain, the space to make a transfer is reduced because it blocks half of the opening to the tub.

**Stall Shower.** A stall shower is safe for use by ambulatory patients and by those who can safely make a transfer onto a slat or bench in the shower stall. The height of the lip should be taken into consideration. If it is too high, the patient may be unable to enter safely. A hand-held shower spray should be installed to direct and bring the source of water closer to the patient. The opening of the shower door must be wide enough to enable a safe transfer to be made. The door can be removed and a shower curtain substituted.

**Sink.** For wheelchair-bound patients, a sink in a countertop is the ideal arrangement. If there is a vanity present under the sink, it should be removed. The countertop should be braced to take at least 250 pounds of weight. The minimum depth should measure 27 inches. Wall-hung sinks, without legs, may be used but are generally not deep enough to accommodate the patient's legs, and therefore the patient will be unable to get close enough to the sink. If removing the vanity is not feasible, the patient will have to work from a side approach. This position requires the patient to have sufficient mobility.

The height of the sink should measure 31 to 33 inches to the countertop. The depth should be no more than 4 inches to allow for clearance underneath without rubbing the top of the thighs.

If a patient is wheelchair-bound, the mirror behind the sink should be lowered to just above the backsplash and to a height of 6 feet from the floor for ambulatory family members. If this is not feasible, a wall-mounted or countertop mirror may be installed. All medicine cabinets and electrical outlets should be relocated to within reach.

Faucet controls must be appropriate for the patient's degree of hand control and must be mounted within the patient's reach. Wing-handle or single-lever controls on sinks are recommended for patients with weak or minimal hand control or for those who cannot perform a turning motion.

**Toilet.** For nonambulatory patients using a commode chair, there must be a minimum of 3 feet of unobstructed space on either side of the toilet for the chair to roll over it. To complete a transfer, there must be a minimum of 30 inches of unobstructed space to place the wheelchair. For elderly patients or those who have difficulty getting on or off low surfaces, an 18-inch high toilet can be installed or a standard toilet can be raised to the proper height. The toilet can be installed on a wood or marble block and the waste pipe extended. A simpler solution may be to purchase a raised toilet seat. Toilet bars may also be used to aid in mobility or to provide stability while on the toilet.

**Roll-In Shower.** Construction of a roll-in shower should be considered for quadriplegic patients or those dependent in bathing activities.

**Safety.** Always use a rubber mat in the bathtub. Remove all scatter rugs without rubber backing to prevent sliding. Wrap or insulate any exposed pipes to prevent scrapes or burns. A towel bar must never be used as a grab bar because towel bars are not properly reinforced to support a patient's weight.

## DOORS

The minimum width to clear any doorway is 32 inches (assuming a standard adult wheelchair is being used). There are a number of different types of doors (single-hung, bifold, pocket, or accordion) that can be used when modifying a space. The type of door can be determined once the size of the room, hallway width, or space around the doorway is known.

The door knob should be mounted at 36 to 38 inches high off the floor. For those patients with weak or limited grasp, a lever-type door handle is ideal. If a patient has no hand control, an automatic door may be necessary.

Door sills are commonly placed on the interior and exterior of the doorways. They must be no higher than a half inch. If they are higher, they may either be removed, and the floor patched flush, or a small wood wedge secured in front of the sill to create a small ramp. For exterior doors, if a sill is removed, weather stripping may be placed on the door to prevent drafts.

For wheelchair-bound patients who live in an apartment, the door peep-hole must be lowered to eye level.

## HALLWAYS

For the wheelchair-bound patient, a narrow hallway can present a difficulty when making a 90-degree turn into a doorway. To improve accessibility, it is best to widen the doorway.

## FURNITURE

Passageways between pieces of furniture must be unobstructed and 3 to 4 feet wide. Likewise, adequate space must be available to enable the patient to transfer to and from the wheelchair and bed, chair, sofa, and so on. Beds, chairs, and sofas must be firm and not too low. Furniture must be secure, with all casters removed, and preferably have rounded edges.

## ENTRANCES

The exterior entrance into the house or apartment building must be accessible and safe. In the case of an apartment building, one must be concerned about all entrances—front, side, back, and garage. Consider also the entrance surface material, the slope to the building, the number of steps, and the presence or absence of ramps.

If there is no elevator, the following solutions may be considered, depending on the patient's level of functioning:

1. If the patient is ambulatory and there are steps, handrails should be installed on both sides.*
2. If the patient is wheelchair bound and able to propel a wheelchair safely, a ramp may be constructed.* A portable ramp must *only* be considered if there are not more than 1 or 2 steps.
3. If the patient is wheelchair bound and unable to propel the chair, a porch lift may be installed.

In an apartment house where there are two sets of doors to create a vestibule, it is safest if both doors swing in the same direction and there is a minimum of 4 feet between the doors.

If the property slopes in front of the house, one may consider regrading to provide a level surface.

## INTERIOR STAIRWAY

Two types of lifts for interior stairways are available—a seat/chair lift and a wheelchair stairway lift. The seat lift is recommended for patients with low endurance or who have lower extremity paralysis, but who are able to perform a safe transfer onto the seat. The wheelchair stairway lift is recommended for patients who are wheelchair bound and who have poor transfer skills.

## KITCHEN

In order to begin planning to retrain a patient in an existing kitchen or to modify that kitchen, one must first discuss the layout and what the patient's (and the family's) daily homemaking habits are. For instance, inquire about who is the primary homemaker, the family's eating habits, what appliances are present and their location, and the amount of storage space located in or near the kitchen.

---

*Guidelines for installing handrails and ramps are available in the publication *Specifications for Making Buildings and Facilities Accessible to and Useable by Physically Handicapped People*, ANSI A117.1-1980, published by the American National Standards Institute, Inc., 1430 Broadway, New York, NY 10018.

The ideal arrangements for an accessible kitchen are as follows:

**Work Surfaces.** The standard kitchen countertop height is 36 inches and is suitable for only the ambulatory patient. For wheelchair-bound patients, countertops should be 31 to 33 inches high. A countertop may be lowered in one section for heavy beating and mixing activities. Work surfaces should be continuous with other areas, such as sink and stove top and open underneath to permit wheelchair accessibility.

**Sink.** For wheelchair-bound patients, the sink should be open underneath. The sink should be no more than 5 to 6 inches deep and the drain should be in a corner (left or right) rather than in the center of the sink. *All drain and water pipes must be insulated to prevent burns and scrapes,* especially if the patient has no sensation in the lower extremities. Single-lever faucet handles are used for patients with poor hand control. Counter space should be provided adjacent to the sink for dishes after washing.

**Range/Stove Top.** Stove tops with open space are ideal for wheelchair-bound patients. Controls should be in front for easy access. If they are difficult to grasp, adaptive equipment may be necessary. Burners that are staggered or in a straight line across are preferable, so the patient does not have to reach over a hot burner to get to the rear burners. Plenty of counter space adjacent to the stove top must be provided on which to place hot dishes from the stove.

**Wall Oven.** A wall oven is best when it is placed at a height accessible to the user. Again, it is essential to have a countertop adjacent to the oven on which to place hot objects.

**Refrigerator.** For wheelchair-bound patients, a side-by-side model is more accessible than the common type with the freezer above the refrigerator. A refrigerator with shelving on the doors is helpful. The refrigerator door should open on the side, adjacent to the countertop, for easy removal of items.

**Storage Space.** Open shelving above or just below countertops, peg boards, easy glide drawers, and lazy susans within cabinets all provide better accessibility to hard-to-reach items. A reacher may be helpful for lighter weight objects.

## CONCLUSION

Quality of life must be the concern of all health-care providers. The physician should assume the primary responsibility for preparation of the patient for discharge home. Review of as few as six areas of function will identify impairments that may need attention. Once identified, these can be minimized with appropriate equipment, home modification, or support services. Conversely, failure to address these impairments will relegate the patient to a life of dependency and despair.

## BIBLIOGRAPHY

Anderson H: The Disabled Homemaker. Springfield, IL, Charles C Thomas, 1981
Cary JR: How to Create Interiors for the Disabled. New York, Pantheon Books, 1978
Hale G: The Source Book for the Disabled. London, Paddington Press, 1979

Klinger JL: Mealtime Manual for People with Disabilities and the Aging. Ronks, PA, Campbell Soup Co, 1978

Martin N, Holt MB, Hicks D: Comprehensive Rehabilitation Nursing. New York, McGraw-Hill, 1981

Rusk HA: Rehabilitation Medicine, 4th ed. St Louis, CV Mosby, 1977

Sargent JV: An Easier Way–Handbook for the Elderly and Handicapped. Ames, IA, Iowa State University Press, 1981

Whitcomb CJ, Benedict P: Your health and safety are your responsibility. Paraplegia News, pp 9–10, Oct, 1985

Winston S: Getting Organized. New York, Warner Books, 1978

## APPENDIX

### BOOKS

American National Standard: *Providing Accessibility and Usability for Physically Handicapped People.* American National Standards Institute, Inc, 1430 Broadway, New York, 1986 (ANSI A 117.1-1986)

Compliance Assistance Service: *The Guide to Disabilities and Barriers and the System of Accessible Design.* Compliance Assistance Service—A Division of Information Development Corp, 360 St Alban Ct, Winston-Salem, NC 27104

Laurie G: *Housing and Home Services for the Disabled.* New York, Harper & Row, 1977

Lifchez R, Winslow B: *Design for Independent Living: The Environment and Physically Disabled People.* Watson-Guptill Publications, New York, 1979

Raschko BB: *Housing Interiors for the Disabled and Elderly.* New York, Van Nostrand Reinhold, 1982

Wheeler V: *Planning Kitchens for Handicapped Homemakers.* New York, NYU Medical Center, (presently out of print)

### CATALOGUES

#### *Institutional*

#### *Assistive Devices*

Fred Sammons, Inc.
Box 32
Brookfield, IL 60513-0032

#### *Equipment*

Activeaid
Box 359
Redwood Falls, MN 56283
800-533-5330

Everest & Jennings, Inc.
3233 East Mission Oaks Blvd.
Camarillo, CA 93010
805-987-6911

Invacare Corporation
1200 Taylor St.
PO Box 4028
Elyria, OH 44036

Lumex
100 Spence St.
Bay Shore, NY 11706
516-273-2200

#### *Equipment, Assistive Devices*

Abbey Medical
17390 Brookhurst St.
Fountain Valley, CA 92728
800-633-9378

Maddak, Inc.
Pequannock, NJ 07440

Med
3223 South Loop 289
Suite 150
Lubbock, TX 79423

J.A. Preston Corporation
60 Page Road
Clifton, NJ 07012
800-631-7277

#### *Consumers*

#### *Assistive Devices*

Capability Collection
Ways and Means
28001 Citrin Drive
Romulus, MI 48178
313-946-5030

Enrichments
PO Box 579
Hinsdale, IL 60521
800-343-9742

### Adaptive Clothing

Laurel Designs
5 Laurel Avenue #7
Belvedere, CA 94920
415-435-1891

Nu Day Creations
Suite 7029
111 East Drake Road
Fort Collins, CO 80525
303-223-5178

Clothing for Handicapped People
The President's Committee on
Employment of the Handicapped
Washington, DC 20210

Products for People with Vision Problems
American Foundation for the Blind
15 West 16th St.
New York, NY 10011

Pirca Fashions
901 Third Avenue
Sacramento, CA 95818

Techni Flair Designer Line
PO Box 40
Cotter, AR 72626
501-435-2000

### Adaptive Clothing (Free Copies of Catalogue)

Fashion Able
5 Crescent Avenue
Box S
Rocky Hill, NJ 08553

### Assistive Devices, Adaptive Clothing (Free Copies of Catalogue)

Comfortably Yours
52 West Hunter Avenue
Maywood, NJ 07607
201-368-0400

Resource Home Health Care/Sears
Department 742 BSC 18 38
PO Box 5544
Chicago, IL 60680

## PAMPHLETS

### Free Copies

*Aids to Independent Living*
Appliance Information Service
Whirlpool Corporation
Administrative Center
Benton Harbor, MI 49022

*Designs for Independent Living*
Appliance Information Service
Whirlpool Corporation
Administrative Center
Benton Harbor, MI 49022

*Fire Safety for You: A Guide
for Handicapped People*
National Fire Protection Association
410 Atlantic Avenue
Boston, MA 02210

*Home Safety Checklist*
Safety for Older Consumers
Consumer Product Safety Commission
Washington, DC 20207

### $2.50/copy

*Home in a Wheelchair*
Paralyzed Veterans of America
4330 East West Highway
Washington, DC 20014

## PUBLICATIONS

*Accent on Living*
Cheerer Publishing, Inc.
PO Box 700
Gillum Road and High Drive
Bloomington, IL 61701

*Access: The Guide to a Better Life
for Disabled Americans,* by Lilly Bruck
Random House
20 E. 50 St.
New York, NY 10022

*Paraplegia News*
5201 N. 19 Avenue Suite 108
Phoenix, AZ 85015

*Sports 'N Spokes*
5201 N. 19 Avenue Suite 108
Phoenix, AZ 85015

*Living at Home After a Stroke*
Be Stroke Smart Series
National Stroke Association
1420 Ogden St.
Denver, CO 80218
303 839-1922

*Mainstream—
Magazine of the Able-Disabled*
2973 Beech St.
San Diego, CA 92102

*Building Without Barriers for the Disabled* (1976),
by Harkness SP and Groom JN
Whitney Library of Design
New York, NY

## SEAT LIFT MANUFACTURERS

American Stair-Glide Corporation
4001 East 138th St.
Grandview, MO 64030
816-763-3100/800-821-2041

The Cheney Company, Inc.
2445 South Calhoun Road
PO Box 188
New Berlin, WI 53151
414-782-1100
1-800-782-1222

Econol Stairway Lift Corporation
2513 Center St.
Cedar Falls, IA 50613
319-277-4777

Flinchbaugh/Murray Corporation
390 Eberts Lane
York, PA 17403
717-854-7720

Iecony Corporation
521 Fifth Avenue
New York, NY 10715
212-563-0123
Attn: Mr. John Seymour

Inclinator Company of America
2200 Paxton St.
Harrisburg, PA 17105
717-234-8065

Toce Brothers
PO Box 489
Broussard, LA 70518
318-856-7241
1-800-842-8158

## PORCH LIFT MANUFACTURERS

American Stair-Glide Corporation
4001 East 138th St.
Grandview, MO 64030
816-763-3100/800-821-2041

The Cheney Company, Inc.
2445 South Calhoun Road
PO Box 188
New Berlin, WI 53151
414-782-1100
1-800-782-1222

Econol Stairway Lift Corporation
2513 Center St.
Cedar Falls, IA 50613
319-277-4777

Ricon Sales, Inc.
11684 Tuxford St.
Sun Valley, CA 91352
818-768-5890

Toce Manufacturing, Ltd
PO Box 489
Broussard, LA 70518
318-856-7241
1-800-842-8158

Giant Lift Equipment Manufacturing Co. Inc.
136 Lafayette Road
North Hampton, NH 03862
603-964-5127
1-800-524-4268

## WHEELCHAIR STAIRWAY LIFT MANUFACTURERS

The Cheney Company, Inc.
2445 South Calhoun Road
PO Box 188
New Berlin, WI 53151
414-782-1100
1-800-782-1222

Econol Stairway Lift Corporation
2513 Center St.
Cedar Falls, IA 50613
319-277-4777

Flinchbaugh/Murray Corporation
390 Eberts Lane
York, PA 17403
717-854-7720

Garaventa (Canada) Ltd
605-202 St.
Langley, BC
Canada V6A 4P4
604-530-5251

## ELEVATOR MANUFACTURERS

Econol Stairway Lift Corporation
2513 Center St.
Cedar Falls, IA 50613
319-277-4777

Iecony Corporation
521 Fifth Avenue
New York, NY 10175
212-563-0123
Attn: Mr. John Seymour

Segwick Lifts Inc.
Foot of Prospect Street
PO Box 630
Poughkeepsie, NY 12602
914-454-5400

Waupaca Elevator Co.
PO Box 246
Waupaca, WI 54981
715-258-5581
Attn: Walt Jome

## EMERGENCY/ALARM SYSTEMS

*Voicemitters*
American Medical Alert Corporation
3265 Lawson Blvd.
Oceanside, NY 11572
516-536-5850
800-645-3244

*Life Line*
Life Line Systems, Inc.
400 Main St.
Waltham, ME 02254
617-923-4141

*Tel-Aid*
Metro Tel Corporation
15 Burke Lane
Syosset, NY 11791
516-364-3377

*Life Aid Corp*
5535 East Osborn #303
Scottsdale, AZ 85251
212-371-2625
602-945-8444

*Life Call Medical Alarm*
800-451-7000

*AT & T Emergency Call System Medical Alert*
800-222-5506

# 4

# Educational Needs of the Patient

SHIRLEY GARNETT
GRACE PHELAN
ANTHONY J. GRIECO

Home care has enjoyed a major resurgence over the past few years and has reclaimed its proper place in the health-care delivery system. Prior to the acceptance of hospitals as a place of healing, rather than as a place to die, families traditionally cared for their sick in the home. The evolution of high-technology hospitals eroded the family's role, as hospital employees assumed the responsibilities of care to a great degree. Today, with the changes in American medical economics and a more consumer-oriented society, coupled with the higher prevalence of chronic disease, patients and their families are again assuming a more active role in care, and the care is moving back into the home setting.

Beyond the traditional personal care activities, such as bathing and dressing, and the additional expected role for those who need to perform their own colostomy care and urine testing, patient and care partner roles at home are now becoming "high-tech." Home blood glucose self-monitoring makes it possible for patients to adjust their own diet, medications, and exercise routine to a remarkable extent in managing diabetes. Patients are at home on total parenteral nutrition, intravenous antibiotics, and chemotherapy. They are even regulating the rate of flow of these fluids themselves, providing an enormous sense of control over their destiny.

Education has always played an important role in the management of patients at home, but today's home educational needs have become much more crucial. The needs extend not only to the patient, but to many of the "others," such as family members, friends, and hired home aides, who will be involved in providing care in the home.

The ultimate goal of patient education is to help individuals gain the knowledge, attitudes, and behavior that will enable them to care for themselves in the best way possible. A planned patient education program is a systematic effort to assess the patient's (and care partner's) knowledge of his health, to provide what he wants and needs to know, and to effect a change in the patient's behavior that continues after his illness ends. The "educated" patient therefore stands to retrieve his health more quickly and is less likely to suffer a recurrence of his illness. He is much more likely to be conscientious about following the prescribed regimen and keeping follow-up visits.

Ideally, a patient should be able to receive enough education so that he can intelligently assume a "partnership" role with his physician. To meet this goal, we should utilize a process that includes (1) assessment of the situation, (2) planning of an appropriate strategy, (3) implementation, and (4) evaluation. The process should not be haphazard, but rather should be systematic and planned. One should not equate this with being overly cumbersome or inflexible. Quite the contrary, the process is quite natural: we size up the situation, plan an appropriate action, put the plan into operation, and obtain feedback about how well it is working.

By a partnership role, we mean that the patient actively participates in his own care under the direction of his physician. The patient, understanding the rationale behind his prescribed treatment, is able to make some informed decisions on what he should and should not do in everyday living; for example, what foods he should eat and what he should avoid. He may be given guidelines by his physician or by the home care nurse for adjusting his medications; for example, he may increase his insulin dosage by certain amounts under certain conditions. This partnership can safely exist only when the patient has the understanding, brought about through education, to apply the physician's directions correctly.

## PLANNING PATIENT EDUCATION PROGRAMS

The individual patient must be the focal point of concern of any well-planned patient education program. Rather than a standard, generic program, it must be adapted in such fashion as the needs of the patient and that of the care partner dictate. Their physical and emotional status and their ability and readiness to learn are first assessed. The program then becomes an educational endeavor planned for the specific patient, having been adapted to the needs and desires of that individual. The content of this educational endeavor can be jointly planned by several health-care professionals, including the physician, nurse, social worker, nutritionist, physical therapist, and pharmacist. The physician should coordinate the education in the same way that he or she coordinates the medical treatment regimen. He should ensure that the patient and care partner learn enough to feel comfortable in their own minds in dealing with the condition or situation. Ideally, learning should allow a partnership role with the physician in making health-care decisions.

## PATIENT RIGHTS—PROFESSIONAL RESPONSIBILITY

The individual has a "right to know" about his condition. The Patient's Bill of Rights presented by the American Hospital Association states as follows:

> The patient has the right to obtain from his physician complete current information concerning his diagnosis, treatment and prognosis in terms the patient can be reasonably expected to understand. When it is not medically advisable to give such information to the patient, the information should be made available to an appropriate person in his behalf.[1]

To have the information given in terms the patient can understand is a constant challenge. It is an all-too-common error for medical personnel when talking with the patient to slip unconsciously into using medical terms with which they are comfortable and familiar, but which are difficult, and at times impossible, for the patient to grasp. There is probably no better way to demonstrate our respect for the patient than by the manner in which our teaching occurs, remembering that one of the original roles of the physician was as teacher.

Rheingold states as follows:

> One must be very careful to fully explain certain terms which may be fraught with frightening associations. Bone marrow examination may mean a search for leukemia unless its use is thoroughly explained. Even electrocardiogram may only mean a heart attack to a patient. These diagnostic tools, like so many others, are used daily by the doctor. If the patient is already anxious, their use must be satisfactorily accounted for.[2]

The difficulty in communication is compounded by the fact that patients frequently do not feel free to question if they do not understand. This hesitation to ask for clarification may be due to many reasons. The patient may feel that the physician is too busy to be bothered with questions; that the physician will consider the questions too trivial; or that the physician will be annoyed at being re-asked a question that has already been partly answered. The members of the home care team might give instructions in a tone of voice and in a manner that implies that the patient should understand and is at fault if he does not. This discourages even the bravest patient from pursuing the questions he would like to have answered. Particularly in the elderly, a lack of questions may mean that the patient actually understood little of what was said—or it may mean that the patient is partly deaf. In a recent experience, a physician gave instructions to a patient to eat some *bran* cereal every morning. When the doctor left, the patient inquired of the family, "Which *brand* of cereal does he want me to eat?"

The policy approved by the House of Delegates of the American Hospital Association in 1981 states as follows:

> The hospital has a responsibility to provide patient education services as an integral part of high-quality, cost-effective care. Patient education services should enable patients, and their families and friends, when appropriate, to make informed decisions about their health; to manage their illnesses; and to implement follow-up care at home. Effective and efficient patient education services require planning and coordination, and responsibility for such planning and coordination should be assigned. The hospital also should provide the necessary staff and financial resources.[3]

Just who is responsible for education of the patient? Patient education must, by its nature, be a shared responsibility, a partnership. It should be shared by the patient, the physician, the patient educator who plans and administers patient education programs, by the nurses in the hospital and in the physician's office, by the nutritionist, by the home care nurses, and by each member of the medical team who comes in contact with the patient. However, we must not diffuse that responsibility to the point where patient education dissolves into the mist of being everyone's concern and no one's responsibility.

Responsible patient education should reflect the fact that knowledge is gained by learning. Simply giving information is not teaching, nor does it imply learning. While there are certain situations in which simply giving information is all that is necessary, for instance in orienting a patient to a hospital stay, it is essential that real learning take place if the patient is to become a partner with the physician in health management. For learning, the patient must be motivated, stimulated, and involved. In truth, we cannot "teach" the patient what he needs to know; we can, however, provide the proper situation and information to promote learning by the patient.

In order to be effective and successful patient educators, we must be adult educators and we thus have a professional responsibility to become and remain updated in the science of adult learning. We should remember that patients are usually ready learners when they are involved in determining their own goals and when they can relate the learning to their immediate needs. Some patients are more receptive if shown that the regimen is flexible enough to permit them to stay in control while adapting to special events or circumstances. For example, the person with diabetes will *learn* insulin dosing if he knows that he can eat birthday cake, yet stay out of trouble by increasing his insulin to prevent the blood glucose level from going up sharply.

In order for the patient to learn, he must be in a state of receptiveness. If he is too anxious, too physically ill, or in a state of denial of his medical condition, our attempts to educate will be too little or to no avail. On the other hand, to cease education because of the patient's denial may actually give the patient the message that denial is appropriate. In the face of denial, education should be altered, not stopped. For example, teaching a patient what he does *not* have or what he will *not* have to do may allow him to begin to accept what his reality is. Similarly, anxiety must be met by a change in our strategy: if the patient is worried about the spread of cancer, we may have to focus his attention onto very practical, concrete goals, such as maintaining nutrition.

While the patient is in the hospital, the patient educators usually assess physical and emotional readiness for learning. If possible, the education sessions are delayed until the patient is ready to learn. This presents a severe dilemma, since in the current economic climate the patient may well be discharged before reaching a state of readiness for learning, while going home earlier increases the need for understanding. Outpatient education and a cooperative care unit where a patient and care partner can learn while being treated seem our best choices to meet the needs of the patient today.

The following is an overview of the steps involved in patient education. The steps—assessment, planning, implementation, and evaluation—are similar to the steps used by physicians in everyday clinical practice. Here, they are transposed from the medical model to the educational process.

## STEPS IN THE PROCESS OF PATIENT EDUCATION

### ASSESSMENT

The first step in the educational process is assessment—sizing up the situation. The importance of this step cannot be overemphasized. Many times when the patient has been labeled as noncompliant, or when evaluation reveals that behavior has not changed, the difficulty can be traced back to an invalid or incomplete assessment.

Involvement of the patient and care partner is the key to accomplishing this step successfully. Involving the patient from the very beginning, allowing him to participate actively in the planning, enables the program to be tailored more appropriately to his specific needs. This takes advantage of the principle that active participation is the major factor influencing adult learning.

Areas that need to be assessed are the patient's knowledge, his educational readiness, the available resources, factors that can influence learning (such as the patient's preconceived notions about doctors and nurses, what they do, and what medicine can accomplish in general), and, not to be underestimated in importance, the patient's and care partner's perceptions of their learning needs, often in terms of what is most acutely felt at that moment.

To assess the patient's current knowledge we can ask questions, engage the patient in conversation, and observe the patient. If it is not convenient for us to actually observe his habits, we should ask the patient to explain what he is currently doing with respect to the perceived learning needs. For example, in planning to intervene in cardiac risk factors we can obtain a diet history from a patient who recently has experienced a myocardial infarction. We will be more successful in eliciting this information if we use nonthreatening, nonleading questions. We must be careful to avoid inferring by our questions that the patient has in some way brought about his illness by his behavior. Although our goal may be to motivate the patient to change his habits, we do not wish to add to the patient's burden of guilt, particularly since excessive anxiety or depression will interfere with the patient's ability to learn.

In assessing the patient's receptivity to learning, we must recognize that physical factors, such as pain and hunger, can negatively influence learning readiness. The patient may be unable to concentrate on learning if the outcome of the illness appears uncertain or unclear. Denial, which may be a helpful or a harmful adaptive defense mechanism, also has a great impact on our planning of the educational process. If the patient is functioning more fully because he denies the severity of his cancer, we need to respect that and be cautious not to tear down all his protection. But, since denial can eventually interfere with the family's ability to provide needed emotional support (because they will be unable to talk honestly with one another about their feelings), we must help them to avoid using this technique beyond reasonable, limited bounds.

It is important to be cognizant of factors that might be limitations to learning, such as impaired sight or hearing. These conditions need not be overwhelming limitations if we can be creative and alter our methods from the more standard approaches. We should take advantage of factors that would facilitate learning, such as the patient's desire for independence, the mastery of past learning experiences (which we should explore in our history-taking), and the presence of an involved family. Since these can have a positive influence on the learning process, we should capitalize on them.

In formulating a realistic and workable educational plan, it is pertinent to assess the patient's socioeconomic status and living conditions. Identification of the patient's primary supporting family and friends, and how they interact, is useful. Understanding the patient's life-style patterns, including work history, leisure and exercise habits, and sleep requirements may be important. The patient's cultural and religious beliefs may also influence the educational plan under development.

In assessing the patient's perception of learning needs, we should avoid imposing our own values and beliefs on the learner. We cannot merely decide what he should know and then implement a plan based on this decision. In some instances the patient may not be aware that he has any learning needs, or he may have different perceptions than we do. By including the patient in the learning process from the planning stage we can more easily develop a plan that is both workable and realistic.

In addition to the patient, there are other resources available to help us with the educational plan. Although this process may sound cumbersome and time-consuming, in reality it is not. It is well worth the effort to assemble the needed data, starting by using information that has been collected previously. For example, the patient's hospital record and the physician's office records will probably contain much of the needed information. We should also utilize data obtained by other health-care team members. They may have a wealth of information to assist us in developing our plan. We can then expedite obtaining the remaining needed information by focusing and structuring our interactions with the patient.

## PLANNING

After the assessment is completed, an educational plan needs to be developed. The educational plan should enhance learning by allowing everyone concerned to have a clear understanding of what is to be done and knowledge of who will be involved, the methods that will be used, and how the effect will be measured. The plan should be able to serve as a contract between the teacher and the learner. This is a continuation of the theme that learning is enhanced by involving the learner as an active participant.

The participants involved in the planning process vary with the nature and complexity of the identified need. In some situations, it may just involve the patient and a health professional. In other instances, in which the needs are greater, the patient, the family, and a wide variety of health professionals may be required. An example of the latter is home care for a stroke patient. The planning team may include the patient, care partner, hired home aide, physician, speech therapist, occupational therapist, physical therapist, and home care nurse. The net effect of effective planning is to save time, because once responsibilities are delineated, duplication of effort can be avoided. The physician and the home care nurse are key players in this delegation of responsibilities.

It is sometimes difficult to determine exactly what should be included in the actual plan. An analysis of the data collected during the assessment phase is helpful. This provides some idea of the amount of education needed. It is sometimes useful to identify the objectives and then to determine which ones are crucial or which are the most important. This is helpful in allowing one to set priorities in the face of age or time constraints. Needs that at first appear to be overwhelming can be broken down into small, manageable steps. In setting priorities in educating a diabetic, we might put giving the injection as step number one, drawing up insulin as step number two, testing blood glucose as step number three, diet instruction as step number four, and an exercise program as step number five, for example.

After identifying what is to be included, it is necessary to identify who will be involved. Once again, in simple educational interactions it may be a single health professional and the patient. Examples of this are medication instruction and the explanation in preparation for a diagnostic test. In other cases, numerous people may be involved. The development of an educational program for a person with newly diagnosed diabetes can include the patient, family, physician, nutritionist, social worker, and nurse. If the patient is a child, the school teacher may also need to be involved.

The involvement of several people in the learning process has advantages and disadvantages. An obvious advantage is that each person can utilize his or her expertise. A difficulty, though, is that unless there is communication among those educating, and unless there is a clear distribution of responsibilities, confusion may result. Consistency is important. It may also be prudent to identify one person as a coordinator of the learning activities. Often, this should be the home care nurse.

The method of interaction will vary, depending on whether the educational need is primarily cognitive, affective, or psychomotor. Each lends itself to a different method. For example, psychomotor skills generally include a demonstration, a "return demonstration," and supervised practice. Explaining how to inject insulin without showing it being done is not very helpful. Cognitive education, on the other hand, lends itself to many different methods, including one-on-one interaction, group sessions, and programmed instruction. To obtain attitudinal changes and handle other affective concerns, support groups or in-depth discussions with the learner may be useful. Whereas one-on-one teaching is superior for individualizing the instruction, the peer support in a group is often very important for the patient and family.

Audiovisual materials can be valuable adjuncts. Although extremely helpful in reinforcing information, stimulating discussion and questions, and in providing repetition, audiovisual materials do not replace live interaction with the nurse or physician.

Also included in the plan should be a determination of when the process should be implemented. The educational process might start in the hospital, for example, and continue at home, or it might be entirely home-based. Discussion with other health professionals may take place immediately before or after a physician's visit or may be scheduled on a separate date. The timing also needs to be coordinated with the patient's educational needs (the question of dining out may arise after the patient improves) and physical needs (the presence of pain, hunger, being late for work).

Last, the actual plan should include appropriate evaluation techniques.

## IMPLEMENTATION

After the plan has been developed, the next step is implementation—putting the plan into operation. Flexibility is needed, since during the implementation process, changes may be appreciated that require significant modifications of the original plan. Attention to verbal and nonverbal cues from the patient is helpful.

In general, it is helpful to start with a review and explanation of what has been planned, giving everyone involved a clearer understanding of what to expect. Explanations should be given in terms that the patient and care partner understand. Abbreviations, technical terms, and jargon should be avoided. Vague instructions to "take it easy" or to "take as needed" may mean different things to different people. Equally vague is telling the patient and care partner that you want to be informed of "any changes." Specific criteria should be identified whenever possible.

Information sheets, for example, medication instruction handouts, are important. Teaching may be neglected because the professional feels that he or she has an inadequate base of knowledge. The use of printed materials can play a role in bridging this gap. It can also be helpful in ensuring that information given by various people is consistent (*e.g.,* a protocol for wound care).

While printed informational materials are often valuable adjuncts to the learning process, they should not be misused. Giving the patient a pamphlet in lieu of verbal instruction does not constitute patient education. These materials should be supplements, not substitutes, for interaction with the appropriate professional.

The environment should be as conducive to learning as possible. Distractions should be limited. For example, we must be certain that the patient is free of pain and can see and hear adequately. A calm, nonrushed, nonthreatening attitude on the part of the educator is an additional prerequisite for learning.

## EVALUATION

Evaluation—obtaining feedback about how well the process is working—is the step that allows us to determine if the learning process that was initiated is actually beneficial. If clearly defined objectives were developed during the planning phase, this process is eased considerably. However, there is a temptation to omit an evaluation process in the belief that it is a complicated and time-consuming process, requiring sophisticated testing techniques. The potentially erroneous assumption may then be made that merely because an educational intervention took place, learning must have ensued.

Planned and ongoing evaluation is essential if we are to document that changes have occurred. The process can range from simple observation to elaborate research techniques. Whatever changes are noted should be documented in the patient's chart so that subsequent teaching efforts can be directed toward reinforcing the learning achieved and building on what has been learned to increase understanding.

In addition to determining whether a behavioral change has taken place, evaluation can also assist in determining the adequacy of the teaching methods used. It can also play a significant role in giving the planners and educators positive feedback and reinforcement.

The choice of technique used is in large part determined by the objective being evaluated. For example, having the patient demonstrate the technique that has been learned is an appropriate way to evaluate a psychomotor skill by allowing the evaluator to identify problems and correct them. Suggestions may then be offered for alternative or easier ways to do the task.

Changes in the cognitive domain can be evaluated by simple questions. Verbal feedback is the predominant method of evaluation used in this area. If questions are used to determine understanding, it is important that they be planned so that they truly elicit the information needed. Questions should be neither too vague (which may be confusing) nor too obvious (so that only a yes or no answer is expected). The questions should be phrased in a way that gives the learner the opportunity to explain.

Content in the cognitive domain can vary from the simple to more complex synthesizing. Once again, we should take our cue from the objective being evaluated. It can range from, "What did you choose for lunch today?" to having the learner problem-solve a scenario that will require that he apply the information he has learned.

Not all verbal feedback must be in the form of questions. Engaging the learner in purposeful conversation can also be an important technique. Being nonjudgmental and asking open-ended questions can be quite helpful.

The area of attitudinal changes is somewhat more difficult to assess. The observation of change in behavior may reflect an attitudinal change.

A major difficulty with evaluation is that we often focus our attention on short-term effects, whereas our goal is long-term behavior change. Actually, this is less of a problem at home when we see patients over a long period of time, than it is in a brief acute hospitalization. Communication among all those who are involved in the patient's care, either verbally or through written documentation, will facilitate true "patient education" and understanding.

## DOCUMENTATION

Documentation that patient education has been performed is mandated for the hospitalized inpatient by Joint Commission on Accreditation of Hospitals (JCAH) standards. If the patient is being educated at home, the same general concepts should prevail. Documentation should describe the education plan developed, the measures taken to meet the identified needs, and the learner's response to them. If additional education is needed, this should be identified as well.

The following is an example of documentation of an education plan:

### CASE STUDY

The patient is a 50-year-old woman, 5'1" and 165 lb, whose mother died of diabetes-related kidney disease. She works as a waitress with irregular hours. She lives with her husband, who is supportive, and the youngest of her three children. She walks one mile to and from work each day.

The medical plan is for the patient to start on NPH insulin twice daily, maintain a 1800-calorie diabetic diet, and follow home blood glucose monitoring before meals and at bedtime. The patient is receptive to learning but is anxious about injecting herself.

The educational plan is to give the patient nutritional instruction regarding the diet and modifications, to teach the technique of blood glucose monitoring and of insulin injection, and to review the symptoms and signs of hyperglycemia and hypoglycemia and the actions to be taken in those instances.

The patient should keep a log of home blood glucose levels and should call if problems arise. Adjustment of insulin, diet, and exercise will be discussed as needed.

## EDUCATING THE PATIENT FOR HOME CARE

Educating the patient, while always important, becomes essential when the patient is being cared for at home. Education becomes the basis for a partnership between the patient and his care partner and his physician, and for providing and communicating important information to the physician to be used as a basis for decisions about treatment. It is an essential part of making home care safe and comfortable for the patient, and of reducing the strain on the family caused by the patient's illness. Clearly then, not only the patient but also his care partner and members of his family should be provided with appropriate education for home care.

What is included in appropriate education? It is important that the patient and his care partner understand the existing condition and how it is expected to progress, the treatment regimen and its rationale, and the tests to be done and how they will affect the patient. Both patient and care partner need to be informed to participate with their physician in the decisions made about treatment and care. They should have "informed choice," which implies more understanding than "informed consent." This implies that the locus of control resides with the patient. Studies have clearly shown that patients who "do" rather than who are "done to" get well better and faster. An "educated" patient and care partner who understand what tests and treatment can do—both good and bad—feel more "in control."

Once the decision for tests and treatment has been agreed upon, the patient and care partner need to understand how to carry out the prescribed treatment regimen.

## TREATMENTS

Proper technique must be taught to the person who will be responsible for carrying out the treatments. Printed instruction sheets should be provided for easy reference. Procedures might include intravenous therapy, care of a Hickman catheter, total parenteral nutrition, injections, dressing changes, or such simple things as good body mechanics, good body position in bed, and turning techniques. However involved or simple, good patient care in the home depends on the education provided the patient and care partner.

## MEDICATIONS

The physician, pharmacist, or nurse should thoroughly discuss both the prescribed and the over-the-counter medications the patient takes. He needs to be aware of the purpose of each medication to increase compliance; of the side-effects, including those that should be reported to the physician; the proper dosage; and when and how each medication should be taken. There is a need to caution against the common error of doubling up if a dose is missed. Drug and food interactions should be discussed. This understanding is important for the safety of the patient. On the other hand, some of the instructions on medications and their relationship to food can be overdone, with the result that the patient may actually *omit* the pill rather than take it with food; there is some sense that something *bad* will happen as opposed to just decreased efficacy of the drug.

Having the patient remember to take his medication and also to remember with certainty whether the medication was actually taken is a major problem, particularly for the elderly. The individual educating the patient should share ideas and resources for tools that can be used to help ensure that medications are taken at the prescribed times. A chart with the medication pictured along with the times it should be taken may be helpful. A small plastic "pill box" with a compartment for each day of the week is available at most pharmacies. Even more elaborate pill boxes are available that have compartments for drug doses to be taken several times during the day so that one can see at a glance whether each dose was taken. An egg carton can be used as a cheap alternative.

## ABUSE AND NEGLECT

Education should outline the level of care one should expect, as well as the avenues for recourse should this level not be obtained. This is part of making home care safe. When asked what she saw as the challenges to the future of home care, Elsie I. Griffith replied

A major problem that may begin to plague home care is the abuse of clients.... Educating the public and physicians about choosing quality agencies and asking the "right questions" may also serve to eliminate the use of poor quality agencies and thus reduce the risk of abuse.[4] Providers should be more concerned about consumer education and should work on new methods for getting the consumer educated about home care.[5]

## RISK OF ABUSE

There are many agencies and even hospitals that provide hired care partners. These hired care partners may be well-supervised, caring individuals who provide excellent personal care. However, there are some hired care partners or even family members who will take advantage of the patient in his dependent condition. The patient may be parted from his prized possessions or sums of money by an unscrupulous care partner who plays on the sympathy of the patient, or who through intimidation arouses fear of reprisal such as placement away from home, inadequate care, or even physical abuse. According to a study done by Cleveland's Chronic Illness Center,[6] one out of every ten elderly persons living with a family member has been abused. Since many cases of abuse may not be reported, the actual incidence of abuse may be much higher.

It is extremely important that whoever arranges for a care partner be sure that the patient understands what should be expected from the care partner and the options should these expectations not be met. Ideally, the patient–care partner relationship should be one that provides fulfillment for both individuals. However, we should be alert for the hired helper who is overly solicitous and fosters overdependence, albeit unwittingly. This can be quite counterproductive to the patient's progress. The potential for distressing situations must never be underestimated.

The physician, nurse, and other professionals involved in the home care of the patient should be alert to such problems. Since the patient understandably will be reluctant to reveal any problem, the physician's relationship of trust with the patient must be used to give him the opportunity to feel safe to reveal care partner problems. In this regard, nothing replaces a home visit and the very direct, specific question, "How's it going with your aide? Is she treating you pretty well?"

## FAMILY STRESS

On occasion it is the patient, not the care partner, who precipitates problems. A patient may make unreasonable demands on a family member who is the care partner. An overstressed care partner may at times become abusive or neglectful. Through education the family can be made aware of what to expect and where to look for the support that may be available. Often the family, friends, or the church or synagogue may provide help.

The physician, nurse, or social worker making the home care arrangements should assess the strain that caring for an ill family member places on all members of the family, and should be aware of the change in family relationships this may bring about. Education can greatly assist the patient and family adjust to the negative situations brought about by illness. For example, we may teach a patient that it is "O.K." to say certain things or feel certain ways, to be angry or sad. The family should be made aware of these feelings and be given the opportunity to discuss them openly without being made to feel guilty for harboring any resentment that resulted from the changes brought about by the illness.

## DYING AT HOME

It is accepted that a goal of education is to reduce stress on family care partners who provide care during illness. Perhaps the greatest stress in illness is the one that education often does not address: education for the patient, care partner, and other family members in preparation for death. Today many illnesses, even terminal illnesses, are cared for in the home. If the wish of the patient is to die at home, the care partner and other family members will need enlightenment as to the process and a dispelling of myths to support them through this crisis. In our death-denying society, death is a subject that is infrequently discussed.

Indeed, it is somewhat taboo. Therefore, we can scarcely expect the patient and the care partner to openly ask for help in preparing for it.

Dr. Elisabeth Kübler-Ross has awakened us to the denial, the anger, and the grief of the dying patient:

> The grieving patient, the patient who cries, not only makes us (physicians and nurses) feel guilty, but he also makes us feel scared about our own ability to sustain a relationship without losing the mask identified with a professional stance. . . . The clergy deserve a significant place not only in helping the dying patient but in serving as a resource to the family and, in addition, to the physician or other health professionals who are troubled by the burden placed on their shoulders.[7]

It therefore becomes the obligation of the physician or nurse to offer suggestions in anticipation regarding when and where help should be sought when the time comes that it will be needed. Without the family having had the opportunity to discuss and ventilate their fears and anxieties, the patient will undoubtedly be rushed to the hospital when symptoms of approaching death begin to appear. This may well put into operation a series of "life-saving" procedures that are difficult to stop once they have been started and may in the final analysis secure only a few days of life for the patient in return for denying him the opportunity to die in peace at home surrounded by those he loved. Permitting the terminally ill patient a dignified and peaceful end at home is an achievable goal of patient and family home care education.

## CONCLUSION

Hospital care works because the professionals are in control. Whether the patient has knowledge and understanding or not, the treatment regimen proceeds as ordered. Out of hospital, the situation is quite different. As Kroenke stated

> . . . The doctor loses therapeutic control. Noncompliance is predominantly an outpatient issue. The Orwellian supervision of diets and drug regimens and patient activities characteristic of the hospital setting evaporates upon discharge. The patient regains autonomy and the management of disease becomes once again a dual venture. The doctor, no longer the "boss," becomes a partner instead. Paternalism decays. Blood pressure and blood glucose levels fluctuate in proportion to the responsibility the patient assumes for his or her health. Thus, ambulatory care becomes a study in the art of negotiation, persuasion, and education.[8]

For home care, this is even more valid, with one major difference. In the home there are two constituencies in need of negotiation, persuasion, and education: the patient and the family. Directing our efforts to education is the only truly effective way to ensure long-term compliance. Adult education is based squarely on the same ideal that the medical regimen rests on at home: a partnership.

## REFERENCES

1. Patients' Bill of Rights. American Hospital Association, Chicago, 1975
2. Rheingold JJ: Patient Compliance. Rx: Patient Education. Proceedings, Southern Illinois University at Carbondale, p 69, 1974

3. Policy and Statement on the Hospital's Responsibility for Patient Education Services. House of Delegates, American Hospital Association, Chicago, 1981

4. Griffith EI: Family and Community Health, vol 8, pp 77–80, 1985

5. Home health care: Answer to a patient's prayers. Consumers Digest 23:38, 1984

6. Haggerty M: Elder abuse: Who is the victim? Grey Panther Network, pp 4–5, 1981

7. Kübler-Ross E: Death, the Final Stage of Growth, pp 11–12. Englewood Cliffs, NJ, Prentice-Hall, 1975

8. Kroenke K: Ambulatory care: Practice imperfect. Am J Med 80:339–342, 1986

**PART 2**

# The Care Givers at Home

# 5
# Professional and Community Resources

MARY K. DETE

Today's home care programs stand ready to provide a wide range of medical and supportive services to the patient in the home. The primary physician will find that there are many talented professional and lay people ready to work together with the physician, the patient, and the care partner.

Perhaps it is nearing 5:30 PM at the physician's office and a long-awaited blood sugar report is called in regarding a brittle diabetic. The physician can call the local home care program and a nurse will soon be en route to the patient's home to instruct the patient in the new insulin dosage, perform a physical assessment, and report any significant findings to the physician. Subsequent visits may be made to complete the necessary teaching, to obtain blood samples, and to teach the patient to use the glucometer.

Or the physician may have been called to the emergency room where an elderly patient has been treated for a fractured humerus following a fall from a step ladder. A home care nurse can be contacted to visit that afternoon or evening to reinforce the emergency room teaching, check the immobilization position needed to protect the fracture, review pain medication instructions, and coordinate the arrangements for homemaker assistance to help the patient with meals, dressing, bathing, and errands. An occupational therapist may be called in a few days to help the patient simplify tasks and perform exercises as directed by the physician.

Perhaps a frail, elderly patient has not been making any progress recovering from a particularly violent bout with gastrointestinal flu syndrome. The home care service can be called upon to administer intravenous fluids and other medications as ordered. The home care nurse will review the care partner's actions and offer suggestions for more efficient bathing, skin and bowel care, diet, and positioning for comfort.

The wide range of conditions that require rehabilitative care respond well to therapy regimens delivered in the home by physical, speech, and occupational therapists. The therapists provide the primary physician with ongoing clinical assessment reports, while performing exercises, teaching safety in the use of required equipment, and applying various treatment modalities such as ultrasound, heat packs, massage, or transcutaneous nerve stimulator units.

## THE HOME CARE TEAM

Home care is the physician-directed, nurse-coordinated delivery of health care and supportive services to the patient in the home. Emphasis is placed on assisting the patient to achieve independence. Home care is a team effort to maximize strengths while reducing weaknesses. The most central members of the home care team are the *patient* and the *care partner*. In the home setting, the home care team's professional members are accepted as "guests" or aides to the patient. The element or perception of *control* that is characteristic of hospital care teams is not true of the home care team. Home care team members are co-workers and, in the best sense, co-team members of the patient and care partner. It is important to remember that not all patients have care partners. Home care, through the availability of homemaker personnel and volunteers, can provide assistance and thus enable the patient who otherwise would be alone to continue to recuperate at home. When cure or full recovery is not possible, the home care team will focus on teaching and shoring up the abilities of the care partner while easing the downhill course of the patient.

The primary physician has the responsibility for prescribing the medical plan of treatment. This written document is the result of conversations with the home care nurse or therapist. Acting on a call or referral from the physician, the home care nurse will contact the patient to schedule a home visit. This visit will provide an opportunity for expanding the baseline data, building on the information already received from the physician. For example, the physician calls to request home care for a 72-year-old widow recovering from a recent anterior myocardial infarction complicated by her chronic arthritis and hypertension. She is aided by a nearby daughter who shops and provides transportation for her.

The physician's phone call to the home care service would request that "the nurse see the patient to check her pulse, blood pressure, respiration; check how she's taking the new medications; help her with her sodium-restricted diet; monitor her progressive exercise program; report pulses below 60 and above 90; and blood pressure readings greater than 160/100; and report any weight gain greater than five pounds."

During the home visit, the nurse will perform a physical assessment and a review of medications, and perhaps begin a food history. The patient will be asked to describe how she has recovered from past illnesses, what her current expectations are, and what problems she is experiencing. The nurse will begin or continue the medication and diet teaching started in the acute care hospital. The reduced activity during hospitalization may have aggravated the long-standing arthritis. Home safety and the way in which the patient performs basic tasks such as bathing, dressing, and cooking will be reviewed. The nurse will stress those items that are to be reported promptly to the physician, explaining the reason for their importance.

After the home visit, the nurse should call to report the findings to the physician and discuss the specific details of what the home care service can provide. This discussion is then transcribed onto a "medical plan of treatment," which will be sent to the physician for review, revision, and signature. If the patient is being referred to a community resource, such as "Meals on Wheels," there may be an additional form for the physician to sign.

The "menu" of services most frequently provided by home care programs is detailed under Home Care Services. An outline of the types of professional and lay people who provide home care, with brief sketches of their functions or responsibilities, is provided under the heading Home Care Team Members and Their Responsibilities.

Following the home visits, respective home care personnel will contact the primary physician to report significant changes in the patient's condition. When these contacts result in receipt of additional medical orders, the physician will receive forms called "supplemental orders" for review and signature.

Home care is a highly regulated health care service. It has its own paperwork burden to satisfy the requirements of safe practice, continuity of care, and the maintenance of a well-ordered legal record of care ordered and given. Third-party reimbursement, primarily Medicare, imposes additional paperwork requirements. Frequently, at the time of arranging home care, the physician may be asked for a variety of orders to cover actual and possible events, for example, what to do for moderate pain, for constipation, nausea, or moderate

## HOME CARE SERVICES

- Nursing care
- Enterostomal therapy
- Physical therapy
- Occupational therapy
- Speech and hearing therapy
- Medical social services
- Home health aide care
- Homemaker care
- Nutritional counseling
- Pharmacy consultation
- Hospice care
- Phototherapy for newborns
- Postpartum, newborn care
- Diagnostic specimen collection (blood, urine, *etc.*)
- Referral to community resources
- Medical supplies
- Durable medical equipment (wheelchair, commode, bed, *etc.*)
- Oxygen and respiratory care therapy
- Self-care instructions
- Home-delivered meals
- Home diagnostic kits
- Friendly visitors
- Transportation services
- Emergency responses communication devices (Life Line, CommuniCall, *etc.*)
- Intravenous therapy
- Chemotherapy
- Bereavement care
- Respite care

respiratory distress. These advance orders not only save time, they also avoid much physical and mental distress for the patient.

Periodically, the physician will receive written progress reports from the home care nurse. Certain payers require that the physician renew the orders for home care on a predetermined schedule, usually at least every 60 days. At the conclusion of home care services, a discharge summary and written discharge instructions for the patient and care partner will be developed, copies of which are sent to the physician and can be helpful for future reference. The physician is thus kept well informed and able to reinforce instructions as needed. Should problems recur in the future, the physician has a ready record of past interventions and their effectiveness. By keeping similar records on file at the office of the home care service, the nurse is better able to respond to calls from the physician to resume care of former patients.

Photographs, taken with the patient's consent, are often obtained to document the efficacy (or sometimes the very slow progress) of specific wound care protocols. The photos may be used as evidence to third-party payers, explaining why the patient cannot reach or see to provide the wound care himself.

The home care team members, under the direction of the physician and coordinated by the nurse, work together to blend their skills and services in what should be an effective and cost-saving manner to meet the needs of the patient and care partner. The following characteristics are typical of the functioning of the home care team:

1. They are advisors to patient care planning and development.
2. They may experience *role-blurring* or cross-training (*e.g.*, a home health aide may perform exercises set up by both the physical and occupational therapists).
3. They may have two services present during the visit (*e.g.*, the nurse assists the patient and performs complex dressing care while the social worker counsels the care partners in use of community resources and ways to facilitate the patient's involvement in self-care).
4. The time of service delivery is matched to the patient care need and preference. (This is in contrast to the active hospital setting, which has less scheduling flexibility.)
5. The patient and care partner are of necessity actively involved in the planning and care because the home care agency team members are not present or available around the clock.

## HOME CARE TEAM MEMBERS AND THEIR RESPONSIBILITIES

This chart presents brief examples of the responsibilities of the respective team members. It is not meant to be an exhaustive listing.

*Physician:* prescribes the medical plan of treatment, including specific medication orders, therapy or exercise orders, safety precautions, activity restrictions, diet specifics, frequency of delivery of service, equipment and supply orders, and nursing care interventions

*Registered nurse:* performs physical assessment; initiates the physician-ordered plan of care; coordinates all services provided; performs preventive and rehabilitative nursing services; administers medications and monitors their effect; performs and teaches stoma care, wound care, bowel and bladder care, and pulmonary toilet; provides counseling and emotional support

*Health care aide:* assists patient with bath and mouth and skin care; assists with dressing, grooming, ambulation, and use of equipment; prepares, serves meals; offers fluids; assists with bathroom needs

*Homemaker:* assists with care of patient's environment, cleaning, laundry; shops, runs errands, prepares meals; offers standby assistance with bathing, dressing, grooming; assists with child care; assists with transportation

*Physical therapist:* evaluates patient's level of function and endurance; instructs patient, care partner, and other team member in carrying out exercise program; evaluates home environment and recommends adaptations for patient safety and convenience; teaches balance and joint mobility exercises; may apply ultrasound, heat, or TENS units as directed; teaches safe use of equipment, splints, braces

*Occupational therapist:* evaluates patient's ability to wash, dress, perform other routine daily functions; teaches patient and care partner to use assistive devices to conserve energy, promote safety; fits patient with splints or braces as needed; teaches and performs active or passive range-of-motion exercises; may apply various modalities to fingers, hands, arms, shoulders to relieve problems; may teach and perform pulmonary hygiene

*Speech therapist:* assists in the diagnosis, evaluation, and treatment of speech, communication, and swallowing disorders; teaches techniques to facilitate improved chewing, sucking, and swallowing; teaches patient, care partner, and other team members exercises and verbal cues to assist patient in speech reeducation

*Medical social worker:* assists patient, care partner, and other team members in understanding the significant social and emotional factors related to health problems and new diagnosis; counsels and instructs in ways to meet patient's social needs; teaches patient and care partner how to utilize community resources; assists in planning for long-term care or respite service in the home

*Dietitian:* evaluates nutritional needs and plans dietary therapy; assists patient, care partner in planning for and accomplishing dietary changes; assists the physician in calculating specific nutrient formulas for patients on parenteral or enteral feedings

*Pharmacist:* advises physician and other team members to provide optimum pain-control, and symptom-control regimens; may provide direct instructions to patient, care partner, or other team members in use of specific drug protocols; may participate in clinical evaluation of patient response to experimental drug therapy

*Durable medical equipment dealer:* recommends specific equipment to facilitate ambulation, safety, comfort, or convenience; fits the equipment to the patient to accommodate height, weight, intended use of the item (for example, a wheeled walker); assists in selection of most appropriate economical respiratory or oxygen equipment; sees to the ongoing maintenance and recalibration of all equipment either loaned or purchased; plays major role in education of patient, care partner regarding various pieces of equipment

*Volunteers:* assist with errands, socializing, transportation to physician appointments, companionship; may perform specific comfort measures; may stay with patient to permit care partners to take time away from home

---

**6.** The services are frequently provided in concentrated periods of time with care partners performing some of the tasks in the absence of the other home care team members.

**7.** The physician relies on the assessment and evaluation reports from nurses and therapists to determine changes in the plan of treatment (*e.g.,* when to alter diuretic therapy, when to increase weight bearing or resistive exercises).

**8.** The nurse/case manager, with the patient, serves as "traffic director" in coordinating the delivery of services and number of services to be provided.

**9.** Unlike the hospital or office setting, in the home attention must be focused on teaching the patient and care partner to recognize early signs of deterioration or undesirable effects to be reported to the physician.

**10.** There is added emphasis on the plans for emergencies (drug reactions, falls, and so on) that patient and care partner will follow.

In the home setting, all team members should tailor the care plans to promote maximum level of patient functioning in the home environment. There should be constant attention to the incorporation of the patient's and care partner's own improvisations whenever possible. There should be a coordinated focus on preparation of the patient and care partner for the absence of the other team members and for working toward identified goals.

The interactive nature of the team members can be illustrated by the example of the speech therapist who develops a communications method using a word or letter board. All persons having contact with the patient are given the explanation for the patient's condition and prognosis. They are then instructed in ways to participate in the therapy to provide necessary stimulation and repetition. They are also taught what not to do so as to prevent well-intentioned "doing for," which would deprive the patient of opportunities for learning and making lasting progress.

Similar to the hospital team, the home care team utilizes one another's skills for problem-solving and for ventilation of frustration when the patient's gains are not forthcoming or when the patient and care partner are not compliant or are passively resistive to the physician's plan of care. In the home setting, there is no "you must," but instead, the approach is one of presenting options and strategies to the patient. The home care team members should use all their talents to win the confidence and cooperation of the patient and care partner in the plan of care. Various scheduling tools are used to keep the patient, care partner, and other directly involved team members apprised of when, why, and who will be visiting the patient. Many agencies use a simple month-at-a-glance calendar page on which they plot the expected visits. They can also schedule activities the patient agrees to do when no services are present (for an example, see Weekly Plan for Unstable Elderly Diabetic Patient Two Weeks Post Total Hip Replacement for reference).

Frequently, home care patients or their care partners are asked to keep records of

## WEEKLY PLAN FOR UNSTABLE ELDERLY DIABETIC PATIENT TWO WEEKS POST TOTAL HIP REPLACEMENT

| *Saturday-Sunday* | *Monday* | *Tuesday* |
|---|---|---|
| Granddaughter home to help with personal care; 10:30 AM take pain medication; 11:00 physical therapist for active/passive range of motion, strengthening exercise, gait training. | 9:30 AM Aide. Bath help, skin care, chores, assist walker. Remind patient to do blood glucose. | 8:30 AM Nurse to review diabetic self-care, foot & skin care, use of Autolet. |
| *Wednesday* | *Thursday* | *Friday* |
| 9:00 AM Aide. Same as on Monday. 10:30 AM take pain medication. Physical therapist also to do transfer training and stair training. | 8:00 AM Nurse to observe insulin and injection prep technique; call for transportation to physician appointment. | 9:30 AM Aide. Same as on Monday. 10:30 AM take pain medication. Physical therapist also to do increase in weight bearing. |

See physician in 2 weeks.

specific events relative to their care. These records are then shown to the primary physician during office visits. Examples of recorded information are the following:

- Daily blood glucose readings
- Daily blood pressure readings
- Weekly weights
- Food and fluid intake amounts
- Time of day/pain or other symptom experienced/action taken/results
- Amount of oxygen used

Much of the success achieved in home care is the result of the blending of the patient's and care partner's ideas with the experience and skills of the home care team. Sometimes trial and error must be the process to find out what works best for the patient. The primary physician contributes much valuable information based on previous acquaintance with the patient.

## WHO PAYS FOR HOME CARE SERVICE?

The primary services that require care to be delivered by a registered nurse, a physical therapist, an occupational therapist, a speech therapist, a medical social worker, or a home health aide are covered by Medicare when the following conditions are met:

1. The patient is a Medicare beneficiary.
2. The care needed is medically necessary and ordered by a physician.
3. The patient is homebound (leaves the home infrequently, accompanied by another; usually the outing requires a taxing effort and is for the purpose of obtaining medical attention).
4. The service is intermittent (more than one visit and usually not daily).

Many private insurance plans cover the services mentioned above. These insurance plans do not always require the patient to be homebound. They may require that home care be in lieu of acute care. Most insurance plans reimburse for home care at 80% of the charge rather than 100%. Medicaid coverage varies from state to state and usually requires that a prior authorization procedure be followed.

Homemaker services, private duty nurses, and respite care are usually not paid for by Medicare, Medicaid, or most private insurances. Instead, these services are paid for by the patients themselves. Occasionally there are programs funded by the local Agency on Aging or United Way that make homemaker services available to patients for a partial fee or no fee if certain financial criteria are met.

Since November 1, 1983, Medicare has offered a hospice benefit that covers the provision of medications, durable medical equipment, medical supplies, respite care, and inpatient hospice care as well as home hospice care and bereavement care.

The home care staff can answer questions regarding the various types of reimbursement available and what the eligibility requirements are.

Durable medical equipment dealers provide printed guides to what equipment and supply items are covered by Medicare, Medicaid, and private insurance plans. These guides are usually available at no charge.

Many drug and nutrition product companies provide a great deal of valuable printed literature with helpful hints for home care. The primary physician is usually visited by company representatives who will provide ordering information.

For many patients the home care nurse will identify the need for referral to a community

## COMMUNITY RESOURCES

| | |
|---|---|
| Alcoholism recovery centers | Equipment loan closets (sponsored by the American Cancer Society, Elks, Moose, other fraternal organizations) |
| Alzheimer support groups | |
| American Association for Retired Persons | Friendly Visitors |
| American Cancer Society | Health education resource center |
| American Diabetes Association | Legal Aide Service |
| American Heart Association | Library services—Books on Wheels |
| American Lung Association | Meals-on-Wheels |
| Arthritis Foundation | Multipurpose center |
| Cancer support groups | Nutrition centers |
| Consumer services | Reach to Recovery |
| Counseling services | Tel-Med (telephone health information service) |
| Day care for adults | |
| Dial-A-Ride services | |

This is a partial listing. The local home care service should be consulted for a more detailed listing, including fees and eligibility requirements.

resource. The primary physician is also frequently the one to whom the patient, family, and care partner turn for guidance in coping with problems.

Community resources are those services available in most towns to help citizens maintain their independence. Frequently, the resources may be provided by a sponsoring organization such as the American Cancer Society. A partial list of community resources is given here. Local senior citizens centers, local Agency on Aging offices, Social Security offices, television stations, and acute-care hospitals develop community resource guides that are available at no charge to the public. There is often a Yellow Pages listing called "information and referral." The information and referral service may also publish a guide to local community resources. The primary physician can find out what guides are available in the community by calling either the local home care program or the discharge planner at an acute-care hospital. Many newspapers publish community service hotlines and other resource numbers.

## CONCLUSION

The primary physician has the resources of the home care team available to assist the patient in the home. A telephone call will put the patient in touch with the home care nurse who, in collaboration with the primary physician, will develop an effective plan of care to assist the patient and care partner in treating various conditions in the home. The home care nurse can coordinate the utilization of appropriate community resources to maximize services and control expense. Together, the physician, patient, care partner, and home care personnel bring continued meaning to the slogan "There's no place like home for your health care."

## BIBLIOGRAPHY

Berkoben RM: Quality Assurance in Home Health Care. Camp Hill, PA, Pennsylvania Assembly of Home Health Agencies, 1976

Cousins N: Anatomy of an Illness. New York, WW Norton, 1979

Cousins N: The Healing Heart. New York, WW Norton, 1983

Dunlop BD: Expanded home-based care for the impaired elderly: Solution or pipe dream. J Public Health 70(5):514, 1980

Ham R: Alternatives to institutionalization. Am Fam Physician 22(1):95, 1980

Home Health Resource Guide. Sacramento, California Association for Health Services at Home, 1985

Information on Home Health Services: A Handbook About Care in the Home. Washington, DC, American Association of Retired Persons, 1982

Johnson M: I'd Rather Be Home. Seattle, Consulting Opinion, 1983

Stanford B: Long Life and Happiness: Taking Charge at 65. Santa Monica, CA, Long Life Center, 1983

Stewart JE: Home Health Care. St Louis, CV Mosby, 1979

Trager B: Homemaker/Home Health Aide Services in the United States. Rockville, MD, Bureau of Community Health Services, June, 1973

Van Dyke F, Brown V: Organized Home Care: An Alternative to Institutions. Baltimore: Social Security Administration, 1972

Weller C: Home health care. NY State J Med 78(12):1957, 1978

Your Home, Your Choice: A Workbook for Older People and Their Families. Washington, DC, American Association of Retired Persons in Cooperation with the Federal Trade Commission, 1984

# 6
# The "Care Partner"

ANTHONY J. GRIECO
WANDA KOWALSKI

Good friends are an essential ingredient for good health.[1]

Hospitals often give the message that power and responsibility are in the hands of the professionals, those who are the givers of care. Dependency is the proper and expected role of the patient, the receiver of care in that situation. These role expectations have been firmly entrenched and certainly need to be reexamined, particularly as we begin to look at the respective roles in the home. Extending the giver/receiver pattern of roles from the hospital into the home does not work as well. Unlike the hospital, with its massive resources and its personnel reserves, the home has few people to shoulder the burden and fewer still to give support to those who are faced with the hard work to be done. A care giver tires after a time, both physically and emotionally, and therefore can function well only as an interim measure. The care giver serves as nurse, homemaker, spouse, head of the household, and more. Each of these roles involves a different degree of physical and, more importantly, emotional attachment or detachment. Some people find these roles to be mutually exclusive. Can we expect everyone to be as loving and caring after having changed stool-soiled linen three times in a day?

Two escapes are possible from the plight of a fatiguing, failing care giver in the home. One option is to hire an emotionally uninvolved, unrelated worker, or series of workers, to give care. As paid, temporary employees of the household, the nurses, aides, companions, or housekeepers can distance themselves from any bothersome turmoil. If they find it too difficult, they can resolve the situation simply by leaving. The alternative to hiring care givers is to establish a caring *partnership* between the patient and the family or friends who will be helping in the home. Caring for a sick person in the home must not be the responsibility of a family member acting as a "care *giver*" if it is to be a successful and fulfilling long-term relationship. The carer must, instead, be a "care *partner.*" A caring partnership means that the patient and the family will be sharing the responsibility, sharing the work, sharing the anguish, sharing the frustration, and sharing the satisfaction. Partnership is the bond that makes the relationship work over a long period of time.

In a caring partnership, who is the boss? Which responsibilities fall to the patient? Which are the care partner's responsibilities? Are the roles fixed? Do they shift or vary? How are decisions reached? How are controversies resolved? Who adjudicates disputes? The answers to these questions for any individual patient–care partner pair should fit into the pattern of problem-solving behavior that has evolved over time in that particular family relationship.

To anticipate the impact that the caring role will have, it is helpful to understand the roles played by the patient and the care partner in the family constellation prior to the illness. To elicit this information, the following questions may be used: Has there been a major shift in roles recently? For example, has the patient been the family strength until this episode of dependency? Has the care partner ever been in the dependency role, cared for by the one who is now the patient? Who are the other supporting members to be called upon for help in the present situation? What contributions or stresses can the additional people be counted on to introduce into the home care situation, based on their past performance?

Looking in as an outsider, the physician or home care nurse will thus find it worthwhile to look at the ways in which problems have been resolved by the patient and family in the past. In some households, the sharing will appear to be a silkenly smooth and calm process. In others, it will be noisily argumentative. The process may lurch and stall before a steady course is achieved. But, if it is true to the normal pattern of behavior of the household and family, it will be a familiar process, with a good likelihood of being successful in reaching its goal—care, with dignity, in the home. If, however, the family's tenor is one of discord and if there are many unresolved issues from years gone by, then the new and more stressful problems brought on by the present illness may not be as amenable to a satisfactory home care solution as they would be otherwise.

The number one task of the caring partnership is giving emotional support. That is a two-way street. The patient's emotional needs are usually obvious to everyone. The care partner's needs are at least as important, but may not be initially appreciated or addressed. The care partner must be given ample opportunity to verbalize her or his frustration within the confines of that role. Often, ventilation and a chance to receive positive reinforcement are all that are needed to reinfuse energy into the process. The common complaints expressed by family or friends caring for patients at home eventually become objections to continuing to function in the caring role.[2] It is part of the job of the physician and, probably to an even greater extent, that of the home care nurse to begin to anticipate some of the difficulties before they occur.

One of the most frequent complaints is that the care partner's sleep is interrupted and disturbed because the patient sleeps poorly and either needs assistance at night or tends to wander, requiring supervision. A second theme is that caring for the patient becomes very inconvenient for the care partner, since it is quite time-consuming. In addition, the physical demands on the care partner may become too straining, such as the need to lift a patient from chair to bed.

Being confined to the home by the constant need to be with the patient restricts the care partner's free time and prevents any social life or recreation. Disrupting the family routine is unsettling and the care partner's own needs are sacrificed as they cannot be met the way they have in the past. The necessity to be at home with the patient causes cancellation of vacation plans. Competing demands on the care partner's time from other relatives and friends become a source of annoyance. The care partner must have adequate recreational time, some privacy, and the opportunity to just relax and do nothing. The physician or home care nurse must help the care partner to plan for these personal needs in advance. It is paradoxical that relaxation must at times be rigidly scheduled and structured for the care partner.

Adjusting emotionally becomes more and more difficult, particularly if arguments arise between patient and care partner. Dealing with the patient's urinary or fecal incontinence is upsetting. It is difficult to accept that the patient's personality may have changed from his or her usual self. As more time is required to be spent caring for the patient in the home, the care partner loses time from work, is forced to stop working, or passes up job opportunities. The financial strain of providing home care becomes a major source of concern. Eventually, the care partner feels completely overwhelmed with worry about how to manage.

Those items fit the concept that it is when the caring relationship is no longer a partnership, in which the patient and care partner give each other emotional support, but converts, instead, into a situation in which one individual is the caretaker and the other is totally the recipient of care, that the stresses rise to a point at which coping becomes tenuous. The problem is particularly troublesome when the care partner is harboring anger but is reticent to ventilate these feelings or is playing the martyr. Some situations in which the physician or nurse may never hear any problems raised are potentially the most explosive and must be dealt with early on.

How can the family's potential ability to cope with the stressful events of home care be assessed in advance? Invaluable clues are available if the physician has had the opportunity to witness how the patient or the family members have adapted to dependency roles during past illnesses.

In order to cope, the family needs to achieve several important goals:[3]

1. The family must become physically independent in the home.
2. They must become competent in applying the prescribed therapeutic regimen.
3. The family must attain adequate knowledge of the patient's health condition.
4. The family must be able to apply the principles of general hygiene to the circumstances of the homebound patient.
5. The family must have a positive attitude toward providing health care.
6. The caring individuals of the family must be emotionally competent.
7. The family must have a stable living pattern.
8. The physical environment must be adequate for the patient's home care needs.
9. When the going gets rough, the help to be used as a "safety valve" must be identified.
10. Community resources must be available to support these needs.

To go further in assessing the family's potential for successfully coping with the homebound patient, we should ask the following questions:[3]

1. Does the family find it easy to recognize the need for help, and do they accept help when it is offered? Have they ever had to ask for outside help in the past? From whom? (Family? Friends? Clergy? Community agencies?) Who do they think will be the most responsive if they want help in the future?
2. Is the family realistic in appraising its situation, including the condition of each family member's health? Does the care partner understand the potential results of his or her actions in providing care? Are the patient's expectations of the care partner reasonable?
3. Do the patient and family have a reciprocal, mutually supporting relationship? How have they helped each other in the past? How has that worked out?
4. Is the overall stress level of the family low?
5. In dealing with stressful situations and life changes in the past, has the family used constructive methods to cope successfully? What have they found to be particularly stressful events in the past? How did they overcome the problems at those times?
6. Do the family members fulfill their expected roles in the household and in society?
7. Is each member of the family, other than the patient, in good health? How much physical care does the patient require? Does the care partner have the necessary physical strength to administer that care?
8. Does the family have a proper balance between the need to have self-confidence and the need to accept their true limitations?
9. Do the family members communicate well among themselves, with brisk interaction, and do they share decision-making as a mutual venture?
10. Has the family been taught the special techniques that will facilitate the care partner role, such as turning, positioning, how to get the patient out of bed, giving injections if necessary? Do they agree to accept these responsibilities?

Those families with predominantly positive responses to the questions listed above have a great probability of coping successfully with the stresses of providing care for a home-bound patient. Their track record predicts that little outside intervention will be needed to support them through the rigors of home care. By contrast, the families with a large number of negative responses to the questions will need extraordinary support. Those families need preventive intervention by all the social agencies, nursing services, and community resources that can be mustered. The earlier that need is recognized and the earlier the appropriate forces can be mobilized, the better the chance of avoiding failure of home management.

The burdens faced by care partners can be divided into three broad categories: dealing with the patient's physical disability, dealing with the patient's intellectual disability, and dealing with the patient's emotional disability. The effect on the family is dramatically different if the problem is only physical, only intellectual, or only emotional, or if it lies in more than one of these areas.

Providing assistance for those patients who are not independent with respect to the activities of daily living, such as bathing, dressing, toileting, mobility, bladder and bowel function, and eating, requires training of the care partner. The care partner should also be taught to derive satisfaction from the signs of physical comfort exhibited by the patient. If the patient, although dependent, can provide positive feedback, this will greatly contribute to the success of the regimen. Knowledge of the negative consequences (*e.g.,* pneumonia, decubiti) that are being prevented by the care partner's actions can also help provide positive reinforcement to a sometimes frustrating and physically demanding job. The care partner's self-esteem will be strengthened as a feeling of accomplishment overcomes frustration and makes the physical labor gratifying.

If, instead, the patient has intellectual impairment as a major problem, the burden and impact on the family providing care are much greater.[4] If the patient's sociability is defective, leading to lack of cooperation, withdrawal, and isolation, the effect on the care partner is loneliness at having lost a friendly, enjoyable, interesting and interested companion. The effect is magnified if, in addition, the patient develops disruptive behavior, becomes verbally or physically abusive, or becomes forgetful or confused. Then, the care partner can have no rest, since constant supervision is mandatory. In such situations the family suffers more than the patient, who is comfortable in the familiar home environment.[5] The partnership fails, evolving into a relationship of a giver and a receiver of services. Depression is the consequence to be anticipated to develop rapidly at that time in the person providing care. The physician can help by clearly sorting out for the family whether this trying behavior is expected to be a temporary result of the disease or whether it must be handled long term.

In being willing to provide home care, modern families are at somewhat of a disadvantage when compared with the situation in previous generations. The smaller family size, the lack of unmarried older children, the need for all members of the family to be employed outside the home, and the splitting of the family to different geographic areas of the country are all currently encountered impediments to family provision of care in the home.

Who actually does provide care at home? It seems clear from the literature[6] that most of the carers at home are women, who represent 70% to 80% of the home care partners. Men requiring home care are more likely to be cared for by a spouse, while women at home are more likely to be cared for by a daughter, rather than by the husband. How does the wife feel at stepping into a long-term carer role for a homebound, disabled husband?

Anger and frustration are frequently expressed by the wives. The myth of the "golden years" remains just that—a myth. In many instances, the husband became disabled shortly after retirement, cancelling any plans that the couple had for enjoying this period in their lives . . . Role ambiguity is also evident as the women shift from the role of wife in a traditional marriage to head of household.[6]

When the patient and spouse are of similar age, the carer, as well as the identified patient, may have physical disease. When the caring spouse begins to complain of personal symptoms, the physician may judge them to be merely reflections of the psychological impact of dealing with the patient's illness. This may be true, since the emotional stresses on the carer can exacerbate prior medical conditions or uncover previously unrecognized diseases. However, the physician must be alert to the fact that the caring spouse may be withholding information regarding his or her own state of health until the patient improves. The spouse may be waiting for the time at which it will be more acceptable to complain of "minor" illness, in view of the primacy of concern with the patient's acknowledged, more serious disorder. The "healthy" spouse may be "waiting in the wings"[7] to become a patient. The physician must seize the initiative and direct active preventive medical and screening health measures toward the caring spouse as a matter of routine. The caring spouse should be encouraged to schedule regular appointments with the physician outside of the home, in the physician's office. This facilitates switching from the caring role into the role of patient.

When the carer at home is a daughter, the level of distress felt in providing for the homebound patient is even greater than the stress perceived by a spouse. The daughter, most often in middle age when faced with the task of providing home care for a disabled parent, finds it difficult to balance the demands of being a wife, mother, and, at the same time, a carer for an elderly, dependent parent.

Daughters seem to be more affected by the restriction on their social life and general quality of life than spouses. Spouses perhaps with age have gradually reduced their outside and social activities and expected that they and/or their spouse would be disabled, perhaps needing care. Daughters having come to middle-age had not expected to have their social life curtailed or to return to the caring role and support elderly relatives.[8]

When the family member who is the primary carer in the home begins to fail in response to the stress, who is available to step in? Do other family members offer to share the burden? In actuality, the opposite is most common. Once one family member accepts the caring role, the other relatives and friends begin to withdraw further and further. Initial offers of help and support evaporate, and the primary carer is left isolated.

There are, of course, no pharmacies available to fill a prescription for "spouses, confidants and friends, p.r.n."[1]

Helping the primary carer at home learn how to enlist the support of other relatives, friends, and neighbors is a challenge that the physician, home care nurse, and social worker must jointly attack. The resentment voiced by the isolated care giver can open deep family wounds and result in family feuds that may engulf even innocent later generations. Group sessions with other people who are facing, or who have faced, the problems of long-term care in the home are more helpful than individual counseling sessions in overcoming the resentment of isolation. The group dynamics should be used to help stimulate the development of the social skills needed to make and keep good friends under adverse conditions.

Groups are also helpful in having the family gain an appreciation of the distinction between the patient's behavior that is the result of a lifelong pattern of behavior and that which is the result of the pressures of the current illness and disability.[9] The group should help the family recognize the ways in which their behavior and their responses to each other and to the patient aggravate rather than help to resolve household conflicts. An important goal of the group is to teach the family healthy manners of response. By helping them to better understand the patient's and their relatives' feelings, fears, and concerns, the primary carer can become more capable of generating more satisfying responses in return.

Extrapolating the successful techniques discovered in the group to their own situation in the home improves relationships within the family.

In view of the natural tendency for the family at large to relinquish responsibility, delegating it entirely to the individual family member who first volunteered to provide temporary service, a yellow flag of caution must be raised at the outset. The physician involved in providing medical care must advise the family not to decide hastily on having the patient move in with one of the daughters or sons. The rash decision, reached with good intent, may become permanent, with irrevocable loss of independence for both patient and family. If it is necessary to have the patient surrender his or her home and live with the next generation of the family, it is important that all the involved parties be advised to discuss mutually agreeable long-term rules about living arrangements, meals, and finances at the very start.[10]

The older patient must be granted the right of active participation in the decision-making process regarding the relocation to a younger family member's home. The conclusion, whether to move or not, must be reached with the patient having been given a real vote. The act of moving itself is traumatic to everyone concerned. In order to maintain self-esteem, the patient must be given the feeling of being in control of the move. An active effort must be made by the physician to alleviate guilt so as to avoid the patient's feeling that the move is forced and that "none of this would have happened if it were not for me."

Following the move, the family faces a hard adjustment. Roles change. Household space becomes limited. The patient may become temporarily more disoriented.[9] The stage of apparent deterioration of cognition shortly after displacement from the original home to the new setting must not be quickly judged to be rampantly racing dementia. The family must be prepared to anticipate increased confusion on the part of the elderly patient as a natural, temporary phase, which will resolve once adjustment is made to the new home setting. In the elderly, slightly confused patient, the responses are analogous to the temporary regression often seen when a young toddler moves to a new home. During this transition, much care and attention must be placed on the location of furniture and rugs in order to avoid accidental tripping and falling. This is a particular hazard at night, when a groggy patient is arising to void and may not immediately remember that the path to the bathroom is not the familiar route that has been followed without conscious thought for so many years.

So far, our concern for the emotional welfare of the care partner has been addressed, since it is the most important determinant of the success of home care. Now, we need to turn our attention to the range of responsibilities and tasks to be carried out by the care partner. Simply listed, they are

Providing emotional support for the patient

Making observations

Providing physical assistance

Performing household chores

Participating in the treatment regimen

Calling for assistance

## PROVIDING EMOTIONAL SUPPORT FOR THE PATIENT

Providing emotional support for the patient is the other side of the coin of the issues discussed so far in this chapter. The care partner, by coming to grips with his or her own feelings and by grappling with the patient's fears, concerns, and worries, brings a lifelong template of behavioral responses to the bedside of the homebound patient. Patterns of words and actions that have been successful recipes for providing comfort to the patient over the years are automatically retrieved and used first. It is when the family's coping begins to falter that the home care professionals, including the physician, nurse, social worker, aide, or housekeeper, must promptly step in.

The professionals, in providing help, do complicate matters. Their presence inhibits the care partner from responding intimately to the patient's needs. The professionals' response to a given distress signal may be culturally different from the response usually triggered in the family. However, by using the techniques mentioned above, including group supports, the family can be given the psychological strength to be able to give emotional support themselves to the patient.

How can the physician help?

The very best doctors . . . share their power with their patients and try to give us the information that we need to control our own treatment.[11]

Whenever I am threatened by panic, my doctor sits me down and tells me something concrete. He draws a picture of my lung, or my lymph nodes; he explains as well as he can how cancer cells work and what might be happening in my body. Together, we approach my disease intelligently and rationally, as a problem to be solved, an exercise in logic to be worked out. Of course, through knowledge, through medicine, through intelligence, we do have some control.[11]

In addition to comforting the patient, the care partner also has a role in "entertaining" the patient. If the patient is a child, the parents, siblings, and friends use entertaining or playing with the child as family activities at the child's level. This plays an important part in calming, reducing anxiety, providing distraction, and reducing fear. Entertainment is no less important for adults. Entertainment is part of normalcy. It diverts attention from the nearly continuous focus on the seriousness of illness and brings back a sense of the importance of recreation and leisure. Likewise, humor can go a long way toward turning an unpleasant situation into something more tolerable.

The vital role that leisure activities play in overcoming the helplessness of facing serious illness has been eloquently stated by a patient:

A year after I had my lung removed, my doctor asked me what I cared about most. I was about to go to Nova Scotia, where we have a summer home, and where I had not been able to go the previous summer because I was having radiation treatments, and I told him that what was most important to me was garden peas. Not the peas themselves, of course, though they were particularly good that year. What was extraordinary to me after that year was that I could again think that peas were important, that I could concentrate on the details of when to plant them and how much mulch they would need instead of thinking about platelets and white cells. I cherished the privilege of thinking about trivia.[11]

The ill patient has an abundance of leisure. But it takes some thought and planning to take advantage of this time productively. Leisure counseling may be needed to change the form of recreation from the pattern followed in that family when all members were entirely well. The leisure activities may need to be less physical and more intellectual or emotional. But they can be physical as well, if adapted to the abilities of the patient and care partner.

## MAKING OBSERVATIONS

Making observations is the second most important role of the care partner, after providing emotional support for the patient. The key to being successful in this task is knowing the patient well. Being familiar with the spectrum of appearances the patient displayed over the years, the care partner is easily able to discern subtle, early changes that signify trouble. It is the care partner, not the professionals, who is most adept at discovering changes in thinking, speech, and behavior. Given instruction, the care partner becomes an excellent resource at noting alterations of many clinical parameters. Rate and regularity of pulse, blood pressure readings, temperature, signs of bleeding, focal weakness, and daily weights are some of the simple items that can be assigned to care partners for routine observation.

## PROVIDING PHYSICAL ASSISTANCE

Care partners expect it to be their responsibility to provide physical assistance to the homebound patient, and they naturally and willingly provide it until it becomes an excessive strain. Aiding the patient in transferring from bed to chair must be taught, preferably in the home, by a skilled individual. Use of a cane, walker, or wheelchair, as well as supporting an unsteady patient in attempts at ambulation, should also be undertaken after instruction. Washing, help with toileting, help with feeding, and other activities of daily living are frustrations until the correct techniques are learned. Giving attention to these needs early, by arranging visits by a home care nurse or therapist, will go a long way toward starting the caring partnership in a successful direction.

An important responsibility of the care partner is to protect the patient. In avoiding falls, the route used to get to the bathroom must be cleared during the night for a patient with nocturia. To avoid medication errors in a confused patient (such as taking the dose twice because of forgetfulness), pill containers can be labeled by the time of day at which the pills are to be used. Preventing the confused patient from wandering is a frequent concern. It can be handled by moving knobs and locks to more difficult to reach locations.[12] The unsteady patient who wants to help with the cooking adds to the workload of supervision by the care partner. Smoking by a drowsy patient poses a significant fire hazard. Driving is a major safety concern if vision or coordination is reduced, and the patient's demand to "just drive in the neighborhood" may lead to confrontations with the care partner. Knowing the patient's condition and personality, the physician should anticipate problems. Taking a strong stand will support the family in these difficult situations. It is much easier for the spouse if the physician or nurse can be blamed for not allowing an activity, but we need to be willing and able to confront the patient directly.

Care partners can quite competently feed patients at home. They not only find this a natural function, but patients are more easily fed by the trusted, attentive, careful family member who is aware of the patient's likes and dislikes and whose verbal and nonverbal communications cajole an anorectic patient into accepting food despite lack of appetite. The care partner is able to spend the time to perform this task at the slow, painstaking pace needed to ensure swallowing, avoiding aspiration and not feeling the need to rush to complete the day's work within a set number of hours on a work shift.

The care partner is the one to encourage the patient to drink adequate amounts of fluids, if that is appropriate, or the opposite, to restrict the volume of liquids ingested, for patients with dilutional hyponatremia such as that due to the syndrome of inappropriate antidiuretic hormone secretion. The care partner may therefore be called on to keep a written record of all the food and fluid taken in by the patient and a record of urinary output and daily weight.

Bathing the patient poses a bit more of a problem. Certainly the care partner is competent to perform this task but, depending on the relationship between patient and care partner, it may entail some embarrassment. Embarrassment is not the problem if the care partner is a spouse, but then advanced age may be a factor, so that limited dexterity of the patient–care partner pair may make it technically difficult to perform this task adequately.

Here, the function is best performed by an offspring of the same gender as the patient. A son bathing a mother is particularly awkward, while a daughter generally accepts bathing either a male or female parent with less objection.

Help with toileting may entail putting the patient on a bedpan, emptying the bedpan, or helping with transfer onto a commode or to the bathroom. Changing the bedclothes or soiled sheets of an incontinent patient is a drudgery that can be minimized by some helpful hints to the family. For example, disposable diaper-like pads can be placed under the patient or pinned on like true diapers; these can be tossed into the garbage bin when soiled and are less disagreeable to deal with than the patient's own clothes, which would require smelly storage until they can be laundered.

Easily accepted care partner duties are dressing and undressing the patient, as well as accompanying or driving the patient to medical treatments.

## PERFORMING HOUSEHOLD CHORES

Performing household chores is simplest for the family to accomplish. Family members who are sometimes unable to assist in the direct care of the patient can often contribute in this area. But that is true only if the patient's personal needs are not overwhelming. Otherwise, the distraction of providing care for the patient may break down the usual routine of washing, shopping, cleaning, and cooking, and these normal, expected chores become the straws that destroy the household equilibrium. Changing the bed linen of an incontinent patient is an example, as discussed above.

The care partner's ability to maintain the household routine must be evaluated periodically. This is most often done by the home care nurse, who can make alternate arrangements if the family begins to falter in this responsibility. If the additional help of a housekeeper does become necessary, the family must be comfortable with this arrangement. Rather than being forced to feel added guilt over failing to cope with the household necessities, the family should be assured that by focusing their attention on the patient's personal needs they will have more fully achieved the higher priority goal.

## PARTICIPATING IN THE TREATMENT REGIMEN

The treatment regimen of medication, dressings, appliances, devices, and diet must be outlined and explained clearly to the care partner. The tasks in this category that are in the purview of the care partner[13] are the following: keeping a record of the amount of urine passed and of bowel movements; obtaining urine specimens and testing them for glucose, acetone, or blood; taking oral or rectal temperature; giving medications; observing the rate, regularity, and ease of respiration; taking the pulse rate, and noting its rhythm variations; changing wound or surgical dressings; giving injections; giving enemas; regulating the rate of flow of home intravenous fluids; and taking blood pressure.

Any or all of these tasks can be delegated to the care partner. The physician's or home care nurse's role is then directed to providing clear, explicit instruction, while liberally sprinkling positive comments of support and encouragement, followed by appropriate evaluation to be sure that the functions are being competently performed. Written information is helpful in answering questions that arise later, when the family is alone and uncertain of some details. Logs, flow sheets, or diaries can be prepared to simplify for the care partner the recording of results of measurements and of medication administration.

## CALLING FOR ASSISTANCE

Not to be underestimated in importance is the care partner's role in calling for help when needed. Guidelines should be discussed at periodic intervals. The degree of calmness or urgency with which assistance should be sought should be identified for several potential scenarios. Whether another family member, the physician, home care nurse, emergency service, or other resource should be called for a particular event should be planned in advance for different events. If the care partner knows that the physician will be available by telephone for advice, and that telephone contact is encouraged at regular intervals, it will help to prevent unwarranted anxiety. We sometimes think of "calling for help" only in terms of the identified patient's physical problems, but certainly calling for help for the care partner's emotional stress is equally valid and acceptable.

In the event of a patient's death, the family must be provided with supportive care after the event. Feelings of guilt and questions about whether the patient would have been better treated in an institution may naturally arise. The family's unique contribution in providing personal attention at home for their loved one must be emphasized and reinforced.

In accepting the responsibility for providing care at home, the family becomes tied down to a varying extent, restricted from leaving the home without advance planning. The severity of the travel restriction depends on the degree to which the patient is dependent on the care partner for safety. In some instances the family cannot leave at all without arranging for a replacement, the way a parent would not leave an infant without having provided for a baby-sitter. In other circumstances, the family is able to leave for short periods without arranging on-site coverage, but they usually must remain within telephone reach.

In being constantly available to the patient, the family is providing an invaluable service, whether or not any actual skillful care is being performed.[12] The family's constant state of being "on-call" is intrinsically stressful. This is quite different, however, from the on-call stress physicians face in professional life, for that is only one role they play. When the care partner is able to play multiple roles—not only as a carer, but with a somewhat intact social life—the position is well tolerated. When the only role possible is as carer, then the "role restriction" culminates in "role fatigue."[14]

The physician should periodically assess the family's ability to continue to provide home care when fatigue is beginning to develop. It is helpful to use the following categories:[15]

1. Is relief unnecessary at this time?
2. Would a temporary relief from the caring responsibilities be beneficial?
3. Will failure of the care partner be likely in the near future without some relief?
4. Is relief urgently needed?

When care partners tire excessively and need relief in the form of more support than can be provided for them in the home, a "respite" is in order. The most effective way to provide the respite is by admitting the patient to the hospital temporarily. This action has been defended on the following grounds:[15]

> The moral argument was that families who were caring for their dependents were families who had accepted their responsibilities. They therefore deserved help....The economic argument recognized the saving...that resulted from family care. Providing holiday relief was a preventive measure, encouraging the family to continue for longer in the caring role.

In hospitalizing for respite care, the patient and family must be braced against twin hazards. The patient must not be permitted to sink into a passive role, relying on the hospital staff and dwindling in independence. If this does occur, the family will find greater difficulty in coping with increased expectations for care after discharge. Rather than a temporary respite, the result would be a termination of the family's ability to provide home care. Therefore, the hospitalization must be for a predetermined number of days. Throughout the hospital stay the physician should describe his or her unhappiness at having disrupted the trends of care that were being provided by the family in the home. The physician should talk about the separation of the patient from the family and home in negative terms, and should contrast the impersonal hospital care with the personalized attention that the family has been providing at home.

The startling finding that elderly people hospitalized for respite care ("social admissions" or "holiday admissions"), without evidence of acute illness at the time of entry, have almost a 9% chance of dying during the period of hospitalization[16] adds more reason for caution in selecting this option.

Rather than hospitalizing the patient to give the care partner a respite, additional services can temporarily be arranged in the home. An aide, companion, or housekeeper may fill some of the needs quite effectively. However, when respite is urgently needed (as discussed under Performing Household Chores, above), a nurse is a better choice.[6] The family member will accept transfer of responsibilities to the nurse more readily and more rapidly. In addition, the nurse can give counseling to the family and provide teaching for the patient and care partner, as well as assess the effectiveness of the ongoing treatment regimen.

Home care usually begins naturally. As time goes on and an illness or disability becomes chronically entrenched, the family's ability to continue falters unless periodic respites are in sight. The sense of "responsibility and duty" then replaces "caring and love"[17] as the family's motivation to care for the ill member. The physician should be attentive to such a change in attitude. The change signifies regression from a caring partnership to a more primitive caregiver–care receiver relationship—a conversion that must be prevented by effective management.

## REFERENCES

1. Eisenberg L: A friend, not an apple, a day will help keep the doctor away. Am J Med 66:551–553, 1979
2. Robinson BC: Validation of a caregiver strain index. J Gerontol 38:344–348, 1983
3. Choi T, Josten L, Christensen ML: Health-specific family coping index for noninstitutional care. Am J Public Health 73:1275–1277, 1983
4. Poulshock SW, Deimling GT: Families caring for elders in residence: Issues in the management of burden. J Gerontol 39:230–239, 1984
5. Meier DE, Cassell CK: Nursing home placement and the demented patient. Ann Intern Med 104:98–105, 1986
6. Crossman L, London C, Barry C: Older women caring for disabled spouses: A model for supportive services. Gerontologist 21:464–470, 1981
7. Klein RF, Dean A, Bogdonoff MD: The impact of illness upon the spouse. J Chronic Dis 20:241–248, 1967
8. Jones DA, Vetter NJ: A survey of those who care for the elderly at home: Their problems and their needs. Soc Sci Med 19:511–514, 1984
9. Hartford ME, Parsons R: Groups with relatives of dependent older adults. Gerontologist 22:394–398, 1982
10. Muir Gray JA: The family doctor's role in the care of the elderly. Practitioner 228:1149–1151, 1984
11. Trillin AS: Of dragons and garden peas. A cancer patient talks to doctors. N Engl J Med 304:699–701, 1981
12. Sheldon F: Supporting the supporters: Working with the relatives of patients with dementia. Age Ageing 11:184–188, 1982

**13.** Webb N, Hull D, Madeley R: Care by parents in hospital. Br Med J 291:176–177, 1985

**14.** Goldstein V, Regnery G, Wellin E: Caretaker role fatigue. Nurs Outlook 29:24–30, 1981

**15.** Packwood T: Supporting the family: A study of the organization and implications of hospital provision of holiday relief for families caring for dependents at home. Soc Sci Med 14A:613–620, 1980

**16.** Rai GS, Bielawska C, Murphy PJ, Wright G: Hazards for elderly people admitted for respite ("holiday admissions") and social care ("social admissions"). Br Med J 292:240, 1986

**17.** Worcester MI, Quayhagen MP: Correlates of caregiving satisfaction: Prerequisites to elder home care. Res Nurs Health 6:61–67, 1983

# 7

# The Family as the Context for Patient Care

PATRICIA MINUCHIN
SALVADOR MINUCHIN

Illness is a family phenomenon. For example, when Barry is diagnosed as diabetic at age 10, it is a major event in the lives of his parents, his grandparents, his 8-year-old brother, and his baby sister. The family, occupied with the usual events of adult careers, managing daily life, and bringing up children, will struggle now with the impact of a chronic illness in their midst. They will develop a routine of diet and medication, explore the degree of responsibility they can safely give the child for his own care, and balance the concern and vigilance directed at this child with the energy and affection that must go to the other children; and all of this must change realistically over time, as medical and family circumstances change.

When the patient is a child, the involvement of the family is obvious, but the ripple effect of illness is just as clear when adults become ill. Jennifer Ames, a 45-year-old wife and mother with a full time job, is at the center of a family that consists of her husband, college-age daughter, son in high school, and widowed father. They have the routines and patterns that go with this stage of life, in which Jennifer and her husband are the strong, decision-making generation, offering both autonomy and protection to the younger and older members of the family. When Jennifer develops cancer, the family reality is dramatically changed. She has periods of incapacitation after each chemotherapy treatment and she finally requires prolonged home care after a serious operation. Who carries on the daily functions of this busy woman, and, even more difficult, what substitutes for her way of injecting humor and mediation into the frequent sparring of father and adolescent son? How does the family calibrate their protection of Jennifer with her need to have some normality of function, even in her incapacitated state? How do the generations reorganize, so that the young and the old are called on appropriately to help out, when the strong middle generation cannot carry on as usual?

For families with parents in home care, medical personnel are a primary resource. They can provide not only information and support but also the kind of specific interventions that expand the family's alternatives and maintain the morale of its members. In order to do that, they must understand something about families under stress. In this chapter, we offer a framework for looking at families. Since the stress of illness and home care is set into the larger framework of normal family life, we begin with some basic concepts of family organization. We move then to more detailed consideration of families under stress, with special emphasis on the impact of illness and on the variety of family patterns for mobilizing resources and coping with change.

## PRINCIPLES OF FAMILY ORGANIZATION

### PATTERNS

We have come to understand that families are organized social systems and that family life is patterned. At any given point, those patterns are describable. They cover the way in which the family manages the routines of daily life, makes decisions, expresses affection, quarrels, and resolves conflict. However spontaneous they seem, those activities have a certain rhythm and form. Every member of the family contributes to the formation of the patterns, and the informal "rules," in turn, shape the way they behave. Like all other members, the person who becomes ill and needs care is an integral part of the family system. Changes in that person's functioning affect family patterns, and the changing patterns affect the further experience of the patient.

### DEVELOPMENTAL STAGE

Each family is unique, but there are commonalities among families at a particular stage of family life, simply because they face similar developmental tasks. Families with young children are inevitably involved in certain parenting issues, such as nurturance and control, the guidance of each child as a separate personality, and the mediation of quarrels and alliances among the children. The children are building their own relationships as siblings, and the adults are involved in the early stages of their work lives, the maintenance of their relationships as husband and wife, and the changed perception of their own parents, who are now grandparents. Single-parent families or others that depart from the nuclear middle-class model share many of these same issues. In this they are all somewhat different from families at different stages, such as families with adolescent children and adults in their forties, or families containing two adult generations and perhaps a third that is aging and in failing health.

Developmental issues, and the family's way of handling them, crosscut the particular challenge of illness and home care. The family of Barry, the 10-year-old diabetic, was involved in the normal adult, sibling, and parenting issues of their developmental stage. The family of Jennifer Ames was involved in work and community obligations, and in the subtle balancing of autonomy and intrusion in all the interactions between family members of different generations. These ongoing issues do not disappear. They interact with the changing demands of the illness, and the challenge to family adaptation becomes increasingly complex. For professional personnel, an alertness to the family's developmental stage provides some framework for understanding their realities and probable resources.

### TRANSITIONAL CRISES

Family patterns are never permanent. Because the family is composed of people who grow and change, and because it is set into a larger social and physical environment, it is an "open system," subject to forces that challenge the established patterns. That is a normal fact of life, periodically experienced by all families simply because new babies are born, children grow older, family members leave home, people retire, and people die. When new circumstances arise, the familiar patterns are no longer adequate, and the family must search for ways of functioning that are more appropriate to the new realities. We describe these periods as transitional crises because they often involve uncertainty and distress, even when the transition is as basically pleasurable as a marriage or the birth of a baby. The basic paradigm for transitional phases indicates a four-stage process: a baseline period of *stability,* in which family patterns are comfortable and adaptive; a *challenge* to the established pattern—for instance, the arrival of a new baby or the departure of a daughter for college; a period of *exploration,* often confusing or tense, in which the family gropes for new relationships and daily routines; and, finally, a *reorganization* of family life that includes the baby or adapts to the daughter's absence, establishing new patterns that work in these circumstances and usher in a new period of stability.

The same paradigm applies to transitions that are not developmental; that come from unexpected events inside or outside the family system. All families face some of these. They include matters like divorce, prolonged unemployment, fires and floods, and serious illness. It is within this framework that we look at the meaning of illness and home care: as a challenge to the family, usually stressful in nature, requiring a recognition of new realities and some reorganization of family patterns on both a practical and emotional level.

## FAMILIES UNDER STRESS

Theories about the relation between stress and physical illness have a long history. They have generally been focused on the individual, establishing the reality of a dysfunctional circle, in which stress and physical symptoms are mutually exacerbating, and exploring the nature of coping mechanisms.[1-8] The literature on family stress suggests, in the same way, that stress is both a cause and effect of illness, and that modes of coping are probably related both to the prognosis of the patient and the psychological survival of the family.[9-12] Current formulations point out that several factors interact with each other, determining the family's experience of stress and their behavior, that is, the reality of the stressful event, the family's interpretation of what is happening, and the family's resources for coping (see the references for discussions of the ABCX Crisis Model,[9, 10, 12, 13] as well as Antonovsky's[1] more individually based concepts of stress, resistance, and "salutogenesis"). In this chapter, we will look particularly at the family's perceptions and resources, but we begin with some consideration of the reality of the disease and the home caretaking task, examining this factor from two points of view: (1) the nature of the illness and (2) the prior role of the patient in the family system.

### THE NATURE OF THE ILLNESS

For obvious reasons, medical personnel think of illness in diagnostic disease categories. The fact that a patient has multiple sclerosis rather than emphysema dictates a certain course of treatment and, in the home setting, a certain routine of medication, professional supervision, and so forth. But the reality for the family exists on another plane. Because both diseases are progressive, periodically incapacitating, and gradual in their course, they may have a similar impact on the family, requiring similar skills and adaptations over time. In an article relevant to both medical and psychological specialists who work with families, Rolland[14] offers a typology for categorizing illness in psychosocial terms. It is geared to the realities a family faces and the forms of adaptation that will be required under different disease conditions. In relation to home care, the *course* of the disease, the expected *outcome,* and the nature and degree of *incapacitation* are particularly relevant considerations.

As Rolland points out, the course of the disease may be constant, progressive, or episodic. A paraplegic condition is constant, for instance, once the initial trauma is past, and the patterns worked out for care and management can hold over time. The family requires stamina, and the threats to adaptation will come from burnout or from family events that challenge the established way of handling the situation (*e.g.,* financial reverses or the illness of a primary caretaker). If the disease is progressive, as in Alzheimer's disease or some forms of cancer, the family faces a series of transitions; they must recognize changes in the capacity of the patient, finding ways to take over and reallocate functions as that becomes necessary. If the disease is episodic or characterized by relapses (*e.g.,* asthma, multiple sclerosis), the patient and family must tolerate an accordion existence, shifting flexibly from one pattern of functioning to another and back again, as circumstances change.

Chronic conditions requiring home care also vary in terms of the expected outcome, for example, the expectation that this illness will or will not result in death. When the disease is life threatening, the family must handle its fears and grief while managing the caretaking tasks, but it must also monitor the quality of life for the patient and other members of the family before the patient dies. In cases where the disease is not necessarily fatal but may shorten life, such as brittle diabetes, the strain on the family takes a different form. The family must deal with their constant fear that mismanagement—or anger or fatigue or time off—threatens the life of a well-loved family member. Parents of chronically ill children are particularly prone to distress, since the always complex tasks of child rearing, which must include some discipline and control, are constantly shadowed by the sense of the child's physical vulnerability.

The nature and degree of incapacitation are other variables that affect the tasks the family must perform and the extent to which the patient can take part in the decisions and routines. The patient with memory loss and speech disturbances presents the family with problems of communication and perhaps decision making; the issues in home care for the patient on kidney dialysis are quite different. In many situations, however, the patient's capacity to function is not totally fixed. It is influenced by the family's expectations and the organization of help *vis-à-vis* autonomy. These vary from one family to another, and may well affect the patient's mood, his or her social integration into the family, and, perhaps, the course of the illness.[15]

In this typology, it is the "grid," of course, that matters. The combination of incapacitation, expected course, and expected outcome defines the objective reality of the physical condition, at least at a general level, and points to the kinds of strengths a family will need in managing home care. In caring for a juvenile diabetic, Barry's family deals with a situation that can be progressive but that is not necessarily incapacitating and that can be controlled, so that it becomes essentially constant and long-term. In caring for Jennifer Ames, the family faces a progressive, fatal illness that is episodically incapacitating, during the chemotherapy and after surgery, and that will enter a terminal phase. In both cases, time is a factor, involving Barry's increasing maturity in the first case and inevitable negative changes in the second.

## THE ROLE OF THE PATIENT IN THE FAMILY SYSTEM

The reality of the disease as well as its characteristics is combined with other family realities, including the position of the patient in the family before the advent of the illness. It is possible to say, of course, that the centrality of the patient is crucial, that the chronic illness of the family breadwinner is more devastating than that of an elderly parent or a child. But that is a poor formulation, not sufficiently helpful for understanding what the family must deal with. It is more accurate to say that the realistic issues are different, depending on unique family patterns and the patient's particular participation before the crisis.

For instance, Jerome Jenks was the 60-year-old patriarch of a family; his wife was active in the community but did not work; the oldest son was married, working, and living independently; and the second son was retarded and living at home. When Jerome required home care as part of a terminal illness, it was obvious that the income of the household would be threatened, that his wife would be overburdened in caring for both husband and retarded son, and that the eldest son and his wife were old enough to be a resource. The other realities, however, were unique to this family, since they resided in Jerome's role and the family relationships. The mutual affection and support with which this couple had surmounted a variety of life crises was now unbalanced. The retarded son, sensing the pain and weakness of a father who had been the strong center of his life, became anxious and unmanageable. Crucial decisions could no longer be made through the usual channels, since Jerome, the patriarch, could not always be consulted in these circumstances and he now lacked energy and certainty even when he was part of the process. These sources of stress were a crucial part of the changed family reality. In Jennifer Ames' family, it was her role as companion to her widowed father, confidante to her young adult daughter, and mediator between her husband and teen-aged son that could not continue in the same form. The family's reality required that they modify the pathways for seeking support and resolving conflict.

In the case of the 10-year-old diabetic, it was clear that the family must monitor diet and medication, working out age-appropriate routines at home and in school. In doing so, they must take account not only of the child's age but of the way he functions in the family, that is, what has been expected of him; whom he obeys and under what circumstances; how he responds to pain, to responsibility, to competition for attention, and so forth. His role in the family's patterns defines the previous reality and the new issues in home care. To the extent that medical personnel can understand not only the illness but also the patient's niche in the family patterns, they are in a better position to assess the nature of the family's stress and to assist them in making realistic adaptations.

## HOW FAMILIES COPE

We come now to the question of how families cope with stress, particularly the stress of chronic illness. The focus of this section is somewhat unusual, in that it highlights *effective* coping patterns. As in most branches of medicine, the customary emphasis in the family field is on pathogenesis: what has gone wrong in the family's way of functioning and what are the available therapeutic techniques for altering dysfunctional patterns? But, as Antonovsky[1] has pointed out, these are not necessarily the crucial questions. Most of us, in modern society, are consistently under stress and, by the known link between stress and illness, should be gravely and continually unhealthy. Yet we are not. So the crucial question revolves around the nature and roots of what Antonovsky has called "salutogenesis." How do people maintain a viable adjustment under stress?

In considering that issue, we will draw particularly, though not exclusively, on an ongoing project with cancer patients and their families in the New York University (NYU) Cooperative Care Unit. For that project, we have selected patients over 40 years of age who come into the unit with spouses as their care partners and who have grown or adolescent children in the geographic area. We have interviewed the patient with his or her spouse, then brought the extended family together for the second and subsequent interviews, focusing each time on the family's experience of the illness, on change, and on coping patterns. These are normal families. They are certainly under stress but they are not pathologic in psychological terms, and their responses clarify the processes we are concerned with.

Normal, viable families show a great variety of mechanisms for dealing with stress. We can make some generalizations about resources and capacities that are useful for any family; these are strong support systems, the financial base for assembling help, flexibility in exploring alternatives, a tolerance for uncertainty and frustration, the capacity to express mutual emotional support within the family, and so forth. But within the broad parameters of such categories, families have different ways of functioning. For medical personnel involved with a family in home care, it is useful to understand how a family defines the situation, mobilizes resources, and calibrates the process of change.

### DEFINING THE SITUATION: CARRYING ON AND EXPLORING CHANGE

When circumstances change, all families explore the balance between carrying on as usual and changing their customary patterns. In our interviews, many families verbalized some version of "We try to keep things as normal as possible," describing both an attitude and some concrete aspects, such as the maintenance of the children's routines or going back to work between chemotherapy treatments, even while they were exploring a reorganization of the way they made decisions, managed the household, and related to each other. Balancing continuity and change is a difficult process, and people bring to it both their understanding of the realities and their typical mechanisms for adapting to change.

Some patients take a very strong position about carrying on their lives as usual. The shading between determination and rigidity, in this attitude, is partly a function of the family pattern. The family may depend on the patient's strength and reinforce the usual functions, or it may monitor excess effort, or it may do both. Different patterns are workable, provided they are comfortable for the family and the illness allows, but the judgment of medical personnel is also important. If the patient can physically carry on, the maintenance of familiar patterns may be viable as well as reassuring and should probably be encouraged. If the patient becomes more incapacitated, or if circumstances are altered, it may be important to help patient and family redefine their reality, relinquishing some established patterns and exploring new ways of functioning.

## MOBILIZING RESOURCES

Faced with serious illness and the need to mobilize their resources, families differ in the way they corral a support network, handle transitions, and delegate responsibility for patient care. Their various approaches may all be viable but they imply different patterns of strength and vulnerability, as the home care situation evolves, and different points at which professional input may be indicated.

### *The Support Network*

Aside from the realities of their particular social situation, each family sees the available network in its own way and mobilizes in keeping with customary patterns. One family is able to use the total outpouring of help from their small-town community, which rallies with fund-raising events, practical help, and emotional support when an accident renders their teen-aged son paraplegic. In other families the boundaries are tight around "family"; whoever is related is a legitimate resource, whoever is not cannot be included. In still others, the unit is even smaller. One middle-aged couple drew the boundaries of their twosome around them like a cloak. They drew closer together when the wife developed cancer, managing the chores in some fashion and fending off their grown children with a determined reliance on their own strength and a liberal dose of humor. These patterns have a long history and they are all functional, as long as the family can cope with the situation and recognize a point of necessary transition. In the last family, if the man's back trouble worsens and the woman becomes bedridden, their definition of acceptable helpers must broaden. In that situation, respected outsiders, such as their medical advisors, can be effective agents of change. They may be able to guide the family in drawing on resources in their own network—people who are willing to help out, although they are not customarily called on. They may also connect the family with community resources, although it is important to understand that some families are blocked not only because they do not have information but also because they have never found it natural to seek such resources. These families need support for changing their ingrained sense of boundaries, as well as concrete suggestions that expand their options.

In situations of home care, the family's relation to the medical establishment is crucial. It is a special case of the family's perception of outside resources, and it exemplifies their sense of where they can put their trust in times of stress. Every physician is familiar with the range of patterns. Some families project unrealistic hope and are overdependent; others accept advice and implement it effectively; still others resist intrusion and project blame. Such patterns do not change easily, but it is the mutual task of family and medical personnel to create a workable liaison between them.

### The Handling of Transitions

The mobilization of resources is not instantaneous; it is a transitional process. It may be accompanied by confusion, conflict, and guilt among family members, and the exacerbation of ordinary developmental issues. When the husband and father of a close, voluble family was diagnosed as terminally ill, the family reacted with turbulent arguments; his wife leaned heavily on their 25-year-old daughter, and the daughter moved out of the house. The reactions may look pathologic, but it is a disservice to label them so, especially in the early phases of adaptation. They are part of a process, and it is important for both medical personnel and the family to see them within that framework, understanding that disorganized exploration often accompanies a challenge to the family's stability and that it may be a precursor to effective adaptation. Interviewed three months later, the 25-year-old daughter described a more mature closeness in family relationships; the family had accepted her new living arrangements and she was now very helpful to both mother and father. The role of medical personnel during these periods of reorganization is partly supportive and partly informational. It is reassuring for families to hear from professional people that their experience is part of a familiar process and that it requires time. It is crucial also that they feel well informed and understand the realities of their situation so that their planning can be knowledgeable.

Families vary in the way they experience trauma and cope with transitions. We know that there are specific points in serious illness when most families feel stressed: diagnosis, surgery, relapse, the assumption of home care, the entry into a terminal phase, and death. But some families rally to these dramatic crises. They mobilize resources and act effectively, making good use of medical advice and outside helpers. Effective in emergencies, their style may be less well suited to the long haul, when other responsibilities must be picked up, caretaking routines maintained, and there is little call to action. The fact that they flounder may be surprising to the physician, who has been impressed by the family's effective behavior under stress, but these families need help in recognizing and using resources for establishing long-term patterns.

Other families, of course, have the reverse pattern. They are immobilized under the first impact of trauma, and the medical establishment sees them as requiring a great deal of help. They may settle well, however, into long-term requirements, where compassion and stamina are at a premium. The role of medical personnel here is more subtle. Arrangements that do not change over time may actually change their meaning, becoming slowly corrosive. While there are no dramatic moments to call attention to the toll, an alert physician or nurse may read the signs of burnout in other family members: exhaustion, depression, an exacerbation of physical symptoms, and so forth. Suggestions for changing the routines, even temporarily, may be helpful, especially when a single family member is carrying most of the caretaking burden.

### Responsibility for Patient Care

In arranging for patient care, families have a variety of possible resources. Some families spread the responsibility, mobilizing community resources and multiple family members. One family organized a network around an elderly man living alone and confined to a wheelchair by arranging for paid helpers for round the clock care, regular visits by each of the out-of-town daughters, and daily phone contact. Satisfactory over a period of several years, that arrangement was facilitated by adequate finances and by such realities in the daughters' lives as supportive husbands, flexible work schedules, and grown children no longer needing close attention. Shared responsibilities spread the burdens and allow for alternatives, but they require some mechanisms among family members for making decisions and resolving conflict.

Such patterns are not possible in all situations and they are not necessarily preferred. In many families, the caretaking function is concentrated in a particular family member. Beyond statistical probability, those roles are carried by the mothers of sick children, daughters of the elderly, and spouses of the middle-aged, although often one offspring is particularly involved with the middle-aged couple. Seen from the family's perspective, the principal caretaker is often the obvious choice—a volunteer who has always been the family helper. Principal care givers are often the family members who contact the medical system, seeking information and advice. Depending on their manner, they are sometimes experienced as a nuisance, since they are, after all, not the patient. But they are frequently the people who will support the patient emotionally, transmit information to other family members, and implement the necessary action. Their access to medical personnel is directly beneficial to the patient, although it may not seem so.

The mobilization of the family around a focal care giver is a common pattern and it is workable, but it has associated risks, especially if the course of the illness is traumatic or long-term. Working with patients who voluntarily come into the hospital with spouses as their care partners, we have seen a fair share of long-term marriages and contented couples. Within that group, there are some potentially overburdened spouses, as well as grown offspring—frequently married daughters with jobs and families of their own—who are stretched by their willing but exhausting responsibility to two generations. With new data on the effects of stress on the immune system, and with evidence concerning the way in which members of a family are psychologically tied together, it is not surprising that caretakers sometimes show an exacerbation of physical symptoms as well as other signs of strain.

The mobilization of resources to deal with the illness and the emergence of family members to carry responsibility are spontaneous processes, neither positive nor negative in themselves. It is the calibration of the pattern that matters—the ability of the family to monitor its arrangements and to read the feedback. The calibration of change is, in fact, the major task for families pushed by circumstances to adapt their patterns.

## CALIBRATING CHANGE

### *The Patient and the Family: Regulating Distance*

How does a family achieve balance? How does it arrive at an appropriate degree of involvement in the illness, neither neglectful nor obsessed, and how does it help the family member who is ill without rendering him or her psychologically helpless? In the parlance of family systems theory, it is a question of appropriate "boundaries" between patient and other family members.

Boundaries refer to the implicit rules that regulate proximity and distance between family members, and to their patterns of interacting and granting each other autonomy. Every family has its characteristic way of setting boundaries and constructing patterns. Some would be described as distant or disengaged, oriented toward privacy and autonomy; others would be described as close knit, embedded, oriented toward communication and monitoring each others' behavior. Those descriptions are not pejorative and they do not indicate pathology, although extremes can be dysfunctional. Most families are somewhere along the continuum, tending in one direction or the other as their dominant style.

When families are under stress and must explore a change in functioning, even viable families may move toward patterns that are not optimal, overshooting in the direction of their dominant style. In relatively disengaged families, members may seem distant or uninvolved. They may not respond adequately to the patient's needs, denying the degree of illness and maintaining unrealistic expectations for the patient's functioning. The input of medical personnel, in these situations, is important. It can bring a more realistic view of the patient's limitations, directing the family toward more adequate and supportive arrangements.

Other families overbalance in the other direction, becoming overinvolved in the illness and overprotective of the patient. They blur boundaries, in effect, so that family life is dominated by this central reality and the patient's life is taken over. For loving families, this effort and concern are understandable, but both clinical experience and research findings document the dangers: a limitation on the autonomy of other family members and a loss of function and energy for the patient, sometimes creating depression and helplessness in adults or a restriction on emotional sturdiness and intellectual independence in children. Even health and survival may be jeopardized. Minuchin, Rosman, and Baker[16] have demonstrated the link between excessively close knit, conflict-avoiding family patterns and the appearance of psychosomatic symptoms (anorexia, asthma, brittle diabetes) in children, and have been able to alleviate those symptoms by helping the family to create firmer boundaries between parents and children. In the same vein, Reiss and his associates[17] have found an unexpected inverse relationship between the survival of patients on kidney dialysis and such factors as close family involvement and strict adherence to medical prescriptions. Their findings do not suggest that concern and adherence to a recommended regimen are negative; rather, they suggest that the degree of involvement must be calibrated. That is a complex process, not only in the family but also in the interface between family and medical system. Unquestioning compliance with medical directives may seem ideal, but it may express itself in obsessive concerns and in rigidities that depower the patient.

In interviewing families, we have seen the many concrete forms that love and concern can take and the potential toll in some circumstances: a family with a gravely ill 6-year-old builds their activities, their meals, their moods around him, so that his 8-year-old sister becomes a shadowy and depressed figure; two grown sons take over medical decisions and household management so thoroughly and efficiently that the parents, in their fifties, function as if they were elderly and the patient's condition worsens steadily. In many situations, family members protect each other by hiding facts or their feelings. It is sometimes the patient who protects others, worrying about their feelings, their health, or their busy lives, and not wanting to be a burden. The very people who are lifelong helpers, making willing care givers for parents, spouses, and children, often draw firm boundaries around themselves when they are ill, making it difficult for family to help them.

The mechanisms for processing change tend to be established in every family, but they vary from one family to the next. In the literature on effective family functioning, there is some emphasis on open communication among members of the family.[18–20] Of course, open communication is a useful characteristic but it does not automatically resolve issues in itself, and it may not be necessary for all family members to be open and expressive. We have found several families in which one member is the emotional switchboard, picking up the evidence of rising tension and activating a process to resolve distress.

Families spontaneously work on these issues, often calibrating with reasonable success despite the difficulty of the situation and the process. The family whose teen-aged son became paraplegic needed to struggle with the stark realities of his limitations, balancing the necessary takeover of functions with the possibilities for growth, purpose, and autonomy. In time, the son finished college and went to work, using his very limited possibilities for physical functioning and his full intellectual capacities for thought and productivity. To accomplish this, family members rose before dawn to wash, dress, feed, and transport him, as well as to attend to their own chores and work responsibilities. The home care situation is a permanent part of their lives but it does not entirely dominate their adaptation. Families often have the strength and repertoire to find a workable pattern, establishing appropriate boundaries, in time, between the patient and the rest of the family. What they require from medical personnel is very clear information about medical care and sufficient understanding of their particular style so that advice is offered in a form that they can use.

### Adjustments Within and Between Generations

Within the family, a patient may simultaneously function as spouse, sibling, parent, and offspring. In other words, he or she may be part of multiple subsystems, each with its customary patterns for functioning and relating. Spouse and sibling units are within the same generation, and patterns here may be deeply ingrained. When one spouse becomes ill, for instance, the couple must often reorganize well-established habits, ranging from the mundane activities of cooking, paying bills, and hauling garbage to the usual ways of making decisions and expressing emotional support. It is difficult for the patient to give up familiar roles, with their often symbolic meaning, and it is equally difficult for the partner to take on new or additional functions. The calibration of what is necessary and acceptable depends on the small signals that regulate "too much" and "too little," and on the willingness of the couple to go beyond their own subsystem, as required, for other resources.

Cross-generational units also face adjustments, and at certain points in the family life cycle these adjustments are particularly complex. When the patient is a young child, it is obvious that the parents will be in charge; whatever changes the family must adapt to, the basic patterns of decision-making and nurturance are not challenged. When the patient is elderly, the distribution of power and support in the family may already have shifted so that it does not challenge family patterns if adult offspring are active in medical decisions and arrangements for home care. But when illness strikes the middle generation, cross-generational issues are likely. Patients who are the parents of adolescents see themselves as the core generation, still responsible for the support and socialization of their children. They are frequently protective of their children, guarding them from details of the illness and their own anxiety, though the children often perceive the situation more clearly than realized and would profit from the opportunity to be more helpful. Increased contact and responsibility can be an active antidote to anxiety and helpless grief. When the patient's children are young adults, the generations are frequently brought closer, with the younger people offering support, practical help, and some participation in crucial decisions about doctors and treatment. The illness often accelerates an issue that comes more naturally at a later stage: the need to balance the increasing power and competence of the younger generation with the sense of threat that the parents may feel about their own competence and centrality. The adjustments are subtle and they are made more difficult by the emotional strain that accompanies chronic illness, but the energy and prognosis of the patient may depend in part on the family's ability to help without taking over the patient's sense of purpose in living. In this process, the medical team can help the family to calibrate their interactions.

## MEDICAL PERSONNEL AND THE FAMILY

We have emphasized certain ideas about families dealing with illness and home care: that they must reorganize their customary patterns of functioning; that they will do this in ways that fit their usual style; and that many different styles of coping can be viable. In this situation of stress, medical personnel can be a major resource, aiding the family in ways that go beyond medical instruction. If they are sensitive to family issues and the complexity of family relations, they may be instrumental in maintaining the family's morale and in mobilizing the healing capacity of the family in the service of the patient. Since that is a difficult task, the following comments may be helpful:

- Know that you inevitably become part of the family system. Like other social systems, families have the power to pull their helpers into preferred pathways. Because that is so, medical personnel may find themselves becoming intrusive and controlling in enmeshed families, and careful or professionally distant in disorganized families. There is no immunity from such experiences, since that is the way a system works, but the medical team will need to be alert to this silent emotional pull.

- Take the time to observe and assess the family. "Diagnosis," in this case, is not a search for pathology. It is an effort to understand the family's organization, developmental stage, and style of coping, as well as the impact of the illness on the system. With that kind of differentiated understanding, it is easier to provide medical information, help the family explore its resources, and suggest alternatives in a way that the family can accept and act upon.

- Accept the style of the family and work with their sources of strength and resilience. Almost all families make some effort to be helpful, in their own terms. It is important to acknowledge the family's efforts and to confirm its members, even if the team will want to suggest alternatives.

- Expect not only distress but also confusion, as the family deals with anxiety and new demands. That is part of a transitional process and may lead in time to effective adaptation. It is not helpful to label the family's behavior as deviant, particularly at points of crisis. It is more helpful to normalize their experience, connecting what they feel to the reactions of other families and to the idea that the process of adaptation is predictable and takes time.

- If therapy seems indicated, it is almost always advisable to frame the problem as a transitional issue, related to the trauma of the illness and the pressures of home care. Families having difficulty are often seen as inherently pathologic, whereas they can more accurately be understood as families under stress, groping for effective ways of coping in a difficult situation. It is usually advisable as well to refer the entire family for therapy, even if only one member seems obviously troubled or asks for help. Illness and home care are a family affair. Difficulties are basically interactional, and the family as a whole is the healing force.

- Supplementary resources for the family should be broadly defined and include the informal network. Medical personnel may think first of organized resources—nursing homes, paid helpers, and so forth—but there are frequently untapped resources in the extended family, among friends and neighbors, or in self-help groups dealing with the same disease. These are often just as beneficial to both patient and family, building more personal ties and long-term supports.

- Understand that the family can be a support for medical personnel. Like family members, professional helpers are subject to burnout, especially if they work with chronic and terminal cases. The use of the family as a framework for understanding and working with the patient is an antidote to depression and helplessness. The family is always healthier than the individual patient. It will always survive, and it will always respond to care and concern.

## REFERENCES

1. Antonovsky A: Health, Stress, and Coping. San Francisco, Jossey-Bass, 1979
2. Dohrenwend BS, Dohrenwend BP: Stressful Life Events: Their Nature and Effects. New York, John Wiley & Sons, 1974
3. Gunderson EK, Rahe RH (eds): Life Stress and Illness. Springfield, Ill, Charles C Thomas, 1974
4. Insel PM, Moos RH (eds): Health and the Social Environment. Lexington, Mass, Heath, 1974
5. Lazarus RS, Cohen JB: Environmental stress. In Altman I, Wohlwill JF (eds): Human Behavior and Environment, vol 2. New York, Plenum, 1977
6. Selye H: The Stress of Life. New York, McGraw-Hill, 1956
7. Selye H: Stress Without Distress. Philadelphia, Lippincott & Crowell, 1974

8. Wolf S, Goodell H: Harold G. Wolff's Stress and Disease, 2nd ed. Springfield, Ill, Charles C Thomas, 1968

9. Hill R: Families Under Stress. New York, Harper & Row, 1949

10. Hill R: Generic features of families under stress. Social Casework 49:139–150, 1958

11. Figley CR, McCubbin HI: Stress and the Family, vol 2. New York, Brunner/Mazel, 1983

12. McCubbin HI, Figley CR: Stress and the Family, vol 1. New York, Brunner/Mazel, 1983

13. McCubbin HI, Patterson JM: Family adaptation to crisis. In McCubbin H, Cauble E, Patterson J (eds): Family Stress, Coping, and Social Support. Springfield, Ill, Charles C Thomas, 1982

14. Rolland JS: Toward a psychosocial typology of chronic and life-threatening illness. Family Systems Medicine 2:245–262, 1984

15. Adams JE, Lindemann E: Coping with long-term disability. In Coelho GV, Hamburg DA, Adams JE (eds): Coping and Adaptation. New York, Basic Books, 1974

16. Minuchin S, Rosman B, Baker L: Psychosomatic Families: Anorexia Nervosa in Context. Cambridge, Harvard, 1978

17. Reiss D, Gonzalez S, Kramer N: Family process, chronic illness and death: On the weakness of strong bonds. Arch Gen Psychiatry 43:795–804, 1986

18. Epstein NB, Bishop DS, Baldwin LM: McMaster model of family functioning: A view of the normal family. In Walsh F (ed): Normal Family Processes. New York, Guilford, 1982

19. Lewis JM, Beavers WR, Gossett JT: No Single Thread: Psychological Health in Family Systems. New York, Brunner/Mazel, 1976

20. Olson D, McCubbin H, Barnes H, et al: Families: What Makes Them Work. Beverly Hills, CA, Sage, 1983

# PART 3

# Providing Care at Home

# 8

# Home Management of Chronic Problems in the Elderly

BARBARA Z. BERK
MICHAEL L. FREEDMAN

With the advent of diagnostic related groups (DRGs) and resource utilization groups (RUGs), elderly people are using hospitals and nursing homes to a lesser extent, and home care has become crucial in dealing with chronic diseases in the elderly population.

The plan of home care for the older patient must be developed and coordinated by a physician, registered nurse, social worker, and other members of the home care team, and services have to be matched with the individual's needs. Also, it may be necessary to have the home maintained with support services such as with housekeeping, homemaking, home attendants, and services such as Meals on Wheels.

In the elderly population there are five common chronic problems that shall be discussed in this chapter: the so-called 5 Is (all begin with the letter i). They are (1) incompetence, (2) immobility, (3) incontinence, (4) iatrogenic disease, and (5) impaired homeostasis. All of these can be managed, at least initially, in the home, before considering institutionalization.

## THE ELDERLY PATIENT WITH INCOMPETENCE

There are various causes of incompetence in the elderly patient. Among them are Alzheimer's disease, multi-infarct dementia, geriatric depression, and benign forgetfulness of senescence. Alzheimer's disease is an organic brain disease characterized by senile plaques and neurofibrillatory tangles in the brain substance.[1] There is gradual progression from forgetfulness to severe loss of cognitive and other high intellectual functions, with loss of ambulation and incontinence.[2] The etiology is unknown, but various theories have been expounded. A recent popular theory has been that a slow latent virus or prion may be implicated.[3]

Multi-infarct dementia has a sudden stroke-like onset with remissions and exacerbations. The patient may be emotionally labile and have risk factors for cerebrovascular disease. Geriatric depression generally has a sudden onset though the patient has a history of memory problems but does not become severely demented. Formal neuropsychological testing can usually differentiate between dementia and depression. In depression, vegetative symptoms frequently occur, mainly sleep and appetite disturbances. Lastly, benign forgetfulness of senescence is a gradual process with only subjective complaints of cognitive deficit. This is commonly seen and can be distinguished from Alzheimer's disease in that with benign forgetfulness details of an event may be forgotten temporarily, while in dementia entire events are completely forgotten and cannot again be recalled.

On first seeing an incompetent patient, reversible disorders of dementia must be sought. After a thorough history and physical examination, including a neurologic examination, are done, laboratory data are obtained. A complete blood count, blood urea nitrogen and creatinine, liver function tests, electrolytes, calcium and glucose, thyroid function tests, $B_{12}$ and folate, toxicology and drug screen, serology, and an electrocardiogram, chest x-ray film and computerized axial tomography will help to rule out hematologic, renal, hepatic, or metabolic disorders, vitamin deficiency, drug or chemical intoxication, tertiary syphilis, arrhythmias, congestive heart failure, subdural hematomas, brain tumors, and normal pressure hydrocephalus, respectively.[4]

Reisberg and co-workers[2] at New York University (NYU) have formulated a global deterioration scale for age-associated cognitive decline and Alzheimer's disease in which they list seven progressively worsening clinical phases (Table 8-1). Stage one has no functional decrement manifest (normal). Stage two has very mild cognitive decline with subjective complaints of forgetfulness (benign forgetfulness of senescence). Stage three exhibits mild cognitive decline having an early confusional phase with earliest clear-cut deficits in which the patient cannot function in demanding situations. He manifests denial and it may be difficult to obtain objective evidence of deficit. Stage four shows moderate cognitive decline, or late confusional stage with memory deficit of personal history, decreased ability to perform more complex tasks, and heightened defense mechanisms. Stage five exhibits moderately severe decline or early dementia where patients become somewhat disoriented and must have some assistance, although they can perform their activities of daily living. Stage six is that of severe cognitive decline, mid-dementia, where the patient requires more assistance with activities of daily living such as bathing and dressing. Also, he may become incontinent. The patient may become unaware of recent events. There are personality and

**TABLE 8-1. GLOBAL DETERIORATION SCALE (GDS) FOR COGNITIVE DECLINE**

| Stage of Decline | Clinical Characteristics |
| --- | --- |
| 1. None | Normal |
| 2. Very mild | Subjective complaints of forgetfulness; poor concentration; benign in 95% in 4 years |
| 3. Mild | Early confusional phase; earliest clear-cut deficits; cannot function in demanding occupational or social situations; denial; benign in 80% in 4 years |
| 4. Moderate | Mild Alzheimer's disease; late confusional phase with decreased ability to perform more complex tasks such as handling money; heightened defense mechanisms; past memory deficits; in 4 years 25% no change, 25% worse at home, 25% institutionalized, 25% dead |
| 5. Moderately severe | Moderate Alzheimer's disease; disoriented; do not know year or season; cannot survive alone; in 4 years, 50% in community, 50% institutionalized or dead |
| 6. Severe | Severe Alzheimer's disease; requires assistance with activities of daily living; incontinence, loss of will power, forgets spouse's name; in 4 years 100% institutionalized or dead |
| 7. Very severe | Verbal abilities and psychomotor skills limited and eventually lost; vocabulary may be one word, "yes" or "okay"; stupor and coma eventually |

(Adapted from Reisberg B, Ferris SA, DeLeon MJ, Crook T: The Global Deterioration Scale for assessment of primary degenerative dementia. Am J Psychiatry 139(9):1136–1139, 1982)

emotional changes with loss of will power due to inability to carry an idea long enough to determine a purposeful course of action. In stage seven of late dementia with very severe cognitive decline verbal abilities are limited and psychomotor skills are eventually lost.[2,5]

An effective treatment for Alzheimer's disease has not yet been found. Perhaps early in the course of the disease ergot alkaloids may improve mood. Recently the use of dietary lecithin to increase the amount of acetylcholine neurotransmitter in the brain has been studied, but seems to be of limited, if any, value.[6]

Many patients with dementia will have a concomitant depression that will worsen the symptoms of the dementia. If the patient has a depression that is secondary to situational stress, psychotherapy or supportive counseling is the therapy of choice early in the disease. However, if the patient has a history of depressive episodes (endogenous depression), electroconvulsive treatment of the nondominant hemisphere appears to be tolerated with good results. The resultant temporary memory loss and confusion should be kept in mind.[6] Antidepressant medications are of value if the elderly patient can tolerate the side-effects of the drugs.

Pharmacologic therapy may play a vital part in controlling agitation and helping the patient sleep. Benzodiazepines have been used to control anxiety and sleep disorders and have been useful in managing irrational behavior. Lorazepam and alprazolam, having no active metabolites, are short acting and allow for greater flexibility in dosage.[6] Neuroleptics such as haloperidol and thioridazine have been effective. It should be kept in mind that elderly patients usually are on other drugs and one should be alert to overmedication or drug side-effects. A frequent side-effect of haloperidol is the development of extra-pyramidal symptoms with increased restlessness. However, there is a low sedative effect. The usual dose of haloperidol is 0.25 mg to 6 mg daily. Thioridazine may cause fainting and dizziness upon arising and is also a frequent cause of ejaculation disturbances in elderly men. Also, there may be mild extrapyramidal symptoms but generally, when properly prescribed, side-effects are minimal. Usual starting dosage of thioridazine is 10 mg at bedtime and dosages are adjusted every two weeks and tailored to the patient's needs. The dose may be increased to 300 mg a day.[6] Haloperidol is not a sedating drug whereas thioridazine is. Thus, if a drug is needed to allow the patient to sleep, thioridazine in low doses should be chosen.

When the diagnosis of Alzheimer's disease is made, even though the patient does not require immediate care, plans should be made for eventual care of the patient either at home or in an institution (see list). The family should seek out the expertise of a lawyer and social worker with experience in this field. Since personal finances often are depleted early in the course of the illness, and Medicare payment is limited, Medicaid may have to be relied on for financial assistance. A lawyer can best advise the family about paperwork, new laws, and rearrangement of finances to protect the financial integrity of the spouse who remains at home. Also, money may be set aside for the purpose of eventual home care.[7]

## WHAT TO DO AFTER THE DIAGNOSIS OF ALZHEIMER'S DISEASE IS MADE: RESOURCES FOR THE CARE GIVER

1. Contact Alzheimer's Disease Foundation or group in your area for general information, educational programs, and support groups.

2. Contact lawyer for expertise about new laws and rearrangement of finances.

3. Contact social worker about insurance and welfare programs and health and support services in the home.

4. Visiting nurse service will assist in determination of level of home care needed and will instruct and supervise the care giver.

5. Gain knowledge about nursing care facilities for when home care is no longer feasible.

Home care provides health and support services to individuals in their place of residence in order to delay the need for residential care. Services included are medical and nursing care, physical therapy, home health aide, housekeeping, homemaking, home attendant, and Meals on Wheels. Home care services are now being vendorized and the vendor agencies are responsible for hiring, training, and supervising home care workers. It is important to be familiar with the various levels of home care services. The housekeeper can be approved for up to 12 hours a week and must be directed by someone in the home. Housekeeper functions include cleaning, laundry, marketing, preparation of meals, and minimal personal care. The home attendant can be approved for up to 24 hours a day. In addition to housekeeping duties, more personal care such as feeding and toileting is offered. Also, with the supervision of a public health nurse, the attendant may also irrigate catheters; change colostomy bags; do simple dressings; measure urine volume, fluid intake, and output; and prepare modified diets as prescribed by a physician. Home health aides are approved if there is a need for skilled nursing. A nurse will assess the patient's needs for the determination of a number of hours needed. Besides the above-described duties, the aides may assist with medication.[8]

In the clinical phase of early dementia up to moderately severe cognitive decline, the patient can usually be taken care of at home by a care giver. This phase begins with forgetfulness, poor concentration, and the inability to function in demanding situations. It eventually leads to inability to perform complex tasks such as handling money. There are deficits in past memory and strong defense mechanisms. The patient eventually becomes disoriented, requires assistance to perform his activities of daily living, and cannot survive alone.

The care giver is usually a family member, but may be a hired aide, and the patient is in his own home or in the home of a close family member. There are various things that can be done in the home in order for the care to run more smoothly. The environment should be simplified so that as the patient develops more cognitive impairment he will be able to function more efficiently. There should be fewer objects to clutter the environment and that have to be accounted for. Safety precautions are of utmost importance. Stairwells should be gated, and access to the stove should not be easy. Also, doors and windows should be locked so that the patient cannot wander away and become lost. The daily routine must be consistent. The patient cannot learn new things, but the things he already knows can be reinforced for him. Memory aids such as signs on the bathroom door with a picture of the toilet, for example, are very helpful. Eventually, as moderate to severe cognitive decline develops, the physical and emotional burdens on the care giver make it necessary to consider institutionalization. The patient becomes more disoriented and forgets his spouse's name. He requires more assistance with his daily activities and eventually becomes incontinent. He may become belligerent and difficult to manage. The care giver may feel isolated and lonely. At first he may try daycare programs or a respite program for a longer stay. The care giver may need to join a support group with other care givers, or get individual counseling. An educational program will help ease the fear of the unknown, the unexpected. It will help the care giver prepare for future stages in the cognitive decline of the patient. The financial burden may be eased with help from the social worker with Medicare and Medicaid and with financial counseling by an informed attorney. Some physical burdens on the care giver can be eased with homemaker services for help in caring for the home. Visiting nurse services care for patient needs such as help with incontinence, bathing, feeding, and other activities of daily living. Also, the primary care giver can get ancillary care givers to relieve him for a few hours or days.

An important decision for the care giver or family of the demented patient is when to institutionalize. Timing of the decision will depend on the ability of the care giver to further tolerate the burden of home care. As the patient becomes more demented he will exhibit more assaultive and threatening behavior toward those around him. There will be a reversed sleep–wake cycle and nocturnal wandering. Eventually the patient will become incontinent and need nursing care.

Careful selection of a nursing home will be dependent on the suitability of the patient for the home and vice versa. The patient must be financially eligible, having the necessary finances or insurance that the home requires. Most institutions will accept Medicaid after finances have been depleted. The patient must be medically eligible for the home so that the nursing care is suitable for his needs. The nursing home should be thoroughly investigated by the family as to its accreditation and licensure. Visiting the institution and speaking with people associated with the home should help in evaluating the quality of care and the safety of the surroundings. Financial arrangements should be well understood and documented in writing so that both sides will be clear as to their responsibilities.

## THE ELDERLY PATIENT WITH IMMOBILITY PROBLEMS

Mobility is the ability to get around in one's environment. It is a function consisting of many component maneuvers that depend on the interplay of physical and cognitive aspects. Factors that compromise performance and ability are depression, knowledge deficit, anxiety, and potential for injury.[9]

Osteoarthritis with cartilaginous destruction of joints and fractures of hips and vertebrae secondary to osteoporosis are some of the disorders that may lead to immobility. People may experience a decline in mobility with aging. This is often the result of multiple chronic diseases and disabilities. However, it is generally felt that if an elderly person is free of disease and continues to be active and exercise, he may avoid or retard the development of an immobile state.

The aging patient should be first evaluated with a complete history and physical examination with emphasis on the neurologic and musculoskeletal aspects. Assessment is needed to determine self-care and home maintenance capabilities.

The physical examination should include the patient's sitting balance; his standing balance with and without his eyes open and on one or both legs; and also his ability to rise from a sitting position. His balance should be evaluated during neck turning and pushing on his sternum to attempt to throw him off balance. Also, he should be asked to lean back, bend forward, and reach up. The range of motion of all joints should be evaluated and any contractures noted. Also, the state of his musculature, especially if atrophic, should be recorded.

The consequences of immobility for the patient include decreased general conditioning and decreased cardiovascular fitness, joint stiffness and contractures, muscle wasting, accelerated osteoporosis with and without fractures, pneumonia, venous stasis, pulmonary emboli, and decubitus ulcers.[9]

The patient who has other people in his household to help him may be more dependent and less mobile than one who lives alone and values his independence. A home visit should provide the best opportunity to see the patient in the environment in which he must function. The home should be evaluated for safety and ease of mobility and these aspects should be optimized. Although decreased mobility is common, this problem can be prevented or slowed down. Problems must be recognized and function optimized. Once limitations have been assessed and areas have been identified where help is warranted, therapy can be considered (see Treatment Modalities for Immobility). Preferably, a specialist in rehabilitation medicine can devise a therapeutic plan and relate this to the therapist. This should include the region to be treated and the type, frequency, and duration of treatment with precautions to be observed. The objectives of treatment are to maintain activities of daily living and achieve functional independence.

Nonpharmacologic methods are the first approach and involve patient education.

### TREATMENT MODALITIES FOR IMMOBILITY

1. Exercises—stretching, range-of-motion
2. Walk programs
3. Heat therapy—packs, paraffin, ultrasound
4. Cryotherapy—whirlpool, packs
5. Splints and braces
6. Traction—cervical or lumbar
7. TENS

8. Assistive devices—crutches, canes, contour pillow, hospital bed
9. Pharmacologic—aspirin or acetaminophen, nonsteroidal anti-inflammatory drugs, intra-articular corticosteroids
10. Surgery—prosthetic implants; fusion of joints for stability

Patients must be taught to modify the use of their affected joints to reduce stress on them and give them optimal periods of rest. Complete bedrest is to be avoided, but appropriate rest intervals are important.

The patient will benefit from physiotherapy and occupational therapy. These therapeutic modalities overlap; each modality looks at the body as a whole entity. However, physiotherapy tends to focus on the lower extremities with goals of transferring or ambulation for the patient. Also, ultrasound, transcutaneous electrical nerve stimulation (TENS), and paraffin are some examples of the modalities used here for pain control. Occupational therapy focuses on the upper extremities and activities of daily living. Patients are taught how to dress, groom, feed, transfer themselves, and perform fine motor coordination.

An important objective of therapy is pain relief. Aggravating activities, as for example needlework, may have to be lessened or discontinued because of involvement of joints in the hands. Moist heat, utilizing warm-water soaks or warm towel wraps, may be applied for 10 to 20 minutes several times daily, and may be used to decrease muscle spasm and help with range-of-motion exercises. Also, hands may be dipped into and coated several times with a mixture of 8 parts paraffin to 1 part mineral oil maintained at a temperature of 126°F to 130°F twice daily. This should be avoided in diabetics, those with sensory disturbances, and those with peripheral vascular disease. Also, ice packs may be used for blocking pain sensation and prior to range-of-motion exercises. Cold therapy is also beneficial for inflamed joints. TENS may be used at home, especially with chronic involvement of the lumbar spine, hips, or knees.[10]

Without exercise there is a 3% to 5% loss of muscle strength a day.[9] Range-of-motion exercises, without excess stress on joints, must be performed in a slow, smooth manner for flexibility and to avoid contractures. Hands may be exercised in warm water. Muscles should be gently stretched to regain lost motion. Gentle knee-flexion exercises can correct and prevent flexion contractures and tighten ligamentous supports. The hips and upper extremities may be flexed, extended, adducted, and abducted. Exercises should be done to help strengthen muscles around various joints. The quadriceps muscles stabilize and support the knees. The quadriceps isometric exercises involve the patient tightening the muscles in extension, holding to a count of five and relaxing, and repeating this at least 20 times twice daily. Hamstring isometrics are done with the leg extended and pressing the back of the heel against the surface of the bed. Isometric exercises also strengthen the abdominal muscles. The patient may place an elastic band around the ankle or knee with the ends held firmly with both hands, while moving the hip joint through its range of motion. This will help to strengthen the muscles about the hip, which is important to future hip surgery. Exercise against gravity puts moderate stress on bones and any weight-bearing activity satisfies that requirement.[9] For osteoporosis, an exercise program, added intake of calcium and vitamin D, and appropriate use of estrogens are protective techniques.[11]

If the patient is able to ambulate, progressive daily walk programs without overtaxing will help promote cardiovascular fitness. Weight reduction is important and this especially affects the knees, because in walking the knee bears weight that is equal to 2 to 3 times that of body weight.

For pain and an anti-inflammatory effect the patient may be given analgesics including preparations of aspirin or acetaminophen with or without codeine. Anti-inflammatory drugs such as ibuprofen (400 mg–600 mg PO qid), sulindac (150 mg–200 mg PO bid), or naproxen (250 mg–375 mg PO bid) can be used. Also, intra-articular corticosteroids such as triamcinolone can be used, no more than 3 to 4 times a year and not less than one month apart.[10]

Hospitalization is rarely necessary since there are numerous aids that can be utilized in the home to facilitate care and increase comfort for the patient. Molded splints are useful to rest joints and alleviate pain, as well as to support a hypermobile or unstable joint and correct deformities. The Orthoplast molded thumb splint is utilized to rest the base of the thumb. Cloth stretch gloves help ease nocturnal pain and morning stiffness of the hands. A wedge pillow is more comfortable than several pillows used to prop up in bed. A contoured pillow (Wall-Pillo) is useful to stabilize and support the neck while sleeping and to prevent stiffness in the morning. The patient may use a soft cervical collar during flare-up of acute neck pain, especially with radicular symptoms. Cervical traction for cervical radiculopathy can be started with physiotherapy in the hospital and continued at home with an overhead traction unit. Positioning is crucial and should be checked. A back brace can be prescribed for excess spinal flexion and as an abdominal support to decrease back pain.

If the patient can ambulate, a cane will broaden the base of support, decrease weight bearing on hip or knee joints, and allow a greater walking distance. If the hands cannot withstand the stress of the cane, forearm crutches can be used. The cane must be appropriately sized for each patient and a tripod cane may be used if balance is a problem. For use of the cane to be effective it must be held on the normal side, which moves in tandem with the affected lower extremity. In this way the tip of the cane and the weak leg are on the floor at the same time.

It is possible to rent a hospital bed that can more easily position the patient and that has a firm mattress. Otherwise, a bed board can improve a not so firm mattress. There are chairs that have devices that help a patient stand from a sitting position. An elevated toilet seat with grab rails on the sides of the commode increases safety and helps achieve functional independence. Other safety measures are nonskid floors and handrails in the halls and stairway. The patient may use large-handled utensils for a better grip and a reacher for high objects.

A long-term home health-care program, as, for example, the Lombardi Program in New York City, is a service that provides health care in the home to patients who might otherwise have to enter a nursing home or health-related facility. Each patient accepted into this type of program receives an individualized coordinated plan of care ordered by a physician. Services may include medical care, nursing care, personal care, medical social worker visits, rehabilitation therapy, medical supplies and equipment, medication, and transportation, as well as other services that assist in keeping the patient at home. Comprehensive care for these patients can be delivered at a cost well below 75% of the cost of a residential health-care facility. The cost is usually paid by Medicaid but rules and regulations are being set up to allow private paying patients to participate in the program.[12]

## THE ELDERLY PATIENT WITH INCONTINENCE

At least ten million people suffer from some form of urinary incontinence. In the geriatric population over age 65, about 10% of the people in the community have urinary incontinence and in institutions this figure is about 50%. Also, about 30% of those over age 80 have acute or chronic incontinence. Recent studies in geriatric patients have shown that this condition is usually manageable and often can be corrected.[13, 14]

The urinary bladder is a hollow organ made up of a serosal layer on the superior surface, a muscular layer termed the detrusor muscle, and a mucosal layer of transitional epithelium. The urethra extends from the bladder neck to the meatus and is composed of two longitudinal smooth muscle layers that form a functional internal sphincter. It is lined proximally with transitional epithelium. The distal urethral lining is stratified squamous epithelium; however, in men, stratified columnar epithelium lines the urethra from the ejaculatory ducts to the distal urethra. The external striated urethral muscle sphincter allows voluntary interruption of voiding and provides a propulsive force for emptying the bladder, although it is not an important factor in continence because it fatigues rapidly when stimulated. Incontinence results from a decrease in pressure within the urethra or from an increase of pressure within the bladder, or from both. To be continent there must be a higher pressure within the urethra than within the bladder. Intraurethral pressure depends on intra-abdominal pressure, striated pelvic muscle tone, urethral and bladder smooth muscle tone, and the thickness of the urethral mucosa, which in women depends somewhat on estrogen. Pressure within the bladder depends on intra-abdominal pressure (less so than does intraurethral pressure), detrusor muscle tone, and bladder volume.[15]

Intact neurologic loops control the above forces in the maintenance of continence.[16, 17] Their net effect is to communicate the status of bladder volume to the brain. The central nervous system interactions are separated into four neurologic loops. Loop I is composed of connecting axons from the frontal lobe of the cerebral cortex and thalamus to the detrusor nucleus in the brain stem, which have an inhibitory effect on the detrusor nucleus. Loop II consists of axons between the detrusor nucleus and the sacral spinal cord. This pathway amplifies reflex contractions from the detrusor muscle back to the detrusor nucleus forming the primary reflex arc of innervation of the detrusor muscle. Loop III consists of sensory input from the detrusor to the spinal pudendal motor nucleus, which inhibits the tonic motor impulses of the pelvic floor muscles to produce passive relaxation during bladder filling. Loop IV is formed from nerves in the anal sphincter and periurethral area, which traverse the corticospinal tract and terminate in the frontal lobe of the cerebral cortex, the thalamus, and cerebellum. This pathway allows volitional control over the pelvic floor muscles and the external urethral sphincter, so that urine flow can be controlled.[15]

When the bladder is distended to about 300 ml, detrusor contraction will occur, amplified by loop II to allow urination. If urination is not desired, loop I (under voluntary control) can inhibit bladder contractions in order to avoid abrupt bladder emptying. Detrusor contractions, when amplified by loop II and not inhibited by loop I, are aided by contractions in the abdominal and pelvic muscles, with relaxation of the bladder outlet and urethral sphincter (loops III and IV), to initiate voiding. There has been advanced understanding of lower urinary tract function by the localization of autonomic neuroreceptors. The sympathetic nervous system is composed of alpha-adrenergic and beta-adrenergic receptors. Alpha-adrenergic receptors in the bladder outlet and urethra increase urethral tone, and beta-adrenergic receptors, mainly in the body of the bladder, aid detrusor relaxation and bladder filling. In addition, parasympathetic cholinergic receptors, found mainly in the bladder, cause detrusor contractions. Voiding is mainly parasympathetically mediated with cholinergic stimuli producing bladder contractions. Sympathetic impulses relax the bladder and aid filling while producing contractions of the urethra and bladder neck.[15]

There are five clinical classifications of urinary incontinence. They are urge, stress, overflow, reflex, and functional. Urge incontinence is accompanied by a strong desire to void prior to and during incontinence. The volume is usually moderate. The usual cause is detrusor hyperactivity where the bladder escapes central inhibition by loop I and contracts repeatedly. Also, a patient with urge incontinence of acute onset must always have inflammation from infection, stone, or tumor excluded.

Stress incontinence is associated with sneezing or coughing, which causes a sudden increase in intra-abdominal pressure. Usually there is a loss of small to moderate amounts of urine. Atrophic vaginitis or urethritis can lead to stress incontinence by affecting the strength and responsiveness of the internal urethral smooth muscle sphincter, and it often can be relieved by application of estrogen cream. Also, in women, weakness of the pelvic muscles from childbirth or obesity causes pelvic floor laxity that leads to urethral hyper-mobility from changes in the posterior urethrovesical angle.

Overflow incontinence occurs when the bladder is overdistended. This may be due to detrusor hyporeflexia. The bladder is hypotonic and does not generate enough pressure to overcome urethral resistance and therefore there is a large residual volume of urine. The patient feels that he must strain to urinate. Detrusor hyporeflexia may be myogenic due to bladder outlet obstruction caused by a markedly enlarged prostate or a fecal impaction, or it may be neurogenic from a herniated disk or peripheral neuropathy. In the latter case, bowel control and perineal sensation are impaired also.[13]

Reflex incontinence occurs when a neurologic impairment, such as a suprasacral spinal cord lesion, results in loss of voluntary control of urination. There is no sensation of impending urination with reflex incontinence and the bladder empties large volumes.

With functional incontinence, the patient is not really incontinent but is unable to get to the toilet in time. He may be confused, restrained, or immobile.[13]

Incontinence may be acute or chronic. Acute incontinence is more often correctable (see Reversible Causes of Urinary Incontinence, listed below). Chronic incontinence, though curable only 20% to 30% of the time, can be managed in the home.

Acute incontinence may be caused by acute confusional states in the elderly. Also, regressive behavior or hostility can manifest itself with acute incontinence. Medications such as diuretics, anticholinergics, sedatives, muscle relaxants, and some antihypertensives may cause acute incontinence. Also, urinary tract infections, fecal impactions, polyuric states, and bladder tumors can present with acute incontinence. Atrophic vaginitis and urethritis, which lead to urethral insufficiency, cause acute as well as chronic stress inconti-nence and can be treated with the use of estrogen preparations locally.

The most common mechanism of chronic incontinence in the elderly is a hyperreflexic or uninhibited bladder and is clinically classified as urge incontinence.[13, 14] Among the causes are stimulation of the bladder from inflammation, radiation, chemotherapy, tumors, or stones, or escape of the bladder from central nervous system inhibition as seen in cerebrovascular disease, tumors, multiple sclerosis, parkinsonism, cervical spondylosis, and normal pressure hydrocephalus. The inhibitory aspects of central nervous system control of voiding are explained in the descriptions of the neurologic loops. Detrusor instability also occurs as a response to an obstructed outlet, as, for example, with an enlarged prostate before overflow incontinence occurs. Also, an individual who has experi-enced incontinence and is fearful of a repeat episode may voluntarily urinate frequently and therefore decondition the detrusor, which leads to a small bladder capacity. Bladder ca-pacity is small but there may be residual urine. Symptoms of detrusor hyperreflexia are urgency, frequency, nocturia, and voiding small volumes.[13, 14]

## REVERSIBLE CAUSES OF URINARY INCONTINENCE

| | |
|---|---|
| 1. Urinary tract infection | 6. Pessary |
| 2. Acute confusional states | 7. Bladder tumor or stones |
| 3. Drugs—diuretics, anticholinergics, sedatives, muscle relaxants, antihypertensives | 8. Obesity |
| | 9. Lack of estrogen in postmenopausal females |
| 4. Fecal impaction | |
| 5. Polyuric states | |

Another mechanism of chronic incontinence is detrusor hyporeflexia, which leads to overflow incontinence. In this condition, the bladder is hypotonic and distended, and a large residual volume of urine exists due to the inability to overcome urethral resistance. Detrusor hyporeflexia can be seen in neurologic conditions such as diabetes mellitus, tabes dorsalis, and alcoholic neuropathy. Medications such as anticholinergic drugs or muscle relaxants commonly precipitate this type of incontinence.

Urethral obstruction is a cause of chronic overflow incontinence. The external sphincter may not properly relax and a functional obstruction may develop. Prostatic hypertrophy, urethral stricture, and pelvic tumors may cause anatomic obstruction.

Many elderly women have a urethra that is too loose, resulting in stress incontinence. Chronic atrophic vaginitis can also lead to chronic stress incontinence. If there is internal sphincter damage from transurethral prostatectomy, men can also develop stress incontinence. During times of increased intra-abdominal pressure, there is a loss of small amounts of urine. However, there is no post-voiding residual.

Elderly individuals may exhibit more than one type of incontinence, which is therefore classified as mixed incontinence.

In order to treat an incontinent patient successfully, the cause of incontinence should be determined. Intermittent incontinence signifies a reversible disorder that may be functional or caused by drugs, whereas established incontinence is due to abnormalities in the detrusor or outlet. The patient or a care giver should keep a record of daily accidents, the circumstances of the accidents, and the amount of urine lost. This record provides a good estimation of bladder status and helps in devising a training schedule. A complete history and physical examination should be performed, and recent surgery and medications should be reviewed (Table 8-2). For example, prazosin, an alpha-adrenergic blocker, can cause stress incontinence by its effect on the urethra. In the physical examination, mental status should be noted. If the patient is confused or immobile, he may not be able to get to the bathroom in time to void. An abdominal examination may elicit a palpable bladder, and rectal examination may reveal a markedly enlarged prostate or a fecal impaction. The

## TABLE 8-2. EVALUATION OF INCONTINENCE*

| Method of Evaluation | Type of Incontinence |
|---|---|
| *History* | |
| Frequent sensation of need to urinate | Urge |
| No sensation of need to urinate | Reflex |
| Occurs only with cough or increased abdominal pressure | Stress |
| Decreased force of stream, dribbling, necessity to strain | Overflow |
| Inability to reach bathroom in time | Functional |
| Amount of urine lost | Small with stress or overflow; small to moderate with urge; large with reflex; variable with functional |
| Dyspareunia (estrogen deficiency) | Stress |
| *Physical Examination* | |
| Confused, immobile | Functional |
| Abnormal gait, motor and sensory deficits | Urge, reflex |
| Palpable bladder | Overflow |
| Prostatic hypertrophy, fecal impaction | Overflow |
| Uterine prolapse, cystocele, signs of estrogen lack | Stress |

*Older people can exhibit more than one type of incontinence and are therefore classified as "mixed."

neurologic examination will rule out central nervous system abnormalities, autonomic nervous system dysfunction, or spinal cord dysfunction. The pelvic examination may reveal a cystocele, uterine prolapse, or atrophic vaginitis. Laboratory data should include a urinalysis and, if indicated, a urine culture and sensitivity. If there is a history of frequent urinary tract infections, an intravenous pyelogram may be done to rule out any obstructive lesions. Blood urea nitrogen, glucose, and calcium are done to rule out a polyuric syndrome. Urodynamic evaluation may be pursued when stress incontinence with outlet obstruction or overflow incontinence is suspected. Cystometry measures lower urinary tract pressure and volume relations by infusing sterile saline into the bladder and recording detrusor contractions and intravesical pressure. Urethral pressure profiles can be done and are more useful in men. Urine flow studies may define outlet obstruction or detrusor inadequacy. In addition, the bladder may be catheterized for residual urine, which is noted in obstructive states.[18]

After the patient has been evaluated and the type of incontinence has been determined, treatment can be begun (Table 8-3). The benefits of drug and surgical regimens must be measured against their dangers.[15] In the home, scheduled voiding routines and disposable undergarment protectors can be used with great benefit. Also, condom catheters may be tried in male patients. The patient should avoid alcohol and caffeine, which cause diuresis.

There are several new drugs being administered to treat incontinence. In detrusor instability, imipramine, 25 mg to 150 mg qd; oxybutynin, 5 mg two to four times daily; and propantheline, 7.5 mg to 30 mg tid, are being used. Also, nifedipine and ibuprofen are currently being evaluated. In addition, alpha-adrenergic stimulants to increase urethral resistance may be useful.[13, 14]

With the problem of detrusor hyporeflexia, bethanechol, 10 mg to 30 mg tid, and phenoxybenzamine, 10 mg to 60 mg qd, have been used, but are often unsuccessful and have a high degree of side-effects. Frequent voidings are very helpful, with Credé and Valsalva maneuvers. Intermittent catheterization may be employed for unacceptable amounts of residual urine.[13, 14] If urethral obstruction cannot be corrected, phenoxybenzamine, 10 mg

## TABLE 8-3. TREATMENT OF URINARY INCONTINENCE

| Cause | Treatment |
|---|---|
| Spastic bladder (detrusor instability) | Bladder retraining<br>Disposable incontinence undergarments<br>Imipramine, 25 mg–150 mg qd<br>Oxybutynin, 5 mg tid<br>Propantheline, 7.5 mg–30 mg tid |
| Hypotonic bladder (detrusor hyporeflexia) | Frequent voidings<br>Intermittent catheterization<br>Disposable incontinence undergarments<br>Bethanechol, 20 mg tid<br>Phenoxybenzamine, 10 mg–60 mg qd |
| Urethral obstruction | Relieve obstruction<br>Disposable incontinence undergarments<br>Sphincterotomy<br>Phenoxybenzamine, 10 mg–60 mg qd |
| Urethral insufficiency | Weight loss<br>Pelvic exercises<br>Pessary<br>Disposable incontinence undergarments<br>Surgery<br>Estrogens<br>Phenylpropanolamine, 25 mg–50 mg bid<br>Imipramine, 25 mg–150 mg qd |

to 60 mg qd, may be tried. Recently, prazosin, an alpha antagonist, has been used with some success.[19] Weight loss and Kegel's exercise can be used for strengthening pelvic musculature.[20] To restore the integrity of the urethral mucosa and resistance to outflow, estrogen[21] in females and alpha-adrenergic agents[22] can be used. Surgery can be done or a pessary inserted for correction of the urethrovesical angle.[13,14] It is rare for a patient to need indwelling bladder catheterization. Disposable undergarments along with good skin care are important to those patients who do not respond to maneuvers or drug therapy. Incontinence is for the most part manageable and need not lead to social isolation of the patient.

## HOME CARE AND IATROGENIC DISEASE

Iatrogenic disease is a major chronic problem in the elderly. This is often due to consequences of therapeutic and diagnostic procedures involving medications and surgery.

There are multiple factors that increase the risk for drug reactions in the elderly. Elderly persons may have multiple disorders that may necessitate the use of an increased number of medications. With greater exposure to various medications there is a greater chance of drug interactions and side-effects. For example, cimetidine inhibits hepatic blood flow and the cytochrome P450 system that metabolizes many central nervous system active drugs, so that there is a greater peak level of the psychotropic drug for a longer period of time when taken with cimetidine. The elderly are at increased risk for adverse drug reactions since with advancing age there is a change in pharmacokinetics.[23,24] Muscle mass is replaced by fat, and fat-soluble drugs last longer in the body. With decreased glomerular filtration rate, drugs will not be excreted in the urine as efficiently as in younger individuals. Receptor sensitivity decreases with age as, for example, older people don't respond as well to beta blockade. However, there are increases in end-organ sensitivity as with opiates and warfarin. About two thirds of all drug reactions are caused by cardiovascular drugs and central nervous system drugs.[25]

The common side-effects of major drug classifications are listed under Common Side-Effects of Major Drug Classes.

Postural hypotension is among the most serious side-effects of drugs. The physician, therefore, must be cautious in prescribing vasodilatory antihypertensives. Diuretic medications can cause a decrease in blood volume, especially if the patient is salt restricted. One must begin with low doses of the drugs and raise them very cautiously. In older individuals blood pressure should not be lowered as aggressively and rapidly as in younger persons. With psychotropic drugs, small doses are usually given at bedtime to avoid postural hypotension.

Anticholinergic drugs, which include antidepressants, antispasmodics, antihistamines, and psychotropics, can cause confusion, urinary retention (overflow incontinence), constipation, and arrhythmias, and can precipitate acute narrow-angle glaucoma.[26]

Practically any drug can cause confusion in the elderly. If a patient complains of confusion after starting a new drug, and even if the blood level of the drug is in the therapeutic range,[6] the drug should be discontinued and the patient observed. Cimetidine, which crosses the blood–brain barrier, is more likely to cause confusion than ranitidine, which does not.

Especially in the elderly, medications such as lidocaine can cause convulsions, anticonvulsants can cause ataxia, and vinca alkaloids and nitrofurantoin can cause peripheral neuropathies; extrapyramidal symptoms[27] are caused mainly by the phenothiazines and butyrophenones. Also, with the major tranquilizers, the elderly develop tardive dyskinesia and akathisia, or motor restlessness, more commonly.[28] Raising the dosage of the medica-

## COMMON SIDE-EFFECTS OF MAJOR DRUG CLASSES

### Postural Hypotension

Antihypertensives
Psychotropics
Calcium channel blockers
Opiates
Antiparkinson drugs

### Anticholinergic

Antidepressants
Antispasmodics
Antihistamines
Psychotropics

### Confusion

Analgesics
Anticholinergics
Antidepressants
Anticonvulsants
Anti-inflammatory agents
Antiparkinson drugs
Barbiturates
Beta blockers
Benzodiazepines
Calcium channel blockers
Cimetidine
Digitalis preparations
Hypoglycemics
Lidocaine
Vincristine

### Neurologic

*Convulsions*
Lidocaine
Antidepressants
*Ataxia*
Anticonvulsants
*Peripheral neuropathy*
Vinca alkaloids
Nitrofurantoin
*Extrapyramidal symptoms*
Phenothiazines
Butyrophenones
Metoclopramide
Antidepressants

### Renal

Aminoglycoside antibiotics
Diuretics
Nonsteroidal anti-inflammatory drugs

### Cardiac

Digitalis preparations
Beta blockers
Calcium channel blockers
Antiarrhythmias
Antidepressants
Psychotropic drugs

---

tion to counteract the symptoms will only worsen the situation. As used in Alzheimer's disease, haloperidol is more likely to produce extrapyramidal side-effects than is thioridazine.

Certain drugs such as aminoglycoside antibiotics, diuretics, and anti-inflammatory drugs compromise renal function, which is already diminished in the elderly. Various drugs with negative inotropic effects, such as beta blockers, calcium channel blockers, and various antiarrhythmics, can cause congestive heart failure in the elderly, who may have compromised cardiac function to begin with. Allergic, hematologic, skin, and gastrointestinal side-effects appear to have equal occurrence in all age groups.

When institutionalized, older persons exhibit more psychological problems. They may be depressed or have delirium and hallucinate in the hospital setting. They are more apt to be immobile and therefore may suffer from pneumonia, thromboembolisms, and incontinence. They also may refuse or be unable to eat (no assistance or no dentures) and therefore may suffer from malnutrition. The use of restraining devices may increase the risk of harm and therefore should be discouraged.[29, 30] On the other hand, overprotection of the geriatric patient may discourage functional independence.[31]

The patient may be unable to reach the bathroom by himself or may not have quick response to his call. This may encourage incontinence.[32] He may fall trying to get over the siderails that are there to protect him from falling out of bed. There may be poor lighting in the room and the patient may not be able to ambulate due to decreased senses. The fragile skin of the elderly person breaks down more easily and eventually ulcerates if not cared for properly.[33]

For the elderly who must be hospitalized, special units such as the New York University Cooperative Care Unit may avoid some of the problems inherent in the usual hospital setting.[34] The patient feels more confident and comfortable with a care partner who is a friend or relative who rooms in with the patient and participates in the whole hospital experience. For the most part, the elderly do respond to therapeutics, and they should not be denied good medical care and therapies should not be omitted because of advanced age.

## THE ELDERLY PATIENT WITH IMPAIRED HOMEOSTASIS

Homeostasis is the ability to maintain a satisfactory internal environment or milieu even though the external environment may not be optimal. This requires a complex association between a central control system and its receptors and effectors. The messages being related go via the nervous system or the endocrine system. All of these elements are affected by the aging process.[35]

There are both internal and external receptors, which, with aging, develop a loss of sensitivity. For example, internal receptors are the baroreceptors that monitor the arterial blood pressure. In the elderly they are blunted and this results in postural hypotension and a dizzy feeling.[36] External receptors are cutaneous receptors in the skin. Older persons suffer a loss of some and a diminished response in the remaining ones. Therefore, they have a poorer ability to recognize temperature changes.[37]

The elderly are at increased risk for hypothermia and hyperthermia. The body core–shell temperature gradient is smaller. There is decreased efficacy of the autonomic nervous system. There are nonconstricting patterns of vasomotor response to cold, causing inability to feel cold and thus to protect oneself.[38] There is inadequate vasodilatation in response to heat so that there is not an efficient decrease in core temperature.[39] Various medications affect the autonomic nervous system.[39] Decreased muscle mass in the elderly leads to less shivering and therefore less heat production. Heat production is hindered by a decreased ability to increase the respiratory quotient in elderly individuals. There is also a decreased ability to increase the cardiac output for heat dissipation. The elderly have a diminished ability to sweat and therefore the heat load persists.[39]

The regulatory centers within the hypothalamus or brain stem lose precision. Therefore, greater deviations from the basal state are needed for the body to initiate action.[38]

The vestibular system interacts with multiple sensory inputs to provide a sense of one's position in space. In the elderly, this system is particularly vulnerable to trauma and medications. An imbalance between the senses and the labyrinthine vestibular system results from an abnormality of any involved components.[40]

Dizziness may be constant or intermittent. Constant dizziness may be caused by depression, various drugs, and systemic illnesses such as metabolic and endocrine disorders. Intermittent dizziness is usually due to visual malfunction, peripheral neuropathy, and labyrinthine vestibular dysfunction, which may be central or peripheral. Central causes (involvement of the vestibular portion of the brain stem) may be due to increased intracranial pressure, acoustic neuroma, vascular insufficiency, and seizures. Peripheral causes (involvement of semicircular canals, saccule, utricle, eighth cranial nerve) may be exhibited as Meniere's disease, benign positional vertigo, acute labyrinthitis, and perilymphatic fistula.[40]

Syncope, or sudden loss of consciousness, is common in the elderly population. Multiple diseases impair cerebral oxygen delivery. With age alone, there is up to a 25% diminution of cerebral blood flow and therefore the elderly have a decreased ability to maintain consciousness. With diseases such as anemia, cardiac arrhythmias, severe bradycardia, congestive heart failure, and chronic obstructive pulmonary disease, oxygen delivery to the

**TABLE 8-4. MANAGEMENT OF DISORDERS OF IMPAIRED HOMEOSTASIS**

| Disorder | Treatment |
| --- | --- |
| Heat fatigue | Cooling, fluids, and electrolytes |
| Heat stroke | Cooling, fluids, and electrolytes; diazepam for prophylaxis of convulsions |
| Hypothermia | Insulate with blankets; rapid local rewarming of areas of frostbite with water baths; suspect and treat bronchopneumonia; check for arrhythmias and metabolic acidosis. |
| Dizziness | |
|   Constant | Treat depression if present. Discontinue psychotropics, ototoxic antibiotics, and cardiac adrenergic inhibitors. Treat any metabolic or endocrine disorder. |
|   Intermittent | Correct refractive error; eye patch for diplopia Treat peripheral neuropathy (if due to vitamin $B_{12}$ deficiency or diabetes mellitus). Patient may use aluminum walker to become aware of spatial orientation transmitted by the trunk and extremities. Check for labyrinthine vestibular dysfunction (involvement of vestibular portion of brain stem or semicircular canals). |
| Syncope | Treat underlying diseases. Eliminate unnecessary drugs. Surgery for aortic stenosis, pacemaker |
| Decreased renin and decreased aldosterone | Maintain intravascular volume with adequate fluid intake; beware of diuretics; for postural hypotension use support hose, arise slowly, sit during micturition. |

brain is further diminished. If an acute illness such as pneumonia or myocardial infarction occurs, this may only manifest itself by confusion or a syncopal episode. The problem of postural hypotension in the elderly, with blunting of compensatory mechanisms, further contributes to decreased cerebral blood flow.[41]

Older persons are more likely to exhibit hyponatremia due to the variation in endocrine gland output.[42] They have a decrease in the secretion of aldosterone, which makes it more difficult to conserve sodium.[43] Also, there is an increase in antidiuretic hormone secretion,[44] making elderly people more prone to hyponatremic syndromes. One should be careful with salt restriction in older patients because hyponatremia may ensue. Usually it is not necessary to restrict sodium to less than 2.5 g per day.

The treatment of impaired homeostasis in the elderly is usually preventive and symptomatic (Table 8-4). Heat fatigue and stroke are treated by cooling, fluids, and electrolytes. In severe cases diazepam may prevent convulsions. Hypothermia is managed by heat conservation and rewarming of frostbitten areas. Also, the elderly patient should be checked for bronchopneumonia and cardiac arrhythmias. Dizziness is managed according to its cause. Offending drugs should be eliminated if possible. Systemic diseases should be controlled and sensory disturbances should be corrected. Depression should be recognized and treated. Labyrinthine vestibular dysfunction, if involved, should be treated.

## CONCLUSION

The elderly patient often can be well managed in the home, even with multiple chronic illnesses. What is necessary is a careful plan taking into account the patient's needs and the environment, and careful coordination with the medical treatment. The physician must always be aware of the danger of medications and treatments and often the key to successful management at home is the discontinuance of medications rather than starting new ones.

## REFERENCES

1. Terry R, Davies P: Dementia of the Alzheimer type. Annu Rev Neurosci 3:77–95, 1980
2. Reisberg B, Ferris SA, DeLeon MJ, Crook T: The Global Deterioration Scale for assessment of primary degenerative dementia. Am J Psychiatry 139(9):1136–1139, 1982
3. Bendheim P, Bolton D: Alzheimer's disease: Is there evidence of an infectious cause? Geriatric Medicine Today 4:93–103, 1985
4. Steel K, Feldman R: Diagnosing dementia and its treatable causes. Geriatrics March:79–88, 1979
5. Diamond E: Testing cognitive function in the elderly. Geriatric Consultant Sept/Oct:21–31, 1985
6. Freedman ML: Organic brain syndrome in the elderly. Postgrad Med 74(4):165–176, 1983
7. Mace N, Robins P: The 36 Hour Day: A Family Guide to Caring for Persons with Alzheimer's Disease. Baltimore, the Johns Hopkins University Press, 1981
8. Information Guide for Helping Families of the Aged Obtain Home Care Services. New York, Natural Supports Program of Community Service Society of New York, 1982
9. Rothschild BM: A physical therapy primer for osteoarthritis. Geriatric Consultant Sept/Oct: 14–20, 1985
10. Quinet RJ: Osteoarthritis: Increasing mobility and reducing disability. Geriatrics 41(2): 36–50, 1986
11. Goodman C: Osteoporosis: Protective measures of nutrition and exercise. Geriatrics 40(4): 59–70, 1985
12. When Illness Strikes. New York, New York City Human Resources Administration Medical Assistance Program, 1980
13. Snustad DG, Rosenthal JT: Urinary incontinence in the elderly. Am Fam Physician 32:182–196, 1985
14. Resnick NM, Subbarao VY: Management of urinary incontinence in the elderly. N Engl J Med 313:800–804, 1985
15. Williams ME, Pannill FC: Urinary incontinence in the elderly. Ann Intern Med 97(6): 895–907, 1982
16. deGroat WC, Booth AM: Autonomic systems to the urinary bladder and sexual organs. In Dyck PJ, Thomas PK, Lambert EH, Beinge R (eds): Peripheral Neuropathy, 2nd ed, pp 285–299. Philadelphia, WB Saunders, 1984
17. Gosling JA, Chilton CP: The anatomy of the bladder, urethra, and pelvic floor. In Mundy AR, Stephenson TP, Wein AJ (eds): Urodynamics: Principles, Practice and Application, pp 3–13. New York, Churchill Livingstone, 1984
18. Hilton P, Stanton SL: Algorithmic method for assessing urinary incontinence in elderly women. Br Med J 282:940–942, 1981
19. Hedlund H, Anderssen KE: Effects of prazosen in patients with benign prostatic obstruction. J Urol 130:275–278, 1983
20. Taub H: Memory span, practice and ageing. J Gerontol 28:335–338, 1973
21. Mohr JA, Roger J Jr, Brown TN et al: Stress urinary incontinence: A simple and practical approach to diagnosis and treatment. J Am Geriatr Soc 31:476–478, 1983
22. Beisland HO, Fassberg E, Moer A et al: Urethral sphincteric insufficiency in post menopausal females: Treatment with phenylpropanolamine and estriol separately and in combination: A urodynamic and clinical evaluation. Urol Int 39:211–216, 1984
23. Crooks J, O'Malley K et al: Pharmacokinetics in the elderly. Clin Pharmacokinet 1:280–296, 1976
24. Greenblatt DJ, Sellers EM: Drug disposition in old age. N Engl J Med 306:1081–1088, 1982
25. Williamson J, Chopin JM: Adverse reactions to prescribed drugs in the elderly: A multicenter investigation. Age Ageing 9:73–80, 1980

26. Feldman RD et al: Alterations in leukocyte B-adrenergic sensitivity in the elderly. N Engl J Med 310:815–819, 1984

27. Critchley EMR: Drug induced neurological disease. Br Med J 1:862–865, 1979

28. Lang A: Tardive dyskinesia. Mid Med Can 39:549–554, 1984

29. Lancet editorial (2). Cotsides: Protecting whom against what? Lancet 2:557–558, 1984

30. Powell C, Edmund L, Fingerote E: Freedom from restraint: Consequences of reducing physical restraints in the treatment of elderly persons. Ann Royal College of Physicians and Surgeons of Canada 16:343, 1983

31. Avorn J, Langer E: Induced disability in nursing home patients: A controlled trial. J Am Geriatr Soc 30:379, 1982

32. Gellick MR, Serrell NA, Gellick CS: Adverse consequences of hospitalization in the elderly. Soc Sci Med 16:1033, 1982

33. Anderson KE, Jensen O, Kvorning SA: Prevention of pressure sores by identifying patients at risk. Br Med J 1:1370, 1982

34. Grieco A, Freedman ML: Cooperative Care: A Model for the Acute Hospital Care of the Elderly. New York, The International Association of Gerontology, 1985

35. Kenney RA: Physiology of aging. Clinics in Geriatric Medicine 1(1):37–59, 1985

36. Gribbin B, Pickering TG, Steight P et al: Effect of age and high blood pressure on baroreflex sensitivity in man. Circ Res 29:424–431, 1971

37. Konshalo DR: Age changes in touch, vibration, temperature, kinesthesis, pain sensitivity. In Bioren JE, Schaie KA (eds): Handbook of the Biology of Aging. New York, Van Nostrand-Reinhold, 1977

38. Reuler JB: Hypothermia: Pathophysiology, clinical settings and management. Ann Intern Med 89:519–527, 1978

39. Heslop HE, Beard ME, Sainsbury R: Heat related illness in the elderly. Geriatric Medicine Today 4 (7):21–24, 1985

40. Greer M: How serious is dizziness. Geriatrics 36(1):34–42, 1981

41. Lipsitz L: Diagnosis and management of syncope. Geriatric Consultant July/August:26–29, 1985

42. Noth RH, Mazzaferri MD: Age and the endocrine system. Clinics in Geriatric Medicine 1(1):223–250, 1985

43. Flood C, Gherondache C, Pincus G et al: The metabolism and secretion of aldosterone in elderly subjects. J Clin Invest 46:960–966, 1967

44. Hellerman JJ, Vestal RE, Rows JW et al: The response of arginine-vasopressin to intravenous ethanol and hypertonic saline in man: The impact of aging. J Gerontol 33:39–47, 1978

# 9
# Arthritis and Rheumatic Disease

STEVEN ABRAMSON
OWEN P. KIERAN

Rheumatic diseases receive comparatively little attention during the physician's formal training in internal medicine. The conditions emphasized are the more glamorous entities, uncommon diseases with complicated names, and curious immunologic aberrations. In contrast, disorders of the musculoskeletal system represent a significant proportion of the physician's experience in clinical practice. The lack of adequate preparation, combined with the sometimes refractory nature of the diseases themselves, has led to a common resignation on the part of both physician and patient. Unorthodox alternatives to medical treatment flourish to an extent unparalleled in clinical medicine. With this in mind it is the goal of this chapter to describe fundamental principles of the diagnosis and treatment of the rheumatic diseases for physicians in the primary care setting. It is hoped that by sharpening our acumen in this field we not only will provide better medical care but also will protect our patients from the abuses of unproven remedies.

## THE APPROACH TO THE PATIENT WITH ARTHRITIS

### INITIAL EVALUATION

Patients with arthritis first seek medical attention because of pain or stiffness in the region of a joint. When accompanied by joint swelling or other signs of inflammation the diagnosis of arthritis is apparent. When the joint symptoms are unaccompanied by objective physical findings, the cause of the patient's "arthralgias" becomes less clear. The physician must consider a variety of articular and nonarticular conditions that range from true musculo-skeletal disorders to unusual infections and occult neoplasms. In approaching such a patient, the following would suggest the likelihood of a primary rheumatic disorder:

1. Worsening of symptoms in the morning. This complaint is characteristic of inflammatory arthritis (particularly rheumatoid arthritis and polymyalgia rheumatica). The fatigue and achiness due to other medical conditions typically worsen during the day or are time-independent.

2. Localization of pain to the joint. While this would seem sufficiently evident to not require mention, it is among the most crucial determinations that the physician must make in early disease, and, surprisingly, it is a common source of physician error. To avoid the potential pitfalls of diagnosis, the clinician must carefully determine by history and physical examination whether the patient's symptoms are primarily articular or soft tissue in origin. Careful palpation of specific joints (including the small joints of the hands and feet, the sacroiliac

joints, and the shoulders) will frequently provide convincing evidence of a primary joint disorder in a patient whose major complaint is generalized achiness. Conversely, symptoms mistakenly attributed to arthritis might represent the bone pain of metastatic disease or the related periarticular pain of periostitis secondary to malignancy.

3. Characteristic joint involvement. Having established that the patient's pain is localized to the joints, the physician can gain much diagnostic insight simply by an analysis of the pattern of joint involvement. It is a common practice of rheumatologists to draw "stick figures" on which they indicate specific points where a patient has joint tenderness, so important is pattern recognition in the diagnostic process. For example, involvement of the first metatarsophalangeal (MTP) joint ("podagra") has been recognized for centuries as gout. Similarly, asymmetric sausage-like swelling of individual toes or involvement of the heel (so-called lover's heel) is strongly indicative of Reiter's disease. Symmetric involvement of the metacarpophalangeal (MCP) and proximal interphalangeal (PIP) joints with sparing of the distal interphalangeal (DIP) joints suggests rheumatoid arthritis while the precisely opposite pattern is highly characteristic of psoriatic arthritis.

4. The presence of a characteristic rash. The primary-care physician can save his patient a specialist's consultation and himself minor embarrassment through an understanding of rashes typically associated with arthritis. The most common of these is psoriasis, which may be complicated by arthritis in 5% of the cases. The psoriatic lesion might be inconspicuous and previously unsuspected, found only after a careful examination of the scalp. A psoriasiform rash on the soles of the feet (keratoderma blennorrhagicum) or the penis (circinate balanitis) might be the main clue indicating a diagnosis of Reiter's disease. Finally, a malar rash, photosensitivity, or a discoid lesion would help establish a diagnosis of systemic lupus erythematosus in a young woman with symmetric arthritis.

## INFLAMMATORY VERSUS NONINFLAMMATORY ARTHRITIS

Once the physician is satisfied that the patient's symptoms are due to arthritis, the task of establishing a specific diagnosis begins. Unfortunately, a precise diagnosis, if not apparent after the initial clinical and laboratory evaluation, may remain elusive for several months. During this time new diagnostic symptoms may evolve; laboratory tests, negative at onset, may become positive; or the joint symptoms may in fact disappear. Therefore, the first task of the physician confronting a new difficult-to-diagnose arthritis is to broadly categorize the condition as either inflammatory or noninflammatory. The latter group of diseases, most commonly degenerative joint conditions, represents no immediate threat to the patient. The processes are usually gradual in onset and localized in nature. In contrast, inflammatory conditions involving the joint may represent an immediate danger to the patient's general health (*e.g.,* sepsis due to an infected joint) or indicate the presence of a systemic abnormality that requires specific therapy. Such a systemic condition may range from an elevated uric acid that requires correction, as in gout, to a more complex dysregulation of the immune system, as in rheumatoid arthritis, which will require the full skills and repeated attention of the physician over a protracted period.

## ROUTINE LABORATORY TESTING

How does the physician differentiate these two broad categories of arthritis? The traditional distinction is based on the findings of synovial fluid analysis: inflammatory synovial fluids, by definition, contain more than 3000 white blood cells per cubic millimeter. Patients with inflammatory arthritis may have elevation of the sedimentation rate or a moderate anemia, indications of the systemic nature of their musculoskeletal symptoms. Therefore, individuals with arthritis and such laboratory abnormalities should have synovial fluid aspiration for diagnostic purposes. The results of this analysis will help the physician determine whether the elevation of erythrocyte sedimentation rate (ESR) and anemia are related to the synovial effusion. Indications for arthrocentesis in other patients with recent onset of joint swelling depends on the physician's degree of certainty with regard to the precise diagnosis. As in all fields, certainty does not always confer accuracy. Therefore, because of the importance of differentiating inflammatory and noninflammatory joint disease, the primary physician will reduce the likelihood of error if the initial evaluation of patients includes synovial fluid analysis. In addition to total white count, other crucial information is also obtained from synovial fluid analysis, such as Gram's stain and culture, examination under polarized light microscopy for crystals of monosodium urate (gout) or calcium pyrophosphate (pseudogout), and glucose (low in rheumatoid arthritis and bacterial infection).

## IMMUNOSEROLOGIC TESTING

The differentiation of the inflammatory arthritides, initially indicated by elevated ESR and synovial fluid analysis, can be facilitated by the appropriate utilization of serologic tests. The availability of an increasing number of tests has led to an improved delineation of diseases with musculoskeletal manifestations and permitted earlier diagnosis in many instances. However, these tests should be used primarily to corroborate clinical impressions based on history, physical examination, and standard laboratory tests as discussed above. The primary care physician should be familiar with the following tests:

### Rheumatoid Factor

The rheumatoid factor as measured by the standard latex fixation test is an IgM immunoglobulin that recognizes a portion of IgG immunoglobulin as its antigen. The interaction of rheumatoid factor with IgG to form immune complexes is believed to contribute to the pathogenesis of the inflammatory process. The rheumatoid factor is detectable in up to 80% of patients with rheumatoid arthritis. Note, therefore, that as many as 25% of patients with *bona fide* rheumatoid arthritis are "seronegative." However, the clinician must be cautious when making this diagnosis and must always remain vigilant for signs indicative of alternative disease possibilities. Conversely, positive tests for rheumatoid factor are not specific for rheumatoid arthritis and may be found in a variety of clinical syndromes, including other rheumatic diseases, sarcoidosis, infection, and chronic liver disease. In addition, up to 20% of normal individuals over the age of 70 may have a positive rheumatoid factor test.

### Antinuclear Antibodies

Antibodies to a variety of nuclear antigens are detectable in many rheumatic diseases. While positive antinuclear antibodies (ANAs) are a sensitive test for the diagnosis of systemic lupus erythematosus (present in 95% of these patients), ANAs may also be seen in rheumatoid arthritis, Sjögren's syndrome, scleroderma, polymyositis, and chronic liver disease. Again, a false positive rate of 15% to 20% may be seen in elderly individuals. Patterns of ANAs are frequently useful in the interpretation of a positive test. The speckled ANA indicates the presence of an antibody directed to a non-DNA nuclear antigen. Most false positive tests are of a speckled pattern. A diffuse or homogeneous-pattern ANA indicates antibodies to a combination of DNA and histone protein. Commonly found in systemic lupus erythematosus, it may also be present in other rheumatic diseases and in drug-induced lupus. A peripheral-pattern ANA is highly suggestive that the patient's serum contains antibodies to DNA. This can be confirmed by specific antibody testing and is strong evidence in support of the diagnosis of systemic lupus erythematosus.

### Histocompatibility Antigens in Rheumatic Disease

In rheumatology, as in all of medicine, the last two decades of the 20th century will witness an increasing utilization of immunogenetic testing to evaluate an individual's risk for disease susceptibility. It is recognized, for example, that one's risk of developing rheumatoid arthritis is enhanced in the presence of the histocompatibility type HLA-DR4, while the presence of HLA-DR2 and HLA-DR-3, as well as HLA-Cw7, confers increased risk for the development of systemic lupus erythematosus. The most impressive association between HLA type and disease is the association between the spondyloarthropathies and HLA-B27. Over 90% of patients with ankylosing spondylitis and 60% to 70% of patients with Reiter's disease have this cell-surface histocompatibility antigen, compared to 8% to 10% of the control caucasian population.

How should the physician utilize these powerful new tools? First, remember that with the exception of HLA-B27, the associations are statistically relevant to large populations but not particularly useful in the diagnosis of disease in the individual patient. For example, the haplotype HLA-DR4 is present in 50% to 60% of patients with rheumatoid arthritis, but may also be found in 25% of the control population. Therefore, the presence of this haplotype is neither necessary nor sufficient for the development of rheumatoid arthritis. Even in the case of the spondyloarthropathies it is not usually necessary to obtain HLA typing. Rarely, when the diagnosis is in doubt, one may order such a test. A diagnosis of ankylosing spondylitis would be unlikely in the absence of HLA-B27; the diagnosis of Reiter's disease in a young woman with an asymmetric seronegative arthritis might become more suspect in the presence of this risk factor. However, the clinician must remain cautious. Remember that the presence of sacroiliitis on x-ray study is a much more useful indication of a spondyloarthropathy; a "confirmatory" histocompatibility antigen confers no greater certainty on the diagnosis. Moreover, the presence of a specific haplotype does not denote disease and indeed may mislead. At the very least, indiscriminate testing may create anxiety in individuals regarding the future development of disease that we cannot at present prevent.

### Antibody Tests in Lyme Disease

Serologic testing for antibodies directed to the spirochete implicated as the etiologic agent of Lyme disease is now available through the department of public health. Since antibiotic therapy has been shown to ameliorate arthritis and prevent the extra-articular complications of Lyme disease, it is essential to recognize this group of patients. Physicians in areas where Lyme disease is reported should consider ordering this test in patients who present with "seronegative" (*i.e.,* rheumatoid factor negative) arthritis, which is typically asymmetric and oligoarticular. A history of tick bite, typical rash, and cardiac or neurologic complications, though not required for diagnosis, should alert the clinician to this possibility.

## PRINCIPLES OF THERAPY IN ARTHRITIS

The proper outpatient management of patients with arthritis consists of anti-inflammatory and analgesic medications, proper exercise and physical therapy, and, in selected patients, reconstructive surgery. Within this framework, attention by the physician to the patient's psychological needs, including the family support structure, becomes essential.

### MEDICAL THERAPY
#### Nonsteroidal Anti-inflammatory Drugs

The goal of medical therapy in arthritis is to reduce pain and inflammation. Virtually all patients therefore are treated initially with aspirin or related nonsteroidal anti-inflammatory drugs (NSAIDs). These compounds, through their inhibition of prostaglandin synthesis, have the capacity to reduce manifestations of the inflammatory response. The marketplace has seen a burgeoning number of these drugs become available during the past decade, which has created confusion and potential pitfalls for the practicing physician. In prescribing NSAIDs the physician should keep the principles discussed below in mind.

**Analgesia Versus Anti-inflammation.** The capacity to reduce pain, common to NSAIDs, is achieved at a dose lower than that required to impart anti-inflammation. This phenomenon has been referred to as the "pain–inflammation gap" and most likely indicates that at high dose these drugs have additional mechanisms of action. It has been demonstrated, for example, that at the high, anti-inflammatory doses, NSAIDs inhibit the activation of white blood cells, such as neutrophils. Physicians recognize this phenomenon, albeit perhaps unwittingly, and will recommend "two aspirin" for a headache as opposed to "12 to 16 aspirin" for arthritis. Similarly, ibuprofen is prescibed over the counter at low doses (Advil, Nuprin) for pain and at significantly higher doses to treat arthritis. The potential consequence of this phenomenon is that physicians and patients may "underdose", accepting pain relief at low dosage of drug while not taking sufficient medication to achieve true control of the inflammatory process. This has become less of a problem with the availability of NSAIDs that are taken only once or twice daily and are thus more likely to achieve consistent anti-inflammatory blood levels. When using drugs with tid or qid dosing schedules, the patient must be instructed to adhere strictly to the full recommended dose. In the case of salicylates, the availability of blood level measurements frequently becomes a useful tool in assessing patient compliance.

The physician must also recognize NSAIDs that are masquerading as analgesics. That is, the marketing of certain NSAIDs (Anaprox, Dolobid, Advil, and Nuprin, for example) emphasizes their use in pain. The unwary physician must recognize such drugs as prostaglandin inhibitors and thus avoid their indiscriminate use in circumstances where aspirin-like drugs would be contraindicated. In fact, NSAIDs should not be analgesics of first choice in the absence of an inflammatory process. This is particularly true in the elderly in whom the risk of toxicity is greater and in whom acetaminophen will often suffice.

**The Choice of an NSAID.** As an increasing number of NSAIDs are approved by the FDA the physician is confronted with having to choose among many drugs that are in fact quite similar. At present (if one excludes phenylbutazone, which should rarely be prescribed), there is no NSAID that has proven either more efficacious or more toxic than another. In general, the newer drugs have fewer side-effects than uncoated aspirin. It is useful to categorize the drugs according to chemical class. Many of the more recently introduced drugs are members of an existing class of compounds. It would seem reasonable, therefore, that should toxicity develop or should the drug not be effective, then the physician might choose an alternative medication from a different class. Again, several principles should be kept in mind. First, it is not uncommon that an individual patient may require a trial of two or more drugs before optimal therapy is achieved. Therapeutic trials should be at least two to three weeks in duration and the drug should be prescribed at full anti-inflammatory doses. Second, clinical experience suggests that selected toxicities vary among the classes of drugs. For example, tinnitus, although a potential side-effect of each drug, is more commonly seen with the salicylates. Central nervous system side-effects such as headache and inability to concentrate tend to appear more often with indomethacin. Finally, diarrhea and flatulence may limit the usefulness of the fenamates. Third, when a side-effect develops, the physician needs to differentiate those toxicities that are related to the inhibition of prostaglandin synthesis from those that are idiosyncratic, as discussed below.

### NSAID Toxicity

*Peptic Ulcer Disease.* The most common side-effects following NSAID use are a direct consequence of their capacity to inhibit prostaglandin synthesis. The gastric mucosa produces prostaglandins of the E series, which reduce gastric acid secretion and promote the formation of a cytoprotective mucus coat. Approximately 1% of patients on chronic NSAID therapy will develop clinically significant peptic ulcer disease. The management of patients with a history of peptic ulcer disease is controversial. The following guidelines are somewhat arbitrary but may prove useful. A recent (under 3–6 months) history of peptic ulcer should represent an absolute contraindication to NSAID use. Such patients should be treated with analgesics alone, combined with intra-articular corticosteroid injections when feasible. In patients whose ulcer history is longer than 6 months and less than several years the drugs remain relatively contraindicated. However, when necessary, NSAIDs may be prescribed cautiously, usually in combination with an anti-ulcer regimen. While such a regimen may include either of the two currently available H2-antagonists, the increasingly popular approach has been to add sucralfate. It should be noted that there has been no convincing study to show that any of these regimens is better than placebo in protecting the patient from the development of NSAID-induced gastric ulceration.

*Salt and Water Retention.* Prostaglandins produced by the kidney promote salt and water excretion. This effect is particularly important in patients whose renal blood flow is compromised by other medical conditions such as congestive heart failure or cirrhosis. Furthermore, patients on diuretic therapy will have reduced renal blood flow and hence be more dependent on prostaglandins to excrete salt and water. Therefore, in selected patients the institution of NSAID therapy may result in fluid retention. This may manifest as weight gain, ankle edema, or frank congestive heart failure. More insidiously there may be an increase in serum creatinine and urea nitrogen on a vasomotor basis. Finally, blood pressure may rise as the only manifestation of this potential side-effect. In response to this NSAID effect, the physician may cautiously try alternative drugs. A controversial literature suggests that sulindac may be the preferred drug in this setting. Alternatively, one may try a nonacetylated salicylate (*e.g.,* Disalcid, Trilisate) that has little or no effect on prostaglandin synthesis.

*Prolonged Bleeding Time.* The inhibition of platelet thromboxane production by NSAIDs may prolong the bleeding time. In the case of aspirin, which irreversibly alters platelet function, this effect may take 6 to 10 days to return to normal. In contrast, the effect of the other NSAIDs on platelet function is reversible; bleeding time will return to normal when the drug is cleared from the blood. This difference may have practical implications when the physician must discontinue therapy prior to surgery. The physician should also know that there is a class of NSAIDs that have no effect on platelet function or bleeding time, the nonacetylated salicylates. These drugs are marketed under the brand names Disalcid, Trilisate, and Arthropan. In selected cases this information can be quite useful, for example when having to use an NSAID in a patient with a bleeding disorder (*e.g.,* arthritis and inflammatory bowel disease). Finally, because of effects on the platelet, NSAID therapy is relatively contraindicated in patients who are anticoagulated. Again, in this setting a case can be made for using the nonacetylated salicylates. However, one must remain cautious since these drugs also decrease coumadin binding to plasma proteins and may thus indirectly affect the prothrombin time.

**The Use of NSAIDs in "Noninflammatory Arthritis."** The most common condition for which NSAIDs are currently prescribed is osteoarthritis, in general a noninflammatory condition. Many of these patients benefit primarily from the analgesic effects of these drugs, in which case alternative therapy would be preferred. What then is the proper role of NSAIDs in degenerative joint disease? Much of such therapy is empirical. There are some patients with osteoarthritis who clearly exhibit an inflammatory component to their condition. For some, the inflammation is episodic associated with superimposed calcium crystal deposition induced arthritis. Episodic NSAID use for several weeks at a time is frequently beneficial in these patients. Intercurrently the patient should be maintained on non-NSAID analgesic therapy. For patients whose disease is less obviously episodic it is recommended that initial control of the symptoms be followed by an attempt to wean the patient from chronic NSAID use. The physician may then uncover an episodic component to the patient's condition that can be appropriately treated as necessary. In general, using such an empirical approach the physician can subdivide his osteoarthritic patients into categories along a spectrum from those requiring only analgesia to those who in fact only do well on chronic NSAID therapy. Given the age distribution of patients with this condition, the physician will do well to minimize unnecessary anti-inflammatory therapy when analgesia will do.

### Corticosteroids

An event that was quickly acclaimed as a landmark discovery in 20th-century medicine was the development of adrenocorticosteroids as therapeutic agents by workers at the Mayo Clinic in the 1940s. So dramatic were the effects in rheumatoid arthritis that following the presentation of the discovery at the national scientific meetings the audiences not only applauded enthusiastically but also stood and cheered. Indeed, the rheumatologist Philip Hench shared the Nobel Prize in 1950 for having introduced this potent anti-inflammatory agent for the treatment of arthritis.

As all physicians recognize, the most dramatic short-term results in the therapy of inflammatory arthritis are provided by corticosteroids. For a minority of patients this class of agents remains the sole therapeutic modality that permits them to function in their activities of daily living. The physician who must use corticosteroids in the treatment of arthritis should attempt to adhere to the following guidelines:

**Dosage.** In most patients 5 mg to 10 mg of prednisone (or equivalent) daily should be sufficient to control symptoms. It is preferred to begin at the lower dose and titrate upward as needed. The goal of therapy should not be to abolish all symptoms; indeed, a patient who is symptom-free due to corticosteroid therapy should have the steroid tapered. In general, prednisone can be tapered by 25% every two to three weeks. Alternate-day steroids in arthritis are not effective.

**Toxicity.** In general the most serious toxicities of prednisone are avoided at doses under 10 mg daily. The patients tend not to become infected, hypertensive, diabetic, or cushingoid in appearance. These, however, are general statements with individual exceptions. For example, although opportunistic infections are rare at these doses, common infections, such as diverticular abscesses, may be masked.

The most serious complications of low-dose corticosteroids are the development of osteoporosis and cataracts. To help prevent the former it is recommended that all patients on corticosteroids receive calcium supplementation of 1000 mg to 1500 mg per day. In selected individuals, serial (*e.g.,* yearly) determinations of bone density by computed tomography scan, where available, are useful in the assessment of progressive osteoporosis.

**Duration of Therapy.** The physician should always attempt to wean patients from steroid therapy. It is believed that these drugs are not superior to NSAIDs with regard to preventing progression of disease. Furthermore, there is circumstantial evidence that steroid-induced osteopenia and attenuation of the integrity of supporting soft tissue structures (including tendons) may worsen the long-term outlook.

The physician must also recognize that the majority of patients begun on steroid therapy rarely are able to discontinue them. It is for that reason that it is appropriate to avoid the institution of these drugs unless the patient's ability to perform daily activities is seriously threatened.

Finally, most rheumatologists recommend that patients who require more than 7.5 mg of prednisone daily are candidates for therapy with disease-modifying drugs such as gold and penicillamine.

## Disease-Modifying Drugs

The care of patients in the primary-care setting requires that the responsible physician recognize which patients should be evaluated for therapy with a disease-modifying drug such as gold or penicillamine. In general, approximately 50% of these patients require such therapy, and the earlier one can institute these drugs, the more likely the patient is to respond. Since these medications (including the recently introduced oral gold) have potentially serious toxicities, it continues to be recommended that they be introduced only when it is apparent that the patient's disease is aggressive. The patient should be referred for evaluation for such therapy under the following circumstances:

1. Failure to respond to an adequate trial (anti-inflammatory doses for 3–4 weeks) of at least three different NSAIDs
2. Dependency on corticosteroid therapy
3. The presence of bone erosions on x-ray film
4. Significant anemia of chronic disease
5. The development of extra-articular manifestations such as nodules, pulmonary involvement, vasculitis, or Felty's syndome

## PHYSICAL THERAPY AND CONDITIONING

### Traditional Physical Therapy

The major goals in the treatment of a patient with arthritis are to preserve strength and range of motion, preserve and if possible increase functional capacity, and decrease pain. These goals must be modified somewhat to accommodate the patient's limited access to equipment and skilled personnel at home.

For convenience of description, a patient's course can be divided somewhat arbitrarily into acute, subacute, and chronic phases. During the acute phase, the relief of symptoms, especially pain, and the preservation of range of motion are the most essential elements in a home therapy program. Cold packs to the affected joint applied for 20 minutes at a time as tolerated are frequently quite effective in at least relieving the intense discomfort temporarily. These may consist of either commercially available cold packs that are chilled in a refrigerator or simply an ice water/ice cube mixture in a plastic bag covered with toweling. The patient at home needs to preserve the range of motion of both the unaffected and the affected joints. This is most easily done by taking the joint through the full range of motion at least once per day. If this is not possible due to significant pain through a part of the range, attempts should be made to perform the motions in a somewhat more restricted range. Somewhat arbitrary figures have been given as far as the numbers of repetitions required, but once per day should be adequate for short periods of time.

The patient, of course, will be his own judge with respect to the degree of discomfort that he can tolerate, and general guidelines are that the pain during the activity should not be severe and that discomfort from the activity should not last more than 24 hours. The joints, aside from the above-mentioned activities, should be rested as much as possible, and various types of splints, depending on the joint, will be useful. The most easily fabricated and tolerated splint is one made from heat-moldable plastic. This can be easily custom made for any patient.

Since the patient may be inactive for a length of time that would result in significant atrophy, it is recommended that he be placed on a program of isometric exercise that will disturb the joint minimally. The most efficient type in this situation is that described by Liberson with BRIME (brief rapid isometric maximal exercises). In this technique, the patient's muscle groups are isometrically contracted for a period of 5 seconds at maximal capacity and then the entire sequence is repeated five times. The end result is an increase in static strength, which is not useful in terms of endurance or bulk but has value in activities requiring short bursts of energy.

As the patient enters the subacute phase in which joints are not overtly inflamed, but in which if a joint is overused a flare-up may result, the patient should begin active exercise of the joint involved, again with limitation of the range as restricted by pain. Additionally, the patient as a whole can become more active and might require an assistive device for mobility. This can range from the use of a cane, which is quite effective in splinting the involved hip, to the use of an electric wheelchair if there has been substantial damage to the weight-bearing structures and both lower extremities. The judicious use of heat, for example, an electric heating pad, can decrease residual symptoms in the affected joints. The patient's exercise program needs to be upgraded and he should begin a mild resistive exercise program, which will be detailed later.

As the patient enters the chronic phase of his disease state, the goals become more comprehensive and should include the resumption of former mobility as well as a return to premorbid strength. The active range of motion should continue and contractures should begin to be dealt with. Before the contracted joint is approached for increasing its range, it should be prepared with the application of heat. A variety of agents can be applied, ranging from a hot water bottle to a hydrocollator pack to a heating pad. Certainly the easiest and recommended choice is a moist electric heating pad on a low setting for approximately 15 minutes at a time. This has a mild anesthetic effect and makes superficial structures such as the Achilles tendon more elastic. The techniques for stretching each joint vary but they all require the application of a prolonged mild to moderate stretch. If possible, they should be followed by a rapid cooling of the structure that is stretched while in the maximal achievable position in an attempt to set the tissue at a longer resting length.

In contrast to the techniques for stretching, which really only vary by joint, the methods for alleviation of pain are manifold. They may include the above mentioned as well as the more mundane, such as the taking of a warm bath or shower to get one going in the morning. More complex but quite effective is the use of a paraffin bath at home with a paraffin–mineral oil solution in 7-to-1 ratio, which is heated to its melting point of 130°F. This particular modality is especially useful in rheumatoid involvement of the hands in which the patient can dip or even immerse the hands in wax and then allow the wax to harden in the air. Wax is allowed to remain while warm (approximately 20 minutes) and then the patient removes the paraffin and is able to perform his exercises better.

The strengthening program should also be increased and more dynamic exercises added to increase the patient's endurance. The most easily performed is a modified program of progressive resistive exercise in which the maximum weight that a particular muscle group can lift through the full range of motion is increased in a graduated fashion as determined by weekly manual muscle tests. This can be done more informally and the patient can be asked to increase his weight use by small increments per week. The weights most conveniently used for the larger muscle groups are fixed with Velcro closures, while the smaller muscles of the hands can be strengthened with the use of a Hand Gym or therapeutic putty. Regardless of the type of exercise involved, the patient is advised to avoid particular movements that cause either severe pain immediately or lesser pain that lasts to the next day. Also, rather than emphasize a particular number of repetitions or sets of exercise, it is much more realistic to advise a patient at home to spend 15 to 20 minutes a day on the exercise program. More recently, aerobic exercise has become an accepted method of treatment in even moderately involved arthritics. Beneficial effects have been noted in general terms of endurance of aerobic capacity and even a decrease in pain without worsening joint complaints. A home aerobic program should be preceded by a supervised stress test in which the patient's training priorities are determined and then a conditioning program of three 20-minute sessions per week by a device such as bicycle ergometer prescribed. The usual target heart rate for a patient is approximately 70% of his age-adjusted heart rate. Of course, if any cardiac symptoms arise, the patient's exercise program should be discontinued and medical attention sought.

## Therapeutic Aids

There are two basic principles governing the provision of equipment for home use. (1) It should be simple and easy to use, and (2) it should be effective for the purpose for which it was prescribed. In terms of splints that the patient can use on an ongoing basis, the ulnar deviation protection splint fulfills both of these. It is lightweight and can be put on by almost any patient even when there are severe hand deformities. Also, in a study in which splinted patients were compared to those without splints in terms of their progression of ulnar deviation at 1 to 5 years, there was significantly less deformity at 1 year in the splinted group. However, by the fifth year there was no significant difference between the two groups. Therefore, it would certainly benefit the patient to wear such splints as often as possible at least for the first few years after the diagnosis of rheumatoid arthritis is made. This applies to other types of splints as well, but one must be somewhat cautious that if too many devices are prescribed none will be used.

Home equipment can be used for other purposes, including the reduction of pain. These include the soft cervical collar, which is used simply to immobilize the neck in patients with both radicular symptoms as well as primary neck pain. Cervical traction units that consist of a weight, pulley system, and a harness to fit the patient's head are also frequently used to relieve neck pain. The applied weight should start at approximately 7 pounds and increase to 15 pounds in a step-wise fashion. They can be used on the order of 30 minutes per day and are most effective when preceded by application of local heat to the neck. Of course, before prescription of such a unit one should review neck x-ray films and exclude any patient with a potentially unstable neck. In the office, the physician should simulate a home traction unit by gently distracting the neck in a slightly flexed position and seeing the effects. Analogous units can be provided for the lower back, including the lumbosacral corset and pelvic traction. The latter, however, is quite cumbersome for home use unless set up by a second person and is probably most useful in simply keeping the patient at a more restricted level of bedrest than would otherwise be obtained.

A different class of home equipment is that used for increasing a patient's mobility. A basic item is a manual wheelchair, which is usually propelled by use of the patient's arms and is quite useful when either pain or weakness prevents normal ambulation. It can be quite effective in a general exercise program since a patient would expend the same amount of energy whether propelling a wheelchair with his arms or walking with a normal gait pattern. Even patients with the use of only one arm can use a modified manual wheelchair. There also are a variety of electric wheelchairs, which range from the more traditional to those that resemble miniature golf carts. These electrically powered chairs are most effective for people with severe upper extremity problems and also those who need to go out of doors for long distances. The electric wheelchair frees the patient from the assistance of an attendant and improves his level of independence immeasurably. There are, of course, drawbacks to such equipment and these include the necessity for ramps and other wheelchair-accessible facilities. Ways to circumvent such a problem in the patient's home with stairs is the use of a Stair Glide, which resembles a small electrically driven platform that allows a patient to go up the stairs, as well as the recent introduction of a stair-climbing wheelchair. For those with less severe involvement, walkers, canes, and crutches can be the means for safe ambulation. Items such as shower commode chairs for use in the bathroom as well as grab bars for bathroom and toilet and raised toilet seats are also essentials for appropriate patients. Hospital beds, be they manual or electric, as well as lounge chairs with spring assists to help the patient upon arising can be extremely useful in allowing patients to have optimal function in a home environment.

In order to improve the patient's level of activities of daily living, there are a variety of dressing aids including dressing stick, a zipper pole, button hooks, sock cone, stocking devices, long-handled shoehorns as well as long-handled reachers, zippered shoes, and Velcro closures for fasteners. Again, the emphasis should not be simply on provision of a great deal of equipment that a patient will not use but rather selective utilization of devices that will be helpful to the patient.

The prescription and details of the home exercise program and equipment require a great deal of skill. Depending on the physician's level of expertise and interest he may be able to prescribe and supervise this without direct on-site supervision. More likely, however, he will use the services of a physical therapist and/or occupational therapist either on an out-patient basis or more appropriately at home to assess the home environment and to modify the program to that which is practical for that situation. The goals of the program as well as the details of the particular exercises and equipment should be made very clear to the patient and should be reviewed several times before the patient is judged to be adequately trained to perform the exercises himself. Periodic reassessments of the patient's status should be made and appropriate modifications made thereof. With proper guidance and instruction the patient's level of function as well as comfort can be increased considerably in his home environment through the use of proper exercise and proper equipment.

### Aerobic Conditioning

There is increasing evidence that aerobic exercise training is of benefit in rehabilitating patients with a variety of medical conditions, including cardiovascular disease, diabetes, obesity, and arthritis. In rheumatoid arthritis, prescribed exercise has traditionally been limited to range-of-motion and isometric exercise. This has resulted in a very low level of physical performance as measured by aerobic capacity. Studies recently published have demonstrated that physician-supervised aerobic exercise training can improve function as well as the self-image of arthritis patients without damaging articular structures.

For many patients, the optimal modality for aerobic training has been exercise in swimming pools. This form of therapy provides an ideal means of providing nonimpact aerobic exercise for patients with arthritis, particularly those with spine and lower extremity involvement. Many chapters of the Arthritis Foundation have developed hydrotherapy programs for patients. For example, the national organization has sponsored the development of an arthritis aquatic program with over 1000 trained instructors nationwide.

## SPECIFIC GUIDELINES FOR MONITORING THE HOMEBOUND PATIENT WITH ARTHRITIS

The management of the patient with arthritis in the home requires a combination of strong family support, the appropriate availability of home health aids as described above, and, where available, the services of a visiting physical therapist to maintain an active exercise program. Home care nurses can be employed to administer parenteral gold when indicated. Commercial laboratories in the community can usually be found to perform venipuncture in the home when blood monitoring is necessary.

The needs of the patient with arthritis with regard to the frequency of physician evaluation, laboratory testing, and hospitalization depend to a large extent on the specific diagnosis. What follows, therefore, are suggested guidelines for the management of rheumatic diseases in the homebound patient based on the condition being treated.

## OSTEOARTHRITIS

Initial evaluation should include complete blood count, erythrocyte sedimentation rate, chemistry profile, and, when available, synovial fluid analysis, to exclude systemic disease. Roentgenograms of involved joints are not usually necessary in a homebound patient unless one is uncertain about the diagnosis (particularly should a septic joint be under consideration).

Physician evaluation in uncomplicated osteoarthritis is required one to two times per year. If the patient is maintained on NSAID therapy, then laboratory monitoring (complete blood count, stool for occult blood, chemistries) should be performed two to three times per year. It is suggested, particularly in the elderly, that these tests be performed within three weeks of initiating therapy in case of idiosyncratic toxicity.

## LOW BACK PAIN

Although most commonly due to osteoarthritis, the syndrome of low back pain deserves special consideration. The pain may originate in the joints, ligaments, or muscles of the spinal column. The laboratory tests, in addition to those listed above for uncomplicated osteoarthritis, would include an alkaline phosphatase, acid phosphatase, and serum protein electrophoresis to exclude bone metastases (particularly prostate cancer) and multiple myeloma. In refractory cases, the testing may require an electromyogram, bone scan, or computed tomography scan with or without myelography.

Conventional therapy consists of strict bedrest for perhaps one or more weeks combined with an NSAID, nonnarcotic analgesics, and possibly a muscle relaxant. Patients should be encouraged to take all meals in bed and to use a bedpan or bedside commode when feasible. Stretching exercises should be introduced gradually, preferably under the guidance of a visiting physical therapist. The therapist can also instruct the patient in the use of home assistive devices such as transcutaneous nerve stimulation as an analgesic modality.

Physician evaluation of the patient with severe low back pain should range from weekly to monthly. Hospitalization may be necessary for the refractory case for 5 to 10 days to treat severe pain or functional incapacity. This is particularly true if physical examination reveals motor neuron involvement. Hospital evaluation with myelogram (preferably with concomitant computed tomography scan) as well as consideration of surgical procedures may be necessary in these cases.

## RHEUMATOID ARTHRITIS AND SERONEGATIVE VARIANTS

Laboratory testing in these patients should include those listed above for osteoarthritis plus those intended to give evidence of the degree of disease activity systemically. Therefore, one additionally obtains C-reactive protein, rheumatoid factor, ANA, urinalysis, and x-ray films of chest and involved joints. The joint x-ray films need not be comprehensive, but rather are selected based on disproportionate signs or symptoms. Selected joints may be x-rayed every 6 to 18 months to assess for the extent of progressive joint erosion.

Office visits depend on the degree of disease activity and range from weekly (for the patient on parenteral gold salts) to every 6 months. In the case of the homebound patient who requires remittive therapy, the following options are to be considered: Gold injections may be administered by a home care nurse and laboratory tests done in the home on a weekly basis. After the patient has been stable for 1 to 2 months, frequency of laboratory tests can be reduced to twice per month. These patients should be examined by a physician on a monthly basis for both evaluation of response and toxicity. Alternatively, one may administer an oral agent (auranofin or penicillamine) that does not require the weekly nurse visit but does necessitate similar laboratory monitoring.

Hospitalization for these patients may be necessary in cases of severe incapacitating flare where rest and intensive (twice daily) rehabilitative programs can be implemented. Systemic complications of disease, including secondary septic arthritis, cutaneous ulcerations, or cardiopulmonary involvement, represent additional possible indications for hospitalization.

## CRYSTAL-INDUCED ARTHRITIS

Laboratory evaluation of these patients includes complete blood count, erythrocyte sedimentation rate, urinalysis, chemistry, and 24-hour urine for calcium and uric acid. In the case of pseudogout (calcium pyrophosphate deposition disease) an evaluation of calcium metabolism is indicated. When possible, a synovial fluid analysis under polarized light microscopy should be performed.

An acute attack is best treated by a short course of anti-inflammatory doses of a NSAID. Therapy lasting less than 1 week is usually without significant toxicity in even elderly patients. In patients intolerant of NSAIDs, colchicine, in the case of gout, or, alternatively, a short course of prednisone (20 mg–30 mg for 4 to 6 days) can be substituted.

Office visits may be weekly for several weeks until the attack is controlled. For the home-bound patient a visit by the home care nurse with reporting to the physician may be substituted in the uncomplicated case.

Hospitalization would be indicated primarily because of uncertain diagnosis where a septic joint is under consideration.

## THE ARTHRITIS FOUNDATION

The services of the local chapter of the Arthritis Foundation can be invaluable to both the physician and patient. For the physician the Foundation can be a source of written educational material that can be distributed to patients. In addition, the Foundation has a strong interest in promoting traditional and proven therapy. Therefore, the Foundation is often helpful in dealing with patients who are inclined to seek alternative and often quack therapies.

The Arthritis Foundation can also be a resource in helping the patient to improve self-sufficiency and independence. They offer self-help advice directed toward pragmatic appliances for the home and personal hygiene. They sponsor programs such as the aquatic exercise program and supportive group discussion as well.

## BIBLIOGRAPHY

Basmajian J (ed): Therapeutic Exercise, 3rd ed. Baltimore, Williams & Wilkins, 1978

Kottke FJ: Krusen's Handbook of Physical Medicine and Rehabilitation, 3rd ed. Philadelphia, WB Saunders, 1982

Ruskin A: Current Therapy in Physiatry, Physical Medicine and Rehabilitation. Philadelphia, WB Saunders, 1984

# 10

# Preventive Health Measures and Screening

## MITCHELL H. CHARAP

## HISTORICAL PERSPECTIVES

Since the turn of the century, physicians in the United States have been actively engaged in disease prevention and health promotion. Physician interest in preventive medicine did not develop by chance, but came about largely because of the tremendous success that public health measures had in reducing the incidence of smallpox, yellow fever, and typhoid, which were major causes of morbidity and mortality in the United States at that time. By 1920, these measures had increased life expectancy in the United States to 58 years, representing a 30% increase over the preceding 50 years.

Mortality in the adult population had shifted from diseases of infectious origin to illnesses such as atherosclerosis, diabetes, renal diseases, and cancer. It is in large part because of these public health successes that home care has come about: people began to live longer and chronic illnesses with their sequelae became commonplace. Physicians in the United States believed that life expectancy could be further increased by utilization of measures that would detect these diseases at an earlier point and thereby lead to reductions in morbidity and mortality.

Several poorly designed studies performed between 1914 and 1922 concluded that the periodic health examination could, in fact, bring about significant improvement in the quality of life as well as prolonged life expectancy. Despite gross inaccuracies in data collection these studies were accepted by the medical profession. The American Medical Association formally endorsed the periodic health examination in 1922 and published several articles detailing the proper examining technique. Later, the National Health Council in association with the United States Public Health Service began a nationwide advertising campaign promoting the periodic health examination.

Over the next 50 years there was a steady increase in interest by both the profession and the lay public in preventive health. With the development of new technology in the late 1940s and 1950s laboratory tests were added to the periodic health examination in the form of multiphasic screening. Pulmonary function tests, electrocardiograms, and even stress tests were added to the list of routine tests to be performed on a periodic basis. Despite the lack of evidence regarding their efficacy, the periodic health examination is more popular than ever; it has become an annual ritual for a significant percentage of the adult population in the United States. In fact, it is the most common single reason people go to doctors, accounting for 7.2% of all office visits.

It has only been within the last decade that physicians have begun to analyze the effectiveness and efficacy of the periodic health examination. The most comprehensive effort was made by the Canadian Task Force, an international group of 51 physicians, who began in 1979 to analyze early detection measures in 78 major conditions. They looked at all the data available on each of these preventable conditions and analyzed the following:

1. The burden of suffering caused by the condition: morbidity, mortality, and cost of treatment
2. The effectiveness of the treatment or preventive measure, that is, the degree to which an intervention does more good than harm
3. The characteristics of early protection procedure: sensitivity and specificity, as well as the safety and accessibility

The result of the work was not surprising. There were few conditions and preventive measures in which sound evidence could justify their inclusion in a periodic health examination. In fact, one of the most important results of the Task Force was in delineating the deficits of information in order to focus future research. Nevertheless, there were a small number of measures that this Task Force strongly recommended, and these were grouped into protective health packages that varied in content and frequency of administration with the age and sex of the individual. Both the American Medical Association and the American College of Physicians developed specific guidelines for periodic examinations based on data from the Canadian Task Force and the American Cancer Society. Thus, in the 60 years since the initial unwarranted enthusiasm for preventive health measures, physicians have now come to realize that there are specific tasks, which when applied in a logical, scientific manner can, in fact, achieve the goals of disease prevention and health promotion.

In the following, basic principles of screening are reviewed and measures are outlined that can be applied to the homebound patient. Most of the general recommendations can be performed in the home without difficulty. It is important to remember that the home patient's needs are no different from the needs of our other patients in most cases. The presence of chronic illness need not impact on all aspects of our approach to these patients.

## BASIC DEFINITIONS

Much of the physician's time is spent in the treatment of diseases that have already progressed well beyond the asymptomatic stage. Patients present to our offices frequently at a point in which a disease has become sufficiently symptomatic for them to perceive the need to seek medical help from a physician. Whether it's diabetes mellitus or alcohol abuse, obstructive lung disease or acute myocardial infarction, our goal is to attempt to control the relentless progression of chronic disorders. We as physicians are at our best in this area with the assistance of new developments in medical technology and pharmacology. However, when we look at the natural course of diseases we know that they pass through various stages. In dealing with seriously ill patients we are engaged in tertiary prevention; that is, the prevention of progressive disability in the setting of a chronic symptomatic disease. However, in our offices or at home we should be engaged in both secondary and primary prevention. *Primary prevention* implies intervening *before* a disease occurs. The best example of primary prevention would be immunizations in the adult. Influenza, pneumococcal, and hepatitis vaccine are all given to prevent diseases from occurring. *Secondary prevention* is the detection and treatment of a disease at an early or asymptomatic state. An example of this would be the Pap smear used in the detection of cervical cancer. Use of the secondary prevention measures in a large population is called *screening* and the use in individual patients is called *case finding*.

The principle justifying the use of preventive health measures by physicians is based on the premise that there is a period of time in which a disease is asymptomatic, and if it is uncovered at that time, a change can be effected in the natural history of that disease, that is, the morbidity and mortality rate can be reduced. The time between the discovery of the disease and the asymptomatic state and its clinical presentation is called the *lead time.* As we shall see in our discussion of specific diseases, the finding of a disease in an asymptomatic state does not necessarily mean that the disease can be cured. Many cancers have escaped cure at a very early point in their evolution. Lung cancer is perhaps the best example of a disease that, even when screened for in high-risk groups, has not demonstrated a significant reduction in morbidity and mortality.

## SCREENING FOR SPECIFIC DISEASES

### BREAST CANCER

Breast cancer is the second most common cause of cancer deaths among women. It is a relatively common disorder, with over 100,000 cases diagnosed each year. Women in the United States have a one-in-eleven chance of developing breast cancer at some point during their lifetime, with the incidence increasing in those over 40 years of age.

The major risk factor for breast cancer is having a mother or sibling who has had breast cancer. Obviously, patients with breast cancer in one breast will have a far greater risk of developing cancer in the other breast when compared with the normal population. Other less important risk factors include older age at first pregnancy (over 30), early menarche, and late menopause. Many home care patients will be on estrogens and calcium for osteoporosis prevention. There is no evidence at the present time that estrogens or birth control pills increase the likelihood of developing breast cancer.

Survival of patients with breast cancer is related to the size of the tumor and the presence or absence of axillary lymph node involvement. Patients with small tumors, less than 2 cm without axillary node involvement, have a 5-year survival over 85% in contrast to those with larger tumors who have positive axillary nodes in which survival decreases to approximately 50% to 60%. These data have been used to justify early screening in that it appears that earlier diagnosis would uncover tumors at an earlier stage and thereby improve prognosis.

There is now evidence from a controlled trial of screening for breast cancer that demonstrates that early detection can improve survival. In 1963, the Health Insurance Plan of Greater New York (HIP) studied 62,000 women between the ages of 40 and 64. They were randomly placed into two groups. The study group was offered four annual screenings consisting of mammography and physical examination. A control group received usual care, that is, mammography for clinical indications and physical examination if requested by the patient. Each group was followed closely for the development of deaths due to breast cancer and deaths due to other causes. The data were analyzed after 10 to 14 years of follow-up. Study-group patients had 38% fewer breast cancer deaths after 5 years of study and 24% fewer deaths in 10 years. Importantly, among the screening-detected cases there was a greater proportion of patients with negative axillary lymph nodes. The study indicated benefit on a statistical basis for women over the age of 50. For women between ages 40 and 50 there was a nonstatistically significant advantage in the study group.

In the HIP study, mammography was the key contributor to increased survival. However, physician breast examination played a complementary role in this setting. Obviously, in the home setting, mammography done on a routine basis would not be feasible. There is evidence from earlier studies that both patient self-examination and physician breast examination resulted in significantly smaller lesions than those noted by the patient by accident. What was also clear from this study was the fact that patients did self-examinations infrequently and without proper understanding of the appropriate technique. It takes but a few moments to demonstrate the proper techniques.

In breast self-examination the patient should examine each breast with the opposite hand either while standing or lying down. The patient should develop a particular order in which she examines the breast, examining all four quadrants. The breast should be pressed gently using circular motions. The physician's breast examination should consist of observation of the woman seated to notice if there are any irregularities in contour and to examine the axilla. With the patient reclined, an examination of all four quadrants should be initiated, as well as an examination of the areola area. The importance of these examinations is increased obviously in a home setting and therefore physician participation and encouragement of the patient should be fostered. If the patient, particularly the middle-aged patient, is unable to do this the care partner should be instructed in doing breast examinations on a monthly basis in addition to the physician's examination.

### Recommendations

1. Physician breast examination should begin at age 35 to 40 and should be continued every year after the age of 40.
2. Patients should be instructed in self-examination by age 35 and be instructed to perform this examination monthly.
3. In patients with a personal or family history of breast carcinoma in a sibling or mother, mammography should be considered despite the hardship of transportation, on an annual basis beginning at the age of 40 or at the time of diagnosis of carcinoma.

There are many questions that remain unanswered with regard to screening for breast cancer. It is uncertain at the present time at what age women should no longer continue to be screened for breast cancer. Patients with large or cystic breasts are difficult to examine, and although they may not be at greater risk for developing breast carcinoma, routine examinations may detect cancer less easily. Therefore, recommendations for mammography may in fact be different in this group.

### COLON CANCER

In the United States, colon cancer is the second most common malignancy affecting both men and women. In 1980 it resulted in 112,000 deaths, which represents 20% of all cancer deaths. Aside from mortality, colon cancer also results in significant morbidity through complications of the disease itself or surgical attempts to treat it.

There is clear evidence that survival in colorectal cancer is dependent on whether there is spread through the bowel wall. Patients with disease limited to the mucosa or extension beyond the mucosa but within the bowel wall have a 5-year survival in excess of 75%. However, with extension beyond the bowel wall the 5-year survival drops dramatically. Those patients with lymph node involvement have a survival of approximately 30%.

To understand fully the recommendations for screening, it is important first to understand the epidemiology and pathogenesis of colon cancer. It is now believed that colorectal carcinoma generally arises from adenomatous polyps and villous adenomas. Polyps are quite common in our population, occurring in over 5% of individuals over the age of 40. Most polyps are markers for cancer because they suggest the possibility of cancer elsewhere in the colon and because they, in and of themselves, have a greater potential for neoplastic development at a future point in time. It is also clear that larger polyps, that is, polyps greater than 2 cm, have a greater likelihood to harbor carcinoma. In addition, pedunculated polyps have a greater tendency to harbor carcinoma than sessile polyps.

The risk of colorectal cancer increases significantly after the age of 40. Aside from polyps, the risk of colorectal cancer increases in patients in whom there is a family history of colon cancer. In addition, families in which there is a history of other adenocarcinomas, such as endometrial cancer, ovarian cancer, and cancer of the stomach, are also at greater risk. The familial polyposis syndromes, such as familial polyposis and Gardner's syndrome, have a marked increase in the incidence of carcinoma. However, most of these patients have had colectomies by the time they reach adulthood. Finally, patients with ulcerative colitis, particularly those with pancolitis, are at high risk after having the disease for 10 years.

In view of its high prevalence and potential curability, if uncovered as a small lesion, colon cancer seems to be an ideal candidate for screening. The two major forms of screening are (1) occult blood detection and (2) proctosigmoidoscopy. There are many unanswered questions about the efficacy and effectiveness of these techniques, which will be outlined below.

Occult blood detection is based on the assumption that colonic cancers and polyps bleed. The most commonly used test, Hemoccult II, consists of a filter paper which is impregnated with gum guaiac, a phenolic compound that turns color with oxidation. Hemoglobin has a peroxidase-like activity; thus, when it is added to the guaiac card with the addition of hydrogen peroxide, the guaiac oxidizes, yielding a blue color. False negative test (*i.e.,* tests that are negative in the face of colon cancer), occur primarily because of a large fluctuation in blood loss from colonic lesions. Blood loss of 20 ml per day is required for positive Hemoccult reaction. Therefore, patients may be bleeding but the test will not be positive. In addition, colonic lesions bleed only intermittently and benign colonic polyps bleed even less. The storage of the stool sample for more than four days can also reduce the peroxidase activity of the hemoglobin and therefore creates more false negatives. Vitamin C, an antioxidant, interferes with the pseudoperoxidase reaction, resulting in more false negatives. False positives also exist and relate primarily to diet. Various food stuffs, including meat, fruits, and uncooked vegetables, contain peroxidases and may lead to a positive stool guaiac. Therefore, it is recommended that patients be on a special diet prior to stool guaiac testing.

Proctosigmoidoscopy has the advantage of direct visualization of an area of the colon that is at great risk for developing colorectal cancer. Occult blood detection and proctosigmoidoscopy should be viewed as complementary procedures in the screening of colon cancer. Hemoccult testing has the potential to pick up lesions more proximal in the colon and sigmoidoscopy has the potential to pick up nonbleeding polyps more distally. The major problem in screening for colorectal cancer relates to the fact that there is no evidence from controlled trials to demonstrate that Hemoccult testing and proctosigmoidoscopy used alone or in combination result in a significant decrease in morbidity and mortality from colon cancer. There are two ongoing trials directing themselves to this issue. However, data are not yet available.

### Recommendations

1. Determine your patient's risk group through careful review of family history and past medical history.
2. In average-risk patients, beginning at age 40, Hemoccult testing should be done annually. The first Hemoccult slide may be obtained during digital rectal examination. Two subsequent slides should be mailed to the physician after being obtained on consecutive days. Stool guaiac testing should not be performed while the patient is on iron, aspirin, ascorbic acid, or cimetidine. If possible, for 48 hours prior to Hemoccult testing the patient should be on a diet free of red meat and fish, raw vegetables, or other substances high in peroxidase activity.
3. One positive test is sufficient evidence to begin evaluation of the patient.
4. Proctosigmoidoscopy should be done every 3 to 5 years.

5. High-risk groups, that is, patients with a prior history of colon cancer or polyps, or with a family history of colon cancer, may require more frequent and more aggressive screening procedures.

The screening procedures can easily be accomplished in the home setting. The following materials are needed:

Gloves

Guaiac paper and solution

Rigid sigmoidoscope

Proctosigmoidoscope cotton swabs

Disposable patient gowns

Sigmoidoscopy can be performed with the patient in the left lateral position in bed, with the physician kneeling on the floor. Because of the bulky suction, insufflation, and light source equipment, it is not currently feasible to use the flexible colonoscope in the home setting.

There is no question that a home sigmoidoscopy is going to be an onerous task at best. There may be times when you will want to do this in the hospital outpatient setting. This can be an opportunity to do other screening procedures such as a mammogram, electrocardiogram, and other such testing.

## CARCINOMA OF THE CERVIX

Although not as common as carcinoma of the breast and carcinoma of the colon, cervical cancer in women is the only cancer in which large population studies have demonstrated a clear reduction in morbidity and mortality resulting from the use of a screening test. It is for this reason that screening for this disease is the most widely accepted component of health maintenance. Unfortunately it is rarely offered to young homebound women, such as patients with multiple sclerosis.

Histologically the outer portion of the cervix is covered with squamous epithelium. The endocervix is lined with columnar cells. The boundary between these two areas is called the *squamocolumnar* junction. With increasing age there is movement of the squamous epithelium inward toward the internal cervical os. It is in this area of dynamic change that cervical cancer occurs. Various lines of evidence suggest that invasive squamous cell carcinoma of the cervix is preceded by progressive evolution of the lesion, with the final outcome being invasive cervical carcinoma in which malignancy extends beyond the basal layer of epithelial cells into the stroma.

Risk for cervical cancer increases with (1) early age of first coitus or marriage, especially if less than age 17; (2) multiple sexual partners; (3) low socioeconomic class; and (4) increasing age.

The Papanicolaou smear of exfoliated cells is the sole screening test for cervical cancer. The major purpose of this test is to detect dysplastic lesions and carcinoma *in situ;* treatment at this stage can result in a 100% cure rate. If one can eliminate these premalignant lesions one would expect a reduction in the incidence of carcinoma of the cervix. In fact, a study from Canada has demonstrated a marked reduction in the incidence of invasive carcinoma of the cervix with the advent of the Pap smear. Associated with this reduction in incidence, there has also been a reduction in mortality.

There has recently been some controversy regarding the interval for obtaining Pap smears. The long lead time between dysplasia and carcinoma is estimated to be between 5 and 10 years, suggesting that the Pap smear need not be done on an annual basis. As a result, most recommendations now separate women into low-risk and high-risk groups. The high-risk group consists of women who have had sexual activity before the age of 20 and have had exposure to multiple male partners.

## Recommendations

1. Pap testing should begin at the onset of sexual activity or at age 18, whichever comes first.
2. Repeat testing one year later should be done on all women.
3. In low-risk groups, repeat Pap smear every three years should be continued until age 65.
4. High-risk women should have Pap smears done annually.
5. If there has been an abnormal smear at any time, repeat Pap smears should be done every 5 years over the age of 65.

### Obtaining Specimens for Pap Smears

In the home, the Pap test can be done without major problem. One will require a vaginal speculum, swabs, both cotton and wooden, two slides, and a spray fixative. In addition a light source must be available so that accurate visualization of the endocervix can be achieved. Specula can be purchased that have a light source attached to them and this may be particularly helpful in the home setting. Likewise, you may want to use a disposable instrument in this setting. The endocervical specimen is obtained using the cotton swab, which is placed into the external os. The other specimen should be taken from the exocervix using another swab or wood spatula. A fixative is then applied to the slides. At the same time this procedure is being done you can obtain a stool sample when doing the rectal examination if that is appropriate. As was mentioned in the discussion of colon cancer, you may want to do this when the patient is in the hospital for another reason.

## CANCER OF THE PROSTATE

Carcinoma of the prostate is a common form of cancer, affecting approximately 1% of men over the age of 65. Digital examination of the prostate is the best screening test for its detection. The initial enthusiasm about prostatic acid phosphatase determination has waned in light of its low specificity. If nodules are palpated, urologic examination is warranted. This examination is performed during the rectal examination.

## TESTICULAR CANCER

Testicular cancer is the most common form of solid cancer in men under the age of 35. It is a treatable disease, with the recent advances in chemotherapy. Although no trial has looked at its efficacy, testicular examination by the physician should be performed on men at risk. Men should be taught to perform monthly testicular self-examination.

## SKIN CANCER

Skin cancer is the most common form of cancer in humans. Although squamous cell and basal cell carcinomas of the skin are extremely common and should be looked for on physical examination, malignant melanoma remains the focus of preventive health measures because it is the cause of significant morbidity and mortality. The physical examination is the screening modality for malignant melanoma. It is essential that physicians recognize the features that distinguish benign pigmented lesions from melanomas. Signs of malignancy include asymmetry, irregular margins, variegated colors, and large size. In addition, any change in a preexisting nevus or the development of a new nevus should alert the physician to the development of a possible melanoma. As with other forms of cancer, the epidemiology of malignant melanoma is important in raising clinical suspicion. Risk factors include (1) light-colored eyes and light complexion; (2) history of severe sunburn, especially in childhood through early 20s; (3) outdoor recreational habits; and (4) individuals with large numbers of nevi in childhood, particularly dysplastic nevi.

Skin inspection should be an integral part of the home care teaching for nurses, aides, and care partners. In addition to looking for unusual or suspicious lesions the skin can be inspected for areas of redness indicating potential skin breakdown. Most decubitus ulcers are preventable if the redness is noted early enough.

## LUNG CANCER

Lung cancer is the most common cause of cancer death in men and women in the United States. Recently lung cancer has surpassed breast cancer in causing cancer death in women. Although the epidemiology of lung cancer and its clear association with smoking and environmental exposure are well understood, screening for the disease even in high-risk patients has not been effective in reducing morbidity and mortality. As was mentioned earlier in this chapter, the effectiveness of a screening procedure is determined by the natural history of that disease. To be effective there must be a time during which the patient harbors asymptomatic disease, which, if treated when asymptomatic, can be cured. Previous screening programs, which have used chest x-rays at 6-month intervals in high-risk populations (*i.e.,* smokers), have not shown that there is statistically increased survival in patients screened versus patients in a control group who did not undergo frequent chest x-ray studies. Lung cancer escapes cure early in its history. At the point at which a patient has a chest x-ray that reveals a pulmonary nodule, even in the absence of symptoms, there is frequently spread of the disease to the lymph nodes.

Cytologic examination increases the sensitivity of screening. There are now ongoing studies to look at the combination of cytologic analysis and chest x-ray in high-risk groups. However, at the present time, the effectiveness of screening approaches to lung carcinoma remains unproved. Therefore, recommendations cannot be made.

## IMMUNIZATION

Immunization of children is a major part of the practice of pediatrics in the United States and in the rest of the world. However, this has not been true in the practice of internal medicine, despite the fact that vaccinations of similar efficacy exist for the adult population. Immunization, in fact, is one of the few areas of preventive medicine in which the occurrence of disease has been shown to be markedly decreased by a preventive health measure. Physicians should therefore develop a routine method of ensuring that patients under their care receive the necessary and recommended vaccinations. As will be seen in the discussion of specific vaccines, the physician's obligation is to understand the epidemiology of the disease in relationship to the specific patient being examined. Chronic disease, age, occupation, and possible environmental exposure should all be evaluated to determine the basic approach to immunization.

## INFLUENZA

Influenza infection typically results in an illness characterized by high fever, sore throat, and non-productive cough. Significant malaise and painful myalgias are also common. The seriousness of influenza infections is based on two factors. First, influenza tends to be an epidemic illness affecting large percentages of the population. Second, frequent lower tract complications (*i.e.,* bacterial pneumonia or viral pneumonia itself) can lead to a major increase in visits to physicians and hospitalization. The vast majority of deaths from influenza occur in patients who, because of their age and underlying problems, are not able to contain the disease. According to the Centers for Disease Control, 90% of excess deaths attributed to pneumonia and influenza in the setting of epidemics occur in persons over the age of 65.

Each year influenza vaccines are developed that contain antigens from strains of influenza felt to be most likely to cause outbreaks of disease. The choice of antigens is derived from information obtained from worldwide influenza surveillance systems. The efficacy of the vaccine is correlated with the development of antibodies. The vaccine is strongly recommended for (1) individuals who are over 65 years of age and (2) individuals with severe underlying medical conditions such as heart disease, chronic pulmonary disease, diabetes, chronic renal failure, and other metabolic diseases.

Side-effects are few and infrequent. Aside from mild tenderness and erythema, which occur in fewer than a third of the recipients, systemic symptoms are very uncommon. Since the vaccine is propagated in egg, individuals who are sensitive to eggs should not be given the influenza vaccine. The increased incidence of Guillain-Barré syndrome following the 1976 influenza vaccine has not occurred with more recent preparations.

## PNEUMOCOCCAL VACCINE

In view of the fact that pneumococcal pneumonia remains the most prevalent community-acquired bacterial pneumonia and that the fatality rate for patients with bacteremia is approximately 20%, extensive efforts have been made to create a vaccine. The most recent development in this area was the replacement of the previous 14-valent products with a new 23-valent product that includes 85% to 90% of the pneumococcal serotypes causing infection in humans.

The incidence of pneumococcal bacteremia increases with age. Therefore, it is recommended that older patients be offered the vaccination. Other risk factors for the development of bacteremic pneumococcal pneumonia or death from pneumococcal pneumonia include patients with functional or anatomic asplenia, congestive heart failure, chronic liver disease, chronic obstructive pulmonary disease, and renal failure. Patients with either naturally occurring or iatrogenically produced immunodeficiency states, such as leukemias, lymphomas, or a patient who is treated with chemotherapy, are also at greater risk of death from pneumococcal disease. However, these patients do not appear to respond to the vaccine as well as non-immunocompromised patients.

Although there have been no large controlled studies to demonstrate the efficacy of pneumococcal vaccine, significant information from retrospective studies has demonstrated that it is safe and effective in 70% of immunocompetent hosts. Transient local side-effects include erythema and induration and some local discomfort, which can occur in up to 40% of recipients. Severe local reactions and fever have been reported in 1%. These severe reactions occur with greater frequency in patients who have received a second vaccination. Therefore, it is not recommended to repeat the pneumococcal vaccination. The vaccine is given either subcutaneously or intramuscularly as a single 0.5-ml dose. The influenza vaccine can be given simultaneously at a separate site without an increase in side-effects.

The pneumococcal vaccine is recommended for (1) all persons over age 65; (2) those patients with chronic conditions, including heart disease, chronic lung disease, alcoholism, diabetes, and patients with asplenia; and (3) closed populations such as nursing homes in which high rates of pneumococcal disease occur.

## TETANUS AND DIPHTHERIA

The routine use of tetanus toxoid has resulted in a marked decrease in the occurrence of tetanus in the United States. In fact, over the last decade the annual rate has been 90 cases. Over two thirds of these cases were in patients who were 50 years or older and had not been adequately immunized. Diphtheria was also a common disease in the United States and because of immunization it is now a rarity, with only 15 cases of respiratory diphtheria occurring in the United States between 1980 and 1983. Although a rarity, most cases that do occur occur in unimmunized or inadequately immunized persons over the age of 20.

Tetanus and diphtheria toxoids are given as a combined preparation in the adult population. It is now recommended that tetanus and diphtheria toxoid be given every 10 years. If a dose is given sooner as part of management of wounds, the booster is not needed for another 10 years thereafter. Local reactions including erythema and induration are common, occurring in over half of those given the vaccine. In addition, mild systemic reactions, including fever and drowsiness, occur frequently. The only contraindication to the tetanus and diphtheria vaccine is a history of a neurologic or severe hypersensitivity reaction after a previous dose.

The above comments regarding the tetanus and diphtheria vaccine assume primary immunization has occurred during childhood. Tetanus prophylaxis in management of a recent wound is beyond the scope of this discussion. It frequently entails the use of tetanus toxoid and tetanus immune globulin, depending on the situation and the immunization history.

In the home setting, the physician must review the chart prior to the visit, to determine the type of vaccines that will be given. The decision will be based on specific patient characteristics and previous immunizations. Although refrigeration is required to maintain influenza and pneumococcal vaccines, short exposure to room temperature will not affect the efficacy of the vaccine.

## SCREENING FOR TUBERCULOSIS

Although the prevalence of active tuberculosis has decreased dramatically during the second half of this century, the disease is still a major health problem in certain populations, in particular the urban poor, recent South American and Southeast Asian immigrants, and the elderly in general. In the United States about 7% of the population are positive reactors to tuberculin skin test. These patients are at risk for developing active tuberculosis. Those at greatest risk are persons who are recent skin test converters or who have a positive chest x-ray film, a home contact with active disease, or immunosuppression. Although the annual risk of activation of tuberculosis is quite small, the cumulative lifetime risk is significant. Fortunately, this risk can be reduced substantially by chemoprophylaxis if the patient is a known converter. Thus, tuberculosis screening is another example of secondary prevention.

The chest x-ray film is a fairly insensitive screening test, with many tuberculin reactors having negative results on x-ray. Therefore, chest x-ray studies should no longer be used for screening. The most effective screening procedure is the tuberculin skin test. It is one of the cheapest, safest, and most easily administered screening tests available. The Mantoux test, using intradermal injection of PPD-S (Tween-80 stabilized, purified protein derivative), is more reliable than the multiple-puncture Tine test. In general, the intermediate, or 5-unit PPD, is used. The test result should be interpreted after 48 to 72 hours. Induration rather than erythema determines positivity, 10 mm or more being positive. The 1-unit PPD is used for people in whom a strong reaction is anticipated.

Negative test results have been documented in up to 20% of patients with tuberculosis. These false negatives are secondary to multiple causes, including incorrect administration of the test, chronic diseases, steroid treatment, intercurrent infection, and recent active tuberculosis. In addition, the sensitivity may decrease with age. A doubtful intermediate strength PPD (*i.e.,* induration of 5 mm to 9 mm) is suggestive of infection with an atypical microbacteria and cross-sensitization to PPD.

### Recommendations

1. All patients in whom tuberculin activity is unknown or previously negative should have a baseline PPD.

2. If the PPD is less than 10 mm, repeat PPD every 2 to 5 years.
3. All reactors and converters should be managed according to the American Thoracic Society Guidelines, which are beyond the scope of this discussion.

In the home setting, the major problem is the reading of the PPD after 48 hours. This task can be accomplished by a trained health-care provider. The patient or family can be taught to mark the area of swelling with a pen if the physician or nurse cannot evaluate the reaction at the precise time. This can then be checked (if it isn't washed off) a day or two later.

## ROUTINE BLOOD TESTS

The use of blood tests or diagnostic procedures without clear indications rarely provides us with information that is helpful in the management of a patient. More often the results offer

RECORD DATES AND RESULTS          HEALTH MAINTENANCE—ADULT

| | Age | | | | | | | | | | | | | | |
|---|---|---|---|---|---|---|---|---|---|---|---|---|---|---|---|
| | Date | | | | | | | | | | | | | | |
| **Immunizations Skin Tests** | Tetanus Toxoid | | | | | | | | | | | | | | |
| | Tuberculin Test | | | | | | | | | | | | | | |
| | Influenza Vaccine | | | | | | | | | | | | | | |
| | Pneumococcal Vaccine | | | | | | | | | | | | | | |
| **Examinations** | Complete Exam | | | | | | | | | | | | | | |
| | Wt. (Ht.          ) | | | | | | | | | | | | | | |
| | Blood Pressure | | | | | | | | | | | | | | |
| | Tonometry | | | | | | | | | | | | | | |
| | Digital Rectal | | | | | | | | | | | | | | |
| | Slide Occult Blood | | | | | | | | | | | | | | |
| | Sigmoidoscopy | | | | | | | | | | | | | | |
| | Physician Breast Exam | | | | | | | | | | | | | | |
| | Mammogram | | | | | | | | | | | | | | |
| | Pap Smear | | | | | | | | | | | | | | |
| **Laboratory** | VDRL | | | | | | | | | | | | | | |
| | Cholesterol | | | | | | | | | | | | | | |
| | | | | | | | | | | | | | | | |
| | | | | | | | | | | | | | | | |
| **High Risk** | | | | | | | | | | | | | | | |

| **Patient Education Topics** | Nutrition & Exercise | Diet (  )          Exercise (  )          Calcium (  ) |
|---|---|---|
| | Substance Abuse & Stress | Smoking (  )     Alcohol (  )     Drugs (  )     Social Support (  )<br>Family    (  )          Sex (  )     Job (  )          Suicide (  ) |
| | Cancer | Breast Self-Exam (  )          Post-Menopausal Bleeding (  ) |
| | Accidents | Safety Belts (  )     Smoke Alarm (  )     Falls (  ) |

*Recommended frequencies and intervals for health maintenance services are not included.

**Figure 10-1** *Physician's progress record.*

us answers to questions we never asked and occasionally lead to expensive and unproductive work-ups that are potentially harmful to the patient. Furthermore, there are no data to suggest that routine blood chemistry, complete blood count, and urinalysis in asymptomatic patients are effective means of disease detection or prevention.

During an initial evaluation of the patient, a complete history is taken and physical examination is performed. It is at this time that baseline blood tests should be done. The tests include a complete blood count, urinalysis, and cholesterol determinations. If these tests are normal, then repeat testing can be done at intervals between 5 and 10 years. In men and women over the age of 40, a baseline electrocardiogram may also be helpful for future comparisons. However, this electrocardiogram need not be repeated unless indicated on the basis of the history. Again, there is no empiric evidence that these are effective preventive health measures. They serve more as a point of reference for future interactions and occurrences in the patient. These routine tests should present no hardship for either patient or physician in the home setting.

## PHYSICIANS AND PREVENTIVE HEALTH MEASURES

One of the major obstacles to successful screening in the general medical population is physicians' failure to utilize them in their practice. For example, in a recent survey conducted by the American Cancer Society, 49% of physicians utilized mammography in their practice and only 11% followed the American Cancer Society guidelines. The physicians' rationale for not complying with the guidelines were varied, ranging from concerns about cost and patient acceptance to risks and overall efficacy. Many of the physicians simply did not understand the purpose of the test. However, there have also been studies to demonstrate that physicians who are aware of the recommendations for screening and who agree with these recommendations still did not utilize them in their practice. It is important to emphasize that the principal problem with screening lies not with the patient or with the recommendations themselves, but with physicians' failure to follow their own recommendations.

There are a variety of different techniques to improve compliance with guidelines for screening. The most frequently used is the checklist, which becomes part of the medical record. A sample of such a list is seen in Figure 10-1. This list provides an opportunity for the physician to note at different ages the screening procedures that have been done, and also gives the physician an idea of the appropriate screening procedures to be done. Reminders generated by computers or by ancillary staff are also effective in increasing physician compliance. However, regardless of the method chosen, reminders must be given at frequent intervals to maintain a high degree of compliance.

# 11

# Diagnostic Monitoring

MARY ELLEN WADSWORTH
ANTHONY J. GRIECO

As the number of people who are cared for at home increases, so too does the need to provide the patient and the family with the knowledge and skills necessary to keep that patient as healthy, safe, and comfortable as possible. The ability to monitor the patient at home for signs of illness or for exacerbation of an already existing problem enables both the patient and the family to exercise a greater measure of control over their situation. Since loss of control is one of the primary causes of stress and anxiety during both acute and chronic illnesses, some of that stress can be alleviated by teaching the patient and family home monitoring techniques. Home monitoring is more than just learning what to observe. Having the family become partners in monitoring requires that they understand why the monitoring is important as well as know what they should do, in the way of taking action, with the information they obtain.

Although home monitoring may relieve the physician of the necessity of seeing some patients in the office very frequently, thereby reducing the expense and hardship faced by the family in arranging transportation for homebound patients, in most instances it will necessitate more frequent telephone contact. If the patient and home care partner are to make observations, keep records, and report changes, they must feel secure in the knowledge that their physician will be readily reachable and responsive. The simple statement, "Call me in two days to report your observations," gives the message that contact is desired, and even demanded.

Home monitoring adds a new dimension to standard professional practice; we will be trusting the assessment and judgment of a nonprofessional person and we will be making decisions about the patient's treatment based on that information. In order for the physician to feel comfortable with this, he or she must be certain that the patient and care partner have been taught properly. When home monitoring works well, it gives the home care partner a more complete picture of the patient's day-to-day pattern, enabling that person to intervene when signs of trouble first arise, rather than waiting to treat a problem until after it becomes obviously serious or an emergency.

In thinking about the homebound patient's need for monitoring we must go well beyond the hospital definition of that word and extend it to a much broader array of observations. Monitoring at home includes not only evaluation by equipment, such as ambulatory electrocardiographic monitors, but also personal observation of physical, emotional, and behavioral changes that may be associated with different illnesses. The person responsible for home monitoring may be the patient himself, family members, friends, professionals, paraprofessionals, or any combination of these. The first steps in arranging home monitoring are to clearly identify who will be the primary individual involved and then to evaluate that person's competence and willingness to assume the responsibilities entailed. The goal of monitoring at home is not just the issue of life and death, which is more relevant in hospital-based monitoring, but has as its primary concern the maintenance of quality of life.

The questions to be answered in arranging for home monitoring are discussed below.

### 1. Who Will Be Responsible for the Monitoring?

In arranging for home monitoring of symptoms, we must be certain that we know who will be responsible for doing the monitoring. The possibilities include the patient, a family member or friend, a hired home aide, or a nurse. In many instances it will be helpful to identify two distinct classes of observations: those to be made by the patient himself and those that should be made by the care partner. The patient will be most reliable in reporting symptoms, while the care partner can be a keen detector of signs, using the classical physical diagnosis definitions.

The individual identified as having the responsibility for monitoring must understand that reporting symptoms and changes is part of that responsibility. There must be clear communication between patient and care partner so that the problem "But I thought *you* called . . ." does not prevent or delay the passage of information to the physician.

### 2. Who Will Do the Teaching?

Once it is determined what type of monitoring will be necessary, the person or persons responsible for teaching the patient or care partner must be identified as well. If the patient has been in the hospital, we cannot assume that education is an orderly, ongoing process. The transition to home can precipitate hasty teaching, with the hospital staff and the primary physician each believing incorrectly that the other has arranged for more detailed instruction. Whether or not the patient and care partner have been adequately educated in the hospital, it is a helpful practice to have a home care nurse visit after discharge to be certain that the monitoring is being carried out properly and to answer the practical questions that should be expected to arise.

### 3. What Observations Will Be Made?

If the patient or care partner does not understand which changes are important and which are not, the physician may find himself or herself on the receiving end of unnecessary telephone calls and the patient and family may become unduly alarmed. On the other hand, changes that are important may not be reported and a serious problem may evolve.

What observations will we ask of them? As an example, if dealing with a patient with cardiovascular disease, the patient and the care partner may be called on to evaluate any combination of the following:

Edema

Shortness of breath

Chest pain

Signs of an impending myocardial infarction

The patient's color

Pulse rate and regularity

Temperature

Lightheadedness

Of course, they might actually be the ones to witness a home cardiac arrest. If that is a significant possibility, consideration should be given to enrolling the family in a certified CPR course for the layman.

## 4. When Should the Observations Be Made?

A "partnership" decision should be reached by the physician, the patient, and the care partner regarding how frequently the observations should be made. This, of course, will depend on what is being observed and the severity of the condition. It may follow the usual pattern of hospital monitoring or be less frequent, as the condition most likely will be less acute. For example, glucose monitoring in the home may be required four to five times per day to establish good control, whereas in other, more stabilized patients, only once or twice a day may be sufficient.

Without having the frequency of observations explicitly defined, some people will, in their zeal, monitor too frequently. For example, most patients do not need their blood pressure checked four times per day. The error of overly protective monitoring tends to occur immediately after discharge from hospital. With little obvious benefit from the findings, enthusiasm may decay into tedium, resulting in too infrequent monitoring over time.

## 5. How Will the Observations Be Made?

How will the observer know whether the pulse rate is too rapid, too slow, or too irregular? Verbal and written information is needed so the observer can make an accurate, reliable assessment. We need to know that the care partner truly understands what we are asking him or her to do. After teaching a skill, even one as simple as taking a pulse, the care partner should be asked to demonstrate proficiency in the skill.

One demonstration of "proficiency" is not enough. Many people are able to imitate a task they have just witnessed but when asked to repeat it from memory after a day or so can no longer perform the task reliably. Performing home glucose monitoring is a classic example of this dilemma. While being taught, patients generally can mimic accurately, but mistakes in technique become apparent rapidly at home. Routine intermittent spot checking to reevaluate such skills is a wise precaution.

## 6. Why Are the Observations Necessary?

Most adults demand some degree of understanding as to why they must perform certain tasks before they will willingly do them. If they acknowledge that they also *agree* that these observations are important, the likelihood of compliance is increased further. Again, involving the patient and family in a partnership role with the physician is key.

## 7. What Should the Observer Do With the Information Obtained?

If the observer feels that the information being collected does not have an impact on the patient's management or well-being, it is unlikely that he will continue to gather the information despite being urged on. We have all seen diabetic patients who come to us with no record of urine testing or of home blood glucose monitoring because they have not known how to use the information.

Sometimes, record keeping is the entire goal of making observations. At other times, medication changes should be made in response to the observations. Even more likely, a telephone call to the physician may be necessary. Some observations will lead to emergency calls.

What constitutes an emergency? Symptoms that require emergency intervention are usually obvious to us. However, a nonprofessional observer at home may not recognize warning signs as easily and may therefore leave the patient in jeopardy. The care partner must know in advance how to make those judgments. We must be sure that the observer knows what to look for, including the specifics that make the distinctions between useful and useless information. Examples help, such as "Chest pain relieved promptly by rest or one to two nitroglycerin tablets is OK, but chest pain that is not relieved by nitroglycerin or is accompanied by the symptoms of a possible coronary require that you immediately call me or the emergency squad." (Signs of a possible coronary are listed below.)

An often overlooked wrinkle in the monitoring plan is preparing the family for reporting the findings to a physician who is covering for the patient's usual doctor. Our patients are well known to us but can be an enigma to someone else, particularly on the telephone. Providing the patient and care partner with a list of the few crucial elements in the history, including the response to drugs and peculiar symptoms experienced in the past, could make the telephone interaction go much more smoothly. Possible examples are, "Always remember to tell any doctor that you get dreadful diarrhea with quinidine," or "A pulse rate of 50 is fine for you, for if we hold your digoxin for a day or two you always slip into heart failure." This is the sort of information that would be helpful for the patient to relate spontaneously to a "strange" physician on the telephone when reporting dyspnea, an irregular pulse, or a few days of anorexia.

In the remainder of this chapter we will present a sampling of patients who commonly have clearly defined needs for home monitoring, with outlined examples that can be of help in instructing patients and care partners.

## THE PATIENT WITH CARDIAC DISEASE

The homebound patient with cardiac disease presents many needs and opportunities for monitoring, whether the patient is restricted to home for another reason but also has cardiac disease or is homebound because of the cardiac disease itself. Faced with a relative who has heart disease, the family often looks upon the observations they must make as meaning the difference between life and death. The physician has the responsibility for providing balance. The family needs to be made aware of the importance of the monitoring, yet not to be made victim of undue stress when accepting this responsibility.

Frequently, home monitoring of the patient with cardiac disease is a dual task, involving a combination of the observation of symptoms and the use of mechanical monitoring devices. An example is having a patient wear a Holter monitor while being responsible for simultaneously recording the day's symptoms in a diary. How often do patients wear the monitor but bring in a blank diary because they did not know how to complete it or did not realize its importance?

Although we are familiar with the observations we ourselves would make and the information we would obtain related to the patient's cardiac status, what do we ask the family to monitor? We cannot just ask them to "report anything unusual" or to watch for signs of dyspnea, edema, arrhythmia, or syncope without ascertaining that they know exactly what we mean.

When asking the patient or care partner to record symptoms, we should have them go through the litany of qualifiers we have been taught to obtain in our own history taking. In addition to discussing each symptom, the following outlines may be adapted as handouts to be incorporated into a home care plan:

Chest Pain
    When does it occur?
        Time of day?
        At night?
        With effort?
        At rest?
        With specific activities?
        With aggravation?
        Is it affected by deep breathing or coughing?
        How often does it occur?

How does it feel?
  Pressure?
  Crushing?
  Aching?
  Burning?
  Tightness?
  Soreness?
  Choking?

Where is the pain?
  Center of chest?
  Right side of chest?
  Left side of chest?

Does it extend to any other area?
  Neck?
  Left or right arm?
  Back?
  Abdomen?

How long does it last?

What relieves it?
  Does it end promptly when stopping your activity?
  Does it stop with rest?
  Is it helped by nitroglycerin?
  Is it helped by an antacid?

Are any other symptoms associated with the pain?
  Nausea?
  Sweating?
  Lightheadedness?
  Faintness?
  Difficulty breathing?
  Change in skin color to paleness?

*Special warnings:* Is the chest pain *new or different* from what has been experienced in the past? If so, report it immediately. If the pain is severe and not relieved by nitroglycerin, seek help immediately.

## Shortness of Breath
When does it occur?
  Time of day?
  At night?
  With effort?
  At rest?
  With specific activities?
  How often does it occur?
  Is it affected by certain positions?

Is it accompanied by any of the following?
  Cough?
  Wheezing?
  Sputum?

Is breathing faster, deeper, or more difficult?

## Swelling
Where is the swelling?
  Feet?
  Legs?
  Face?
  Hands?

Is it pitting?

When is it present?
Morning on arising?
At end of day?

Is it getting better or worse each day?

Has there been a change in weight?

## Pulse

What is the rate per minute?

Is it strong or weak?

Is it regular or irregular?

Are pulses present at
Both wrists?
Both feet?

(Note that apical pulse may be required.)

## Respirations

What is the rate per minute?

Is it quiet or noisy?
Any wheezing?
Any rattles?

Is the breathing deep or shallow?

What is the breathing like while the patient is sleeping?

What is the breathing like after a standard degree of exertion? As a baseline, a familiar task should be used, such as climbing one flight of stairs at home (it should always be the same stairs).

## Color

Does the patient appear
Pale?
Grayish?
Bluish?
Flushed?

Is there any redness of the skin?

Any jaundice?

## Lightheadedness

When does it occur?

How does it feel?
Do you feel faintness?
Do you feel a spinning sensation?
Do you have blurry vision?

What relieves it?

Is it associated with any of the following?
Nausea
Headache
Chest pain
Palpitations

## Possible Coronary

Chest pain that is persistent

Chest pain that is more severe than usual

Chest pain not relieved by nitroglycerin or rest

Spread of pain to the jaw

Pain accompanied by sweating

Pain accompanied by dizziness

Feeling of doom

Pain accompanied by nausea and vomiting

Appearance of pale color

## Intake and Output

Fluid intake includes
> Water
> Juice
> Coffee
> Milk
> All other liquids
> Jello
> Sherbert
> Ice cream

A measuring cup should be used to determine the capacity of the home fluid containers, such as
> Glasses
> Mugs
> Bowls

Output includes
> Urine
> Vomitus
> Diarrhea

In addition to the personal observations outlined above, mechanical devices may be needed to record additional information. Home blood pressure monitoring is quite simple. Most patients acquire the skill to read systolic and diastolic pressure quickly. For those who are insecure, the digital readout home sphygmomanometer is an effective alternative.

Heart rhythm or pacemaker function can be monitored by telephone transmission of electrocardiogram to the physician's office or to a centralized service. The telephone device can double as a "symptomatic incident recorder" when we have a patient who has infrequent arrhythmias that do not appear on a routine 24-hour ambulatory electrocardiogram. By this simple home technique, a frantic rush to an emergency room to document an arrhythmia can be avoided.

## THE PATIENT WITH VASCULAR DISEASE

The homebound patient with peripheral vascular disease is at risk for developing problems secondary to inactivity. Observations that may be needed are similar to those described for the cardiac patient above, including the following:

## Leg Pain

Where is the pain?
> One leg?
> Both legs?
> Calf only?
> Thigh? Back? Foot?

How far can the patient walk before pain develops?

Is pain relieved by stopping?

Does pain occur at rest?

Does pain occur when walking indoors or outdoors, or both?

## Swelling of Legs

Do the legs swell at the end of the day?

Is swelling present on arising in the morning?

What is the location of the swelling?
Right or left foot or both feet?
Right or left ankle or both ankles?
Right or left leg or both legs?

In addition, the patient or care partner may be asked to note the following:

Change in temperature of the extremity
Localized heat
Localized coolness

Pulses of each extremity

Change in color of an extremity
Redness
Bluish color
Pallor

Skin irritation, open areas

## THE PATIENT WITH GASTROINTESTINAL DISEASE

The homebound patient with gastrointestinal disease is, in many ways, easier to monitor than the cardiovascular patient because changes that would indicate potential problems are not usually so subtle. The patient and care partner might be instructed to observe any of the following items, for which the following outlines can be adapted as aids in reporting:

## Abdominal Pain

Where is the pain located?
Chest?
Upper abdomen or lower abdomen?
Near the umbilicus?
Left side or right side of abdomen?

Does it spread to the back?

Is it related to
Mealtimes?
Any particular foods?
Alcohol intake?

Does it occur at night, awakening patient from sleep?

Is pain relieved by
Food?
Milk?
Hot or cold liquids?
Antacids?

Is pain associated with, or followed by, diarrhea?

What does the pain feel like?
Burning?
Aching?
Cramping?
Tightness?
Knife-like?

## Change in Bowel Habits

How often does a bowel movement occur?

At what time of day do the bowel movements occur?

Any night-time bowel movements?

What color is the stool?
   Lighter than usual?
   Darker than usual?
   Black?

Is the stool soft, hard, watery?

Does it vary with food intake?
   Does milk or dairy product affect the bowels?

Is there any red blood in the stool?
   Is blood mixed with the stool?
   Is the entire stool red?
   Is the stool normal but with blood on toilet tissue?
   Is the stool normal but with blood in toilet bowl?

Is the stool malodorous?

Does the stool float or sink in toilet bowl?

## Difficulty in Swallowing

Is there any difficulty swallowing solid foods?

Is there any difficulty swallowing liquids?

Is there any pain on swallowing?

Does choking occur?

Is there any regurgitation of food?

Do you experience heartburn?

Do you belch?

Do you get hiccups?

In addition, the patient or care partner may be called on to record the following items:

   Food intake at each meal, particularly as related to symptoms

   Stool occult blood

   Daily weight

   Episodes of nausea

   Episodes of vomiting, including description of vomitus

   Fever

   Increased abdominal girth (note any change in belt size)

## THE PATIENT WITH DIABETES

The diabetic patient at home has many glucose monitoring needs. The old-fashioned urine glucose testing has been largely supplanted by fingerstick blood glucose measurements, particularly for those people with type I diabetes, but also for some people with type II diabetes.

Checking for the immediate effect of a particular diet change or insulin dose by blood glucose self-measurement gets the patient involved and deepens understanding of the intricacies of diabetic control more effectively than any lecture or class. The idea of puncturing fingers is not appealing, but the hesitancy is quickly abolished as the patient is won over to true partnership in treatment. The increase in safety is obvious, since the guesswork is eliminated and an answer is rapidly available as to whether malaise is due to hyperglycemia or hypoglycemia. Thus, the ability to initiate correction is literally in the patient's hands. Changing insulin dosage upward or downward, evaluating the effects of exercise on glucose control, documenting hypoglycemia and treating it promptly, adding or subtracting foods, all become as easily accomplished at home as in hospital, and actually become easier in many instances; the middlemen have been eliminated, so the sources of error are reduced.

Some diabetic patients wrongly assume that the symptoms of hypoglycemia or hyperglycemia are to be tolerated as part of the illness. They may not recognize these symptoms as indicating that something is wrong with their regimen. The following outline may help them to recognize the common manifestations and bring them to our attention:

## Symptoms of Hyperglycemia

Increase in thirst

Frequent urination

Slow healing

Skin infections

Vaginal itching

Pain or burning sensation on urination

Pain in the legs

Sleepiness

Decrease in energy level

Difficulty concentrating

Blurring of vision

Dryness of the lips

Dry skin

Weight loss

## Symptoms of Hypoglycemia

Weakness

Dizziness

Tingling of the lips or tongue

Headaches

Faintness or actual fainting

Nightmares

Cold sweats

Sudden awakening from sleep

Shakiness

Episodes of confusion

"Anxiety attacks"

Extreme hunger

## Symptoms of Either Hyperglycemia or Hypoglycemia

When does it occur?

What is its relation to the following?
Diet
Medication
Activity
Exercise

How often does it occur?

What relieves it?

## THE PATIENT WITH INFECTIOUS DISEASE

The person at home who has an infection, whether acute or chronic, requires close monitoring, since a subtle change may indicate a more serious problem. The patient or care partner may be instructed to look for any of the following:

### Wound or Skin Infection
Any drainage from the wound? If so, what color is the drainage?
    Colorless?
    Straw colored?
    Pink?
    Bloody?
    Yellow?
    Green?
    Pus?

Any odor at the wound?

Has any swelling appeared at or around the wound?

Does the wound have any redness?

Is the wound painful?

Has the size of the wound increased?

Is there any fever?

Is the wound warm?

### Respiratory Infection
Any cough?

Any sputum production?
    Color of the sputum?
    Amount of sputum?
    Tenacity of sputum?
    Blood in the sputum?

How many breaths are there per minute?

Is the breathing regular?

Any fever?

Is the throat sore?
    Does the throat look red?
    Do the tonsils appear enlarged?
    Do the lymph glands in the neck appear enlarged?

Any earache?

### Urinary Tract Infection
What is the color of the urine?
Is the urine clear or is it cloudy?
Does the urine have an odor?
How frequent is the need for urination?
Is there any pain on voiding?
Is there any pain in the back or flank?
Is there any abdominal pain?
Is the urine pink or bloody?
Any fever?

The patient or care partner should be made aware that an elderly or debilitated person may not experience fever in conjunction with an infection, so monitoring symptoms and signs as listed above becomes even more important in that instance. Other general, vague complaints that the family should note as possible signs of infection include

General malaise

Tiredness

Decreased appetite

Unexplained rise in blood glucose

Dizziness

Headache

The statement, "I just don't feel good."

A home care nurse or laboratory can be called on to go into the home to obtain blood samples or cultures of wound drainage, urine, or other secretions as indicated.

## THE PATIENT WITH UROLOGIC DISEASE

The homebound person with urologic disease may require monitoring of, and care for, an indwelling catheter, or may have a neuromuscular disorder that needs individualized instruction. Generally applicable observations include

Incontinence

Weight change

Dehydration

Flank pain

Pain on voiding

Increase or decrease of urine volume

Urinary frequency

Edema

Blood pressure

Urine dipsticks may be used by the patient or family to monitor urinary $p$H, blood protein, and nitrite in the same fashion that a diabetic patient is called on to monitor urinary glucose. In addition, they may need to strain the urine for stones or obtain clean-catch specimens for culture.

## THE PATIENT WITH RESPIRATORY DISEASE

Respiratory disease, like cardiovascular disease, can be very frightening to the patient and care partner, particularly when difficulties arise at night. Making regular observations brings a sense of control to the situation and helps to avoid panic. Therefore, it is beneficial for the family to have responsibility for the following determinations:

What is the rate of respirations?

Are the respirations regular?

Is the breathing deeper or more shallow than usual?

Is any wheezing heard?

Is there any cough?

Is it a dry cough?

Does the cough produce any sputum?
What is its color?
How much is produced?
What is its consistency?
Is any blood in the sputum?

Any fever?

Any chills?

Any shortness of breath?
What seems to provoke it?
What seems to relieve it?
Is it related to position?
Is it related to activity?

Any chest pain?
Where is it located?
Is it affected by deep breathing?
Is it affected by coughing?

Does the patient appear to have any cyanosis?

What is the patient's weight each day?

What is the pulse rate?

The patient or care partner may be called on to obtain sterile sputum samples. Although beyond the scope of this chapter, but applicable in special circumstances, the family may need to use an infant apnea monitor, watch for aspiration, or use tracheal suctioning, a respirator, or oxygen-delivery system. It may be helpful to have instruction in the Heimlich maneuver.

## THE PATIENT WITH NEUROLOGIC DISEASE

Neurologic illness presents a situation somewhat different from that associated with many other clinical disorders managed at home. The patient with neurologic disease is less likely to be aware of subjective symptoms; therefore, the care partner must be responsible for detecting and reporting changes. This puts a greater burden on the family for monitoring symptoms and signs. The following guidelines may be helpful:

### Speech
Is the patient able to speak?

Is the speech clear and intelligible?

Is there any slurring of speech?

Is there any hesitancy or seaching for the correct word?

Are there any mistakes of one word for another?

Is the speech garbled?

Is speech mainly in English or in a native language?

### Understanding
Does the patient reliably understand everything said?

Does the patient follow oral directions correctly?

Does the patient follow visual directions correctly?

### Gait
Is any assistance needed in walking?

Is balance good?

Is there any tendency to sway toward one side?

Is there any shuffling of feet?

Do the legs buckle on standing or walking?

Are the legs stiff?

Are the legs wider apart than usual in walking?

Is the stride longer or shorter than usual?

## Orientation

Does the patient know where he is?

Does the patient know the day, month, year?

Does the patient recognize you and visitors?

## Pupillary Reflexes

Are the pupils equal in size?

Do they constrict in response to light?

Are the pupils large (dilated) or narrow (constricted)?

## Motor Power

Is the grasp strong and equal in both hands?

Do both arms and both legs move appropriately?

Other items of importance include the description of seizure activity, changes in level of consciousness, alterations in vision, ability to swallow, and appropriateness of behavior.

## THE PATIENT WITH DEPRESSION

Monitoring the emotional health of the homebound patient is an important task relegated to the care partner, who is in the best position to provide early detection of signs of depression. To gather such information in systematic, reproducible fashion, the following lists of questions may be of help:

## Mood

Is the patient happy?

Is the patient sad?

Are moods constantly changing?

Are there abrupt changes in mood?

How is the "energy level"?

Are there spells of crying?

Does the patient appear

Angry?

Anxious?

Fearful?

Apprehensive?

Does the patient appear to have a feeling of panic?

Does the patient seem to feel a sense of guilt?

Does the patient appear mournful?

## Personality

Is the patient socializing?

Is the patient withdrawn?

Is the patient too talkative?

Does the patient joke appropriately?

Is there too much joking?

Does the patient seem aloof?

Is the patient very demanding?

Is the patient verbally abusive?

Does the patient seem too complaining?

Is the patient hostile?

### Activity

Is the patient physically active?

Is the patient hyperactive?

Is the patient inactive?

Does the patient sleep well?

Does the patient seem sleepier than usual?

Is the patient having difficulty falling asleep?

Is the sleep fitful?

Since it is so important to arrange intervention when depression is prolonged or serious, any talk of suicide must be considered reason for prompt professional action. In dealing with patients who have this as a potential problem, we should probe to determine whether the care partner has detected clues of worsening depression, such as giving away personal belongings, saying good-byes, discussions of death, or, paradoxically, sudden appearance of out-of-character happiness after a long episode of depression. Those must be considered possibly emergency situations demanding evaluation and intervention, with the patient not permitted to remain alone until a professional assessment has been made.

## CONCLUSION

The goal of home monitoring is to have the patient and care partner be aware of problems that may arise in the future. They should be taught the ritual of systematic observation. By recognizing, recording, and reporting changes regularly, they can avoid being in the position of overlooking what would otherwise be unexpected findings that may signify important new developments. To accomplish this goal, we need to think of the people at home as extensions of ourselves and to simplify our instructions so that the family can understand (1) who will be responsible for the monitoring, (2) who will do the teaching, (3) what observations will be made, (4) when the observations should be made, (5) how the observations will be made, (6) why the observations are necessary, and (7) what the observer should do with the information obtained.

The disadvantages of monitoring in the home are significant. The monitoring may be less accurate than that performed by professionals. It may be neglected in the pressures of day-to-day responsibilities. Communication with the physician may be a problem unless a mechanism is clearly outlined. More physician time is consumed by communicating with the patient and family and assuring that the education has been sufficient to ensure that the data are representative and correct.

Those disadvantages are more than outweighed by the definite advantages. The records produced are indicative of actual daily conditions, not artificial situations (as in diet-restricted and activity-restricted hospitalized patients). As the patient and care partner become more involved, deeper understanding of the treatment regimen makes informed decision-making achievable. A conscientious observer feels "in control" and becomes a real partner in care.

# 12

# Cardiac Disease

LISA E. BABITZ
MARTIN L. KAHN

Cardiac care is usually envisioned as a high-technology endeavor requiring the sophisticated environment of an intensive-care unit. However, once the disease is identified and the associated problems are defined, careful planning can facilitate stabilization and maintenance of even the very tenuous cardiac patient in the home setting. Although skillful home care may require some extra effort on the part of the physician, the incentives in terms of shortening acute hospitalizations and minimizing the frequency of readmissions are readily apparent in today's economic climate. A physician knowledgeable in home care can design a package of support services and equipment that can provide the necessary close monitoring of potentially life-threatening conditions without requiring an overwhelming burden of home or office visits.

Determination of home care needs is best approached by evaluating the signs and symptoms manifested by the individual patient as well as the prognostic and risk factors attendant to the specific cardiac diagnosis and underlying state of health. It is beyond the scope of this text to address the diagnosis and acute management of the compendium of cardiac diseases. Rather, we will approach our discussion from the standpoint of the problems common to a broad spectrum of cardiac diseases. These include congestive heart failure, low cardiac output syndromes, angina, arrhythmias, and thromboembolic disease. Each discussion will commence with hospital discharge and focus on initial planning as well as follow-up requirements.

## CONGESTIVE HEART FAILURE

### DISCHARGE PLANNING

#### Education
The key to optimal management of congestive heart failure is education of the patient and the care givers. An uninformed patient is likely to be a noncompliant one. Prior to discharge, the physician should initiate a discussion of the need to avoid volume overload by careful diet and faithful medication compliance. This discussion can then be reinforced by the nursing staff and dietitians.

#### Diet
Although most physicians recognize the need for some degree of sodium restriction in their congestive failure patients, many are unprepared to answer the myriad of questions that can arise. Patients and care partners often require advice on a meal-by-meal basis,

making their education a time-consuming task. Most hospitals have a clinical nutritionist or dietitian on staff who specializes in patient education and is accustomed to reviewing diets and dietary questions. These services should be routinely requested in all newly diagnosed cardiac patients. If dietary consultation is unavailable, the physician can provide his patient with an exhaustive variety of pamphlets that detail practical approaches to the salt-restricted diet. The following are resources for patient education pamphlets about sodium-restricted diets:

Consumer Information Center
Dept. EE
Pueblo, CO 81009

American Heart Association
7320 Greenville Avenue
Dallas, TX 75231

Sodium, HFE-88
U.S. Department of Health and Human Services
Public Health Service
Food and Drug Administration
5600 Fishers Lane
Rockville, MD 20857

While discussing sodium restriction, the physician should introduce the topic of salt substitutes. Many of the commercially available products contain potassium salts; patients with a moderate degree of renal failure and those already on potassium replacement or potassium-sparing diuretics should be cautioned against those salt substitutes or need to have serum levels carefully monitored while using them. Nonpotassium salt substitutes derived from herbal seasoning combinations can be found on the market or can be home-made, following recipes in the dietary pamphlets.

Education alone is not sufficient to ensure compliance. The dietary regimen should be modified to meet the patient's needs and abilities. A severe salt restriction is likely to be ignored if the food is unpalatable. Likewise, some authorities now believe that intensive salt restriction can lead to hyponatremia in certain geriatric patients.[1] In general, a no-salt-added diet of 4 g of sodium daily is sufficient in many congestive failure patients, with more severe sodium-restricted diets (1 g–2 g) reserved for the most refractory individuals.

Severe congestive failure may also mandate fluid restriction in order to avoid dilutional hyponatremia and volume overload. By starting with a daily fluid allowance of between 1200 ml and 1500 ml (240 ml = 8-oz cup) and titrating according to serum sodium measurements and daily weights, an appropriate fluid guideline can be established for the individual patient. Careful monitoring and recording of daily fluid intake and urinary output will be necessary. Fluids for consumption can be measured in standard household measuring cups, and toilets can be equipped with calibrated collection containers. Compliance can be encouraged by discussing techniques for thirst management with your patient; these include chewing gum and lozenges.

Appropriate supportive resources can also improve compliance. A homebound person who normally prepares meals from canned foods or orders fast-food delivery may need assistance with shopping or meal preparation in order to restructure the diet. If no family care partners are available, home health-aide services may be required.

### Activity

Congestive heart failure *per se* requires no particular activity prescription; rather, limitations will be determined by the patient's underlying cardiac diagnosis and condition. During periods of severe decompensation bedrest is felt to be beneficial. Since patients with severe congestive failure may have an increased risk of thromboembolic disease, prophylactic mini-dose heparin (5000 units subcutaneously bid) should be instituted upon initiation of bedrest. The patient or care partner can be instructed in administration techniques either prior to hospital discharge or by a visiting home care nurse. For the visually impaired, the visiting home care nurse can prefill syringes on a weekly basis.

After an acute hospitalization, a patient is likely to be deconditioned and the more elderly patients may be bedbound. All patients should be encouraged to ambulate as early in the hospitalization as feasible in order to minimize thromboembolic complications and to regain muscle tone. The geriatric patient with his decreased muscle mass[2] may require a physical therapy consultation for supervision and safe progression toward the premorbid level of mobility. In fact, physical therapy for passive range of motion can be begun at the bedside in the coronary care unit to avoid contractures and loss of mobility in the arthritic or frail elderly. Physical therapists can also assist the physician in assessing what mobilization aids a patient might require in terms of crutches, canes, walkers, braces, and orthopedic shoes.

In those situations where a patient is medically ready for discharge but still has not attained the expected degree of mobility, home physical therapy is available on a short-term basis. This service is generally provided through the same agencies that provide visiting nurse services and is financed in much the same manner. When prescribing home physical therapy, the physician will be expected to specify the therapeutic goal; consultation with the in-hospital therapist who has worked with the patient can often provide the realistic prognosis and expected duration of treatment. If such advice is unavailable, as in the situation in which the physical therapy is initiated in the home setting, the premorbid level of functioning can be used as a guideline for prognosis. In general, any active exercise program prescribed for a cardiac patient must start slowly and progress gradually with careful pulse and blood pressure monitoring. The home physical therapist generally makes only a few home visits but trains the care partner and the patient in the necessary daily exercises. Physician encouragement may improve patient participation.

### Medications

The in-hospital medication regimen required to stabilize a patient must be simplified as much as possible prior to discharge in order to encourage compliance. By consulting the nursing staff, the physician can be alerted to difficult schedules, such as a 2 AM dose, and revise the schedule to fit the patient's waking hours. For patients with cognitive difficulties or those who are bedbound, doses can be timed to fit the hours when a care partner is present to assist with preparation or administration. If medically acceptable, once-a-day or twice-a-day medications can decrease the frequency of "missed" doses. Written charts, coordinating doses with daily events such as meals or bedtime, can assist the memory (see Sample Daily Medication Chart). Such charts can be preprinted, with details filled in on a case-by-case basis.

For patients unable to read the prescription label due to illiteracy, foreign language, or visual deficits, pill samples can be glued to the medication chart to facilitate identification.

### SAMPLE DAILY MEDICATION CHART

| | Time: Breakfast (8 AM) | Lunch (noon) | Dinner (5 PM) | Bedtime (9 PM) |
|---|---|---|---|---|
| Medication: | | | | |
| Digoxin | X | | | |
| Furosemide | X | | | |
| Isosorbide dinitrate | X | X | X | X |

Patients with severe visual impairment or moderate cognitive deficits might be capable of self-administration if a care partner sets out the scheduled doses in a compartmentalized box such that each compartment represents a different medication interval. Compartmentalized pillboxes are available at pharmacies, but even hardware storage boxes can be adapted. Pillboxes with built-in alarms are even available.

Nursing staff frequently assists with discharge medication instructions, including medication charts, particularly when alerted to the need by the physician. In those situations where the patient may require initial supervision or assistance with preparation of medications, a visiting home care nurse service referral can be made. Although the home care nurse cannot be present to administer all of the required doses, he or she can visit once or twice weekly to review instructions and set aside designated doses to be self-administered at later times. The visiting home care nurse can also provide intramuscular injections when required on an infrequent basis. (A more detailed discussion of the visiting home care nurse service is presented under Home Management below.)

## HOME MANAGEMENT

Once the cardiac patient has left the hospital, optimal recuperation and health maintenance are dependent on the quality of the support systems available to him and the knowledge of how to utilize them properly. The necessary manpower and equipment must be tailored to the individual, ideally through foresighted planning prior to discharge.

The health-care team for the homebound patient consists, at a minimum, of the patient and the physician. If the patient is capable of self-sufficiency in attending to the activities of daily living (hygiene, dressing, meal preparation, cleaning, *etc.*), is able to follow physician instructions, and is medically stable enough to require infrequent physician visits, this limited team may be adequate. The homebound patient can be assisted in self-sufficiency by the availability of such services as grocery and pharmacy deliveries and Meals-on-Wheels, a subsidized hot meal delivery occurring weekdays, except holidays. An occupational therapist, available through the rehabilitation or physical therapy department of many hospitals or home care vendors, can recommend modifications of the home environment and special equipment to facilitate self-sufficiency in the physically disabled.

The crucial factor for the isolated homebound patient is a means to communicate in an emergency; a telephone is optimal but a brief daily visit from a concerned friend or neighbor might suffice. Telephones can be adapted for those with visual or auditory impairments. Outreach programs are available in certain communities whereby a homebound individual is telephoned every day. If the person fails to respond, a designated contact person or emergency service is contacted. Certain programs equip patients with an alarm device to wear; when triggered by the patient in an emergency, a central switchboard is signaled and can institute a response protocol. A social worker can best advise on the available resources in your community.

Patients who are unable to meet all of their care needs may require the health-care team to be expanded to include one or more care givers; the type of care necessary will determine the composition of the team. Skilled nursing tasks require the services of a nurse unless a family member can be trained to do these tasks, under skilled nursing supervision. Unskilled health-care tasks and assistance with activities of daily living can be assumed by a family member or a home health aide, depending on available manpower and financial resources.

The visiting home care nurse service provides skilled nursing services on an intermittent care basis. In the context of a patient with congestive heart failure, the home care nurse could monitor weight and vital signs, auscultate lungs, counsel regarding medication and dietary regimens, and notify the physician by telephone of any acute change in conditions that might require intervention. In addition, the home care nurse can initiate appropriate intervention, on a physician's orders, such as medication adjustment or intramuscular furosemide. Since the visits are seldom more frequent than once or twice weekly, except in situations of acute, short-term need, a patient requiring more frequent services might need a private duty nurse or a skilled nursing facility. Sometimes a family care partner can be trained by the nurse to perform certain skilled nursing tasks. Home health aides are usually not permitted to perform skilled nursing chores.

### Home Monitoring

The crucial signs to monitor in the homebound congestive heart failure patient are weight, pulse, blood pressure and respiratory rate, pedal edema, and rales. The crucial symptoms are dyspnea, orthopnea, malaise, decreased appetite, and change in anginal pattern. The key to successful home care is to be able to monitor these signs and symptoms from a distance via reliable observers (patient, care partners, and nurses), with physician home visits kept to a manageable frequency or reserved for crises.

All patients and care partners should be apprised of their ideal or "dry" weight, usually established during the acute hospitalization. At discharge, their home should be equipped with a scale and they should be encouraged to obtain and record daily weights. For greatest reliability of measurements, weight should be recorded at the same time each day. Bed-bound patients can be weighed on a chair scale or sling device but these might be too costly or unwieldy for most home environments. With improved nutrition after the acute illness, some slight weight gain should be anticipated. However, the patient or care partner should report any steady or rapid weight gain to the physician. The physician can then assess the significance (fluid versus fat) in the context of the other signs and symptoms. If the weight gain is in excess of 2 lb per week or is accompanied by edema, rales, or orthopnea, suggestive of congestive failure, the diuretic dosage should be increased until the dry weight is achieved. At the same time, the dietary regimen should be reviewed to ensure that dietary indiscretion was not the origin of the fluid gain.

Weight loss in excess of the established dry weight is an ominous sign and should also be reported to the physician. Such loss may result from excessive diuresis or "cardiac cachexia," a potentially terminal condition. By reviewing medication regimens, serum electrolytes, blood urea nitrogen, and dietary intake, the probable cause can be determined and addressed. Remember that many medications, even when present at levels within the therapeutic range, may cause anorexia.[3] Compromise may have to be made between clinical volume status and liberalizing the diet if cardiac cachexia supervenes.

Pulse, respiratory rate, and blood pressure can be monitored by a trained care partner, but pulmonary auscultation is usually reserved for the home care nurse. The physician should be notified of any tachycardia, tachypnea, or rales and, again, should assess them in the clinical context in order to determine a course of action. Gradual onset of tachycardia, tachypnea, or rales accompanied by weight gain may be treatable by increasing the diuretic dosage. If the tachypnea is marked, an intramuscular dosage of furosemide, administered by the visiting home care nurse, may provide relief within 15 minutes. The time of onset of an oral dose is approximately 1 hour. When intramuscular administration is unfeasible, liquid preparations of furosemide may provide a rapid onset of action, usually within 15 to 30 minutes.

Sudden onset of tachycardia may require an electrocardiogram to assess for arrhythmia, particularly in a patient with no prior history of tachyarrhythmias. If the home is not equipped with a transducer to transmit an electrocardiogram over the telephone, an office visit may be required. Certain commercial laboratories will perform electrocardiograms in the home. The currently marketed transtelephonic electrocardiograms transmit only one lead and therefore are only appropriate for determining rate and rhythm. Sudden onset of tachypnea and dyspnea may represent arrhythmic or ischemic acute myocardial dysfunction, pulmonary embolism, or pneumonia. This differential requires an electrocardiogram, as well as cardiac and pulmonic auscultation by the physician, (*i.e.,* a home visit). Abnormalities in the latter may suggest the need for a chest x-ray, a procedure requiring departure from the home.

Gradually progressive orthopnea can be treated at home with diuretic adjustment. Patients with severe congestive heart failure and chronic orthopnea may require a mechanized "hospital" bed for elevation of head and feet if adjustment of their regular mattress is insufficient. The cost of a hospital bed can be covered by both Medicaid and Medicare when prescribed by a physician. Patients with chronic hypoxia or those who become acutely hypoxic with exacerbations of congestive heart failure may benefit from home oxygen if their condition does not otherwise require hospitalization. Oxygen is also covered by Medicaid and Medicare, if the room air $pO_2$ is less then 55 mm Hg. A caveat: home oxygen should not be instituted in hypercapneic patients unless a safe flow rate that does not depress the respiratory drive is established under closely monitored hospital conditions.

## *Medication Monitoring*

Patients with congestive heart failure who are on diuretics will need periodic electrolyte, blood urea nitrogen (BUN), and creatinine measurements to evaluate for potassium depletion, hyponatremia, and prerenal dehydration. Patients on digitalis compounds will require periodic monitoring of serum levels, particularly whenever there is an alteration in renal function (digoxin clearance), hepatic function (digitoxin clearance), or the addition of medications, such as quinidine and verapamil. In addition to routine periodic screening, episodes of anorexia, nausea, decreased oral intake, generalized malaise, arrhythmias, and exacerbations of congestive failure are all indications for blood testing. Digitalis has been associated with delirium in elderly patients, even at nontoxic levels.[3]

## LOW CARDIAC OUTPUT SYNDROMES

Low cardiac output can be caused by a variety of cardiac diseases, including valvular dysfunction, cardiomyopathies, and chronic arrhythmias. Management of the homebound patient with low cardiac output requires careful attention to any signs and symptoms suggestive of inadequate perfusion of the head, kidneys, or extremities.

## DISCHARGE PLANNING

### *Education*

The patient and care partner should be made aware of the nature of the cardiac condition that will cause periods of inadequate perfusion and understand how these episodes might be manifested. They must understand the reasoning behind restrictions in physical activity so that they do not try to overexert beyond the capabilities of the already limited cardiac output.

Due to the complexity of the regimens required and the numerous potential complications, the patient or care partner should be taught to keep accurate daily records, including weights, vital signs, fluid intake and output, medications, and laboratory test results. In addition to assisting the physician, this home "charting" may play a psychological role by lessening the sense of helplessness.

### *Diet*

Dietary restrictions will depend on the concomitant cardiac conditions. In general, diets must balance the inability of the heart to handle large volume loads against the tendency to further decrease the cardiac output by decreasing preload volume from dehydration. Optimal volume requirements can be established in the hospital setting, particularly during pulmonary artery pressure monitoring of intracardiac pressures. Translating these volumes into dietary sodium and fluid restrictions may require multiple readjustments while monitoring BUN and creatinine measurements of renal perfusion, systemic blood pressure, peripheral perfusion, and symptoms of fatigue and dyspnea. Requirements may fluctuate with the patient's underlying condition and degree of activity. Because of the tenuous nature of this condition, the homebound patient is likely to require assistance in maintaining a strict diet, particularly if easy fatigability is a prominent feature.

### Activity

The patient and the care partner must be educated in regard to any limitations on physical activity posed by the low cardiac output. Guidelines can be established prior to discharge by either progressive physical therapy with vital sign monitoring or submaximal exercise stress testing. Symptoms of excessive fatigue, inadequate cerebral perfusion, claudication, dyspnea, or angina suggest functional limitations. Severe functional limitations, to the extent that the patient may be unable to perform activities of daily living, mandate home assistance.

### Medications

The patient with low cardiac output can be managed on a variety of medications, including the diuretic and ionotropic preparations mentioned in the discussion of congestive heart failure, earlier in this chapter. Afterload-reducing agents may be of particular benefit to these patients in improving renal and peripheral perfusion. Afterload-reducing agents include the vasodilators, such as hydralazine. Captopril and prazosin perform both afterload and preload reduction. Nitrates are predominantly preload reducers.

Afterload-reducing agents should be begun at low doses with close attention to pulse and blood pressure. This is best initiated prior to discharge from the hospital, but can be done in the home setting with home care nurse monitoring. The increase in pulse rate often encountered with these medications is not usually a problem with the patient who is already mustering all cardiac reserves to offset the marginal cardiac output. However, these patients often have very low baseline pressures and therefore any further reduction in blood pressures may be detrimental. In general, we would not start an afterload-reducing agent or increase the dosage in any patient with a systolic blood pressure less than 110 mm Hg or a resting pulse of greater than 100 beats per minute. If the systolic blood pressure falls to less than 100 mm Hg during therapy, the medication should be discontinued.

The medication dosage can be gradually increased until the desired effect, improvement in symptoms or reduction in BUN, is accomplished. Each dosage increment requires close monitoring of vital signs. In those patients with severely impaired cardiac output, optimal medication adjustment may best be accomplished in the hospital under pulmonary artery pressure monitoring to assess precise preload and afterload requirements.

### HOME MANAGEMENT

The patient impaired by low cardiac output is likely to require assistance with household chores as well as monitoring the disease process, particularly if poor cerebral perfusion or exertional fatigue is a prominent feature.

Care partners should follow the patient's blood pressure, pulse, and weight on a daily basis. Hypotension, tachycardia, and weight gain can all be evidence of worsening cardiac output and should be reported to the physician; the physician must set individualized guidelines for these parameters. Asymptomatic hypotension can be managed in the home setting by medication adjustment while monitoring the electrocardiogram and BUN and creatinine on a daily basis to detect any evidence of inadequate renal or coronary perfusion. Such evidence would be strong provocation for hospitalization so that inotropic therapy could be instituted under invasive monitoring conditions. Likewise, hypotension accompanied by syncope, presyncope, angina, or cerebral insufficiency requires immediate hospitalization.

Tachycardia requires an electrocardiogram to assess rhythm. Sinus tachycardia may suggest a chronotropic response to further deterioration of cardiac output, excessive afterload reduction, or volume depletion. A physician's home visit for examination will be required to assess these possibilities. Volume depletion can be restored by liberalizing fluid intake or reducing diuretic dosage. The dosage of the afterload-reducing agent can be gradually reduced until the tachycardia resolves. In the face of an unchanged electrocardiogram with no evidence for recent infarction, a new decline in cardiac performance is suggested by a drop in blood pressure, a new gallop, new onset of resting sinus tachycardia, elevation of jugular venous pressure, new onset of peripheral edema, or rales. Such a decline in cardiac function may require readjustment of the entire therapeutic regimen to meet the requirements of the new cardiac condition.

Weight gain suggestive of fluid retention might be from excessive sodium or water intake or from decreased renal perfusion. Review of the BUN and creatinine can help distinguish these two etiologies. An increased BUN and creatinine may respond to more afterload reduction. A stable or decreased BUN accompanied by weight gain may suggest the need for gentle diuresis and stricter dietary compliance. Vigorous diuresis in the home setting is dangerous in the low cardiac output patient due to the tenuous perfusion and the inherent risks of further diminution of cardiac output by compromising preload; it should therefore be avoided. Cautious home diuresis is accomplished with very gradual diuretic dosage increments while monitoring daily supine and sitting blood pressures, daily weights, and every-other-day BUN, creatinine, and electrolytes. Significant orthostatic hypotension or a weight loss of more than 1 lb per day requires slowing of the rate of diuresis.

The patient and the care partner should be familiar with the symptoms of worsening ventricular performance and report them to the physician. In addition to those detailed in the section on congestive heart failure, they include decreased exercise tolerance, change in anginal pattern, intermittent confusion or neurologic deficits, worsening claudication or peripheral cyanosis, and symptoms of uremia, such as malaise, anorexia, and nausea. Occurrence of any of these symptoms requires a physician examination, electrocardiogram, and blood tests for electrolytes, BUN, creatinine, and digitalis levels. Consideration should be given to other underlying conditions, such as infection, which might compromise an already limited cardiac performance. Infarction, unstable angina, inadequate cerebral or peripheral perfusion, symptomatic uremia, and digitalis toxic rhythms, including high degrees of atrioventricular block and ventricular tachycardia, all require evaluation for hospitalization. Other etiologies might be remediable in the home setting with adjustment of medication or diet; however, in the very tenuous patient, hospitalization is recommended.

## ANGINA

### DISCHARGE PLANNING
*Education*

The patient with angina should be taught, in terms tailored to his understanding, what angina represents, what causes it, what it can lead to, and what can be done to alleviate it. Although he may initially feel overwhelmed and helpless, particularly after an acute infarction, he should be made to understand that he can influence his own illness by modification of his behavior and life-style. The influence of cigarette smoking, diet, emotional stress, exercise, hypertension, and diabetic control should all be reviewed. Although the homebound patient is unlikely to be preoccupied with returning to work, he will be concerned about prognosis and limitations.

Many hospitals have patient education programs, which can begin as early as on admission to the coronary care unit. If such a program is unavailable, or supplementary to it, educational pamphlets can be provided for the patient and care partner. The American Heart Association is one of many resources for obtaining such material. Nursing staff and dietitians can review particulars regarding medications and diet, as well as general patient questions. However, the patient is more likely to engage in life-style modification if it is reinforced by the physician.

### Diet

Most physicians encourage their angina patients to follow a fat-controlled, low-cholesterol diet. In addition to utilizing the skills of the hospital nutritionist for patient education, many pamphlets are available from the American Heart Association and other sources. Do not neglect to discuss the adverse effects of excessive caffeine intake and review what substances contain it; coffee and tea are obvious sources but many patients are unaware that chocolates and many soft drinks also contain caffeine.

### Activity

The proper activity prescription for postinfarction patients has been detailed in multiple cardiology texts and is beyond the scope of this chapter. Most homebound patients are not engaging in vigorous exercise such as jogging or returning to work; nevertheless, they require guidelines tailored to their anginal pattern and premorbid level of functioning. Physical therapy with vital sign monitoring early in the hospitalization can help to establish functional activity guidelines. Submaximal stress testing may better delineate activity prescriptions for the more active homebound patient. The physician should not neglect to counsel the patient on such issues as sexual activity and the need to avoid isometric exercise such as weight lifting (heavy groceries, laundry, furniture). Activity restrictions may require a previously independent homebound individual to obtain assistance in the home.

### Medications

The commonly used antianginal agents (nitrates, beta-blockers, and calcium channel antagonists) should be employed in the simplest possible regimen required to maximize angina-free exertion. Complex regimens requiring doses more frequently than four times a day are likely to be forgotten by all but the most compulsive patient. The patient should be taught to use sublingual nitroglycerin tablets only when seated or supine in order to avoid the induction of syncope and falls; this is particularly dangerous for the isolated homebound and the elderly osteoporotic patient. Long-acting oral capsules of isosorbide dinitrate may not be well absorbed by the elderly patient with gastric hypoacidity. Beta-blockade may be unattainable in the elderly patient[4] and side-effects such as fatigue or confusion may supervene. Calcium channel antagonists have also been associated with confusion in the elderly.

## HOME MANAGEMENT

The homebound angina patient has a built-in warning system when his condition is becoming decompensated—worsening angina with respect to frequency, duration, intensity, and unprovoked pain. The patient and care partner must be aware of the particular manifestations of the individual's anginal syndrome and should alert the physician to a change in pattern. They must also be taught to call an ambulance directly for prolonged angina unrelieved by nitroglycerin, particularly when accompanied by nausea, diaphoresis, palpitations, or presyncope.

Patients on beta blockers should be taught to check their pulse rates daily and report bradycardia, particularly when symptomatic, to the physician. Any pulse irregularity should be confirmed by an apical pulse. Patients on nitrates should have blood pressure determinations, particularly after a dosage is increased. Automatic sphygmomanometers with digital readouts are available for those unable to manipulate manual pumps and stethoscopes. Visiting home care nurses can also monitor vital sign responses to medication adjustments.

## ARRHYTHMIAS

## DISCHARGE PLANNING

Many arrhythmias accompanied by cardiovascular compromise require stabilization in a hospital setting. Once corrected or controlled, the patient will be discharged on a variety of medications to prevent recurrence. Adequate home management requires strict medication compliance and close rate and rhythm monitoring. Discharge planning for the home-bound must include provision for periodic in-home electrocardiograms, either by telephone transmission or home visits by a commercial laboratory.

### Education

The patient should be familiar with the symptoms that herald his arrhythmia and have emergency assistance telephone numbers readily available. It is also valuable to have the patient carry a card detailing what maneuvers were successful in controlling his arrhythmia in the past. The necessity for medication compliance must be stressed, but he should also be informed of the common side-effects and encouraged to notify the physician about difficulties prior to discontinuing a medication.

### Diet

Substances felt to exacerbate a particular arrhythmia should be avoided. These might include caffeine for a patient prone to paroxysmal atrial tachycardia or alcohol for a patient with alcoholic cardiomyopathy. Patients on diuretics should be counseled to maintain adequate potassium intake.

### Activity

If certain activities predispose a patient to an arrhythmia, he should either be cautioned to avoid them or be advised on appropriate prophylaxis.

## HOME MONITORING

The patient or care partner should monitor the pulse daily and whenever the patient experiences presyncope, palpitations, or any other manifestations associated with arrhythmic episodes. The physician should be notified immediately of any suspected irregularities of pulse or any typical symptoms. In situations of syncope, presyncope, chest pain, or history of ventricular tachycardia, the care partner or patient should alert an emergency ambulance immediately and afterwards call the physician. Patients with particularly unstable arrhythmias who live alone would be excellent candidates for the self-triggered alarm devices discussed earlier in this chapter.

### Home Treatment

If an arrhythmia responds readily to carotid sinus massage or Valsalva maneuver, the patient and care partner can be taught these techniques with the proviso that if they do not work immediately, assistance must be summoned. If exacerbation of an arrhythmia is unaccompanied by symptoms of cardiovascular compromise, the physician may be able to make the appropriate medication adjustments in the home setting. For example, in a patient with an increased ventricular rate and chronic atrial fibrillation, an increased digitalis dosage may return the rate to an acceptable range. An intervention done in the home does, however, require a physician visit to assess accurately for signs of compromise.

In patients requiring medication adjustments for poorly controlled arrhythmias, Holter monitors can be applied in the home and used to assess the efficacy of the therapy.

## PACEMAKERS

### DISCHARGE PLANNING
*Education*

Both the patient and physician should become familiar with the type of pacemaker implanted, the initial rate setting, and the recommended monitoring protocol. The patient should be alerted to the recommendations for antibiotic prophylaxis during dental and invasive procedures as well as the need to avoid magnetic fields and microwaves.

### HOME MANAGEMENT

Initially, the physician and patient should be vigilant for evidence of local infections at the surgical site, inappropriate stimulation of skeletal muscle inducing chest wall contractions or hiccoughs, and pacer failure resulting in recurrence of the original presenting symptoms. Afterwards, at intervals dictated by the particular device, the pacer must be evaluated for battery charge, appropriate sensing, and appropriate capture.

The pacemaker rate changes as a function of battery voltage; therefore, graphing the rate over time since implantation yields a visual depiction of the decay of battery charge. Any sudden drop in rate suggests impending failure and demands close surveillance or replacement. The rate of a "fixed-rate" pacemaker can be determined by simply counting the spikes on the electrocardiogram. However, in a "demand-mode" pacemaker, the pacer impulse rate may not be apparent unless the patient's intrinsic heart rate is below the sensing setpoint. For the purpose of rate determination, the demand-mode can be temporarily converted to a "fixed-rate" mode by placing a magnet over the pacemaker. Homebound patients can be equipped with a telephone transducer that converts the electrical pacemaker impulses into sound tones for transmission to the medical facility for rate measurement.

## THROMBOEMBOLIC DISEASE

Several cardiac conditions, including valvular disease, severe cardiomyopathy, and unstable arrhythmias, carry a risk of thromboembolism. Warfarin anticoagulation, with its requirement for close monitoring, requires painstaking discharge planning for the homebound patient.

### DISCHARGE PLANNING
*Education*

The patient must be made aware of the reasons for anticoagulation and the effect that it will have on his blood clotting. The need for close monitoring with blood tests must be emphasized, as well as the need for rigorous compliance. The potential for interactions with other medications must be stressed and the patient should be particularly warned against self-medication with aspirin, nonsteroidal anti-inflammatory agents, and over-the-counter cold remedies.

## Diet

The patient should be counseled to avoid fluctuations in consumption of green leafy vegetables and other foods rich in vitamin K once his warfarin requirements have been established. Remember that a multiple vitamin preparation can be a surreptitious source of vitamin K. Alcohol intake should be restricted.

## HOME MANAGEMENT

Home monitoring can be facilitated by having the patient keep a diary of medication doses and prothrombin times. The patient should always take his medication at night so that prothrombin times can be obtained in the mornings. Many commercial laboratories will make home visits to obtain prothrombin times.

In general the prothrombin time should be kept toward the lower end of the therapeutic range, approximately one and one-half times control, in order to minimize bleeding complications. Any alteration in warfarin dose should be followed by a prothrombin time measurement three days afterward to assess its effect. After discharge from the hospital, a prothrombin time should be checked at least twice in the first week to ensure that it is stable on outpatient regimens. Thereafter, it can be checked once a week until stable and eventually on an every-other-week basis. Any addition of medication, such as antibiotics, to a patient's regimen requires an evaluation of prothrombin time to assess for interaction with the anticoagulant.

## REFERENCES

1. Franklin SS: Geriatric hypertension. Med Clin North Am 67(2):402, 1983
2. Adams GF: Essentials of Geriatric Medicine, 2nd ed, p 14. Oxford, Oxford University Press, 1981
3. Goldberg PB, Roberts J: Rational drug regimens for the elderly patient. Med Clin North Am 67(2):323, 1983
4. Franklin SS: Geriatric hypertension. Med Clin North Am 67(2):412, 1983

# 13

# Bladder Management

PABLO A. MORALES
EDUARDO M. FARCON
JOHN WHELAN

Home care of the patient who leaves the hospital with uncontrolled urinary leakage, inability to void or completely empty the bladder, or dependence on catheters, urinary collecting appliances, or prosthetic devices can pose an overwhelming problem for the patient, family, and nurses. Failure to cope with such difficulties can lead to social unacceptability, loss of employment opportunities, and, at worst, deterioration of the urinary tract.

Planning for home management should begin before the patient leaves the hospital. The patient should be familiarized with the measures that will have to be continued after hospital discharge. The family's willingness to participate in the continued care should be clarified and their capability to administer such care verified. If the family cannot assume the responsibility, arrangements should be made for assistance from other health-care providers.

This chapter will discuss the common diseases causing bladder disturbances that require continued care after the patient leaves the hospital environment and provide guidelines to aid in the implementation of the treatment modalities that will have to be continued at home. Likewise, we will address urinary problems of the home patient, the largest group that does not necessarily need hospitalization. In fact, this is our largest audience.

## DISEASES OF THE BRAIN

### CEREBROVASCULAR DISEASE

Occlusive cerebrovascular disease can affect neurons in the cerebrum or brain stem concerned with urinary bladder innervation. The most common bladder symptoms are frequency, urgency, and urge incontinence. Voiding usually occurs in a coordinated manner, that is, the urethral sphincters relax during detrusor contraction, the normal physiologic response to bladder distention.

Management is usually with anticholinergic drugs combined with intermittent catheterization if needed. If incontinence persists, despite pharmacologic agents and intermittent self-catheterization, condom catheters may be used for men and undergarments with absorptive lining for women. Many of the elderly men with this disease have enlarged prostate glands and may need transurethral resection of the prostate to improve bladder emptying if retention persists.

## PARKINSON'S DISEASE

Patients with Parkinson's disease, with loss of function of the basal ganglia, develop frequency, urgency, and urge incontinence. A number of these elderly patients also have prostatic enlargement, and urinary retention can be easily precipitated by the administration of L-dopa and other antiparkinsonian drugs. Because these patients may not verbalize their symptoms, you should routinely inquire about retention and, if appropriate, measure post-void residuals.

Anticholinergic drugs are usually helpful; surgical relief of prostatic obstruction may be needed to improve bladder emptying.

## BRAIN TUMOR

Bladder disturbance can occur in patients with brain tumors in certain locations, specifically the paracentral lobule. The urinary symptoms include frequency, urgency, and urge incontinence. Anticholinergic drugs are usually prescribed to alleviate the symptoms.

## DEMENTIA

The etiology of dementia includes aging, severe head injury, or encephalitis. Presenile dementia may result from Alzheimer's disease, normal pressure hydrocephalus, and syphilis. Urinary frequency, urgency, and urge incontinence are the usual bladder manifestations in this large group of patients. The incontinence may be due to direct involvement of the cerebrocortical areas concerned with bladder control or may be due to inattention to personal hygiene and inability to physically move to the toilet.

Condom catheters are usually satisfactory for men, and undergarments with absorptive lining for women, although indwelling catheter drainage is an option, especially for women. Anticholinergic medications to treat the frequency and urgency should be avoided.

## MULTIPLE SCLEROSIS

Up to 90% of patients with multiple sclerosis will sooner or later show signs of bladder involvement. The clinical course of multiple sclerosis is often characterized by remissions and exacerbations, but the urinary symptoms are usually progressive. Demyelinization of localized patches of white matter located in proximity to cortical and subcortical areas controlling the bladder and in the lateral and posterior columns of the spinal tract give rise to a variety of symptoms such as frequency, urgency, urge incontinence, hesitancy, and complete or partial urinary retention.

The treatment is symptomatic and includes anticholinergics, alpha blocking agents, polysynaptic blocking drugs, and intermittent catheterization. If this is not successful in achieving control, indwelling catheter drainage may be necessary for some female patients. A more aggressive approach is intestinal conduit urinary diversion which may benefit some good risk patients. Absorptive undergarments and condom catheters can be of help in other situations. The artificial urinary sphincter and external sphincterotomy, however, are rarely indicated in multiple sclerosis.

## DISEASES OF THE SPINAL CORD

### SPINAL CORD INJURY

The type of bladder dysfunction in spinal cord injury depends on the level of the lesion. Patients with lesions located above the conus medullaris will void reflexly without voluntary control. The urethral sphincters usually do not coordinate with the bladder musculature and tighten during detrusor contraction, sometimes preventing voiding or causing incomplete bladder emptying. These patients suffer from both incontinence and retention.

A condom catheter is generally needed to control the incontinence in men. If total or partial urinary retention persists, intermittent catheterization combined with the use of the condom catheter will be needed. Surgical reduction of the outlet resistance by transurethral incisions of the vesical neck and prostatic urethra, together with external sphincterotomy, will improve bladder emptying and is an option for patients who decline, or are unable to perform, intermittent catheterization. This is often a decision reached by the patient, family, and nurse. Women who have tried intermittent catheterization and absorptive pads unsuccessfully may need indwelling catheter drainage.

When the lesion is in the conus medullaris or cauda equina, voiding is accomplished by abdominal muscle contraction, or Credé maneuver. These patients may have a dribbling incontinence (overflow) or stress-type incontinence.

The treatment is aimed toward improving bladder emptying by scheduled voidings every 3 hours, aided by manual or muscular compression on the bladder and intermittent catheterization or transurethral incision of the vesical neck and prostatic urethra if unable to void or empty the bladder completely. Indwelling catheter drainage is an option for women where intermittent catheterization is not feasible. The condom catheter and absorptive pads have a role in alleviating the incontinence problem.

## MYELODYSPLASIA

Myelodysplasia is defective closure of the neural groove and presents as occult spina bifida, meningocele, and myelomeningocele with most of the defects occurring in the lumbosacral vertebrae. The incidence of bladder dysfunction depends on the severity of the malformation, and the type of dysfunction is dependent on the location of the lesion. Loss of volitional control as a result of a hyperreflexic bladder is seen in 25% to 30% of the children, while complete absence of bladder contraction (areflexia) has been noted in as many as 60%. In 75% of the children, the sphincter is partially or completely denervated.

The treatment is a combination of intermittent catheterization and pharmacotherapy. Absorptive diapers for girls and younger boys and urinary collecting appliances for older boys are resorted to in many cases. Some patients are suitable candidates for the artificial urinary sphincter if bladder capacity and compliance are adequate. Deterioration of the upper urinary tract manifested by progressive hydronephrosis and hydroureter can occur early or later in life and is usually the consequence of poor detrusor compliance. Cystoplasty to augment the bladder has been beneficial in such cases.

## DISEASES AFFECTING THE PERIPHERAL INNERVATION OF THE BLADDER

### DIABETES MELLITUS

Bladder dysfunction in diabetes mellitus is due to peripheral neuropathy that impairs conduction in the sensory axons. The patient fails to recognize bladder distention, and, as a result of ensuing chronic overdistention, the bladder musculature is damaged and detrusor contraction weakened. As residual urine accumulates, the patient experiences difficulty in initiating micturition, and later develops overflow incontinence or urinary retention.

The treatment focuses on improvement of bladder emptying. The patient is advised to observe scheduled voidings every three hours and intermittent catheterization is advised if there is significant residual urine, which should be checked periodically if you suspect problems. Another option for men is surgical lessening of the outlet resistance by transurethral incisions of the vesical neck and prostatic urethra or transurethral resection if the prostate is enlarged.

## GENERAL CONDITIONS

In addition to the specific diseases mentioned, there are other problems of a more general nature that can lead to incontinence. One of the more common of these is mobility; for physical reasons the patient may just not be able to make it to the toilet. The patient may move slowly or have osteoarthritis, or the toilet may be down a long dark hallway. The answer for these patients may be a commode or urinal.

Similarly, some patients may be sedated as either a side-effect of medication or as a primary goal of treatment. Often these patients are too sleepy to recognize a full bladder with ensuing incontinence. Medication side-effects are always a concern. Any patient who was previously continent and becomes incontinent after starting a new medication should have that possibility looked into. In general, any process that affects the patient's overall status may affect the patient's ability to remain continent. Some of the simple obvious causes should be investigated because of the ease in remedying the situation.

## BLADDER MANAGEMENT IN THE HOME SETTING

The bladder problems that require continued care in the home can be categorized into the following two groups:

1. Problems of bladder storage manifested by urinary frequency, urgency, and urge incontinence
2. Problems of bladder emptying manifested by total or partial urinary retention

The various treatment modalities available for these problems include

1. Urethral catheter drainage
   a. Intermittent catheterization
   b. Indwelling catheter
2. Pharmacologic therapy
3. Urinary collecting appliances
4. Urinary diversion
5. Artificial urinary sphincter

## URETHRAL CATHETER

The use of a urethral catheter becomes necessary in the following situations:

1. Total or partial urinary retention or incontinence of patients who are seriously ill or severely handicapped
2. An alternative option for patients who undergo or decline surgery for relief of outlet obstruction or when such surgery has been unsuccessful
3. When upper urinary tract deterioration or vesicoureteral reflux is demonstrated in certain patients with neurogenic bladder

### Intermittent Clean Catheterization

Intermittent clean catheterization is the most popular form of catheter drainage. It has been demonstrated that with intermittent catheterization the urinary tract can be kept sterile, or at least left only with a minor degree of urinary infection. Moreover, patients can continue with normal sexual function and be spared the psychological trauma of being attached to a catheter and a leg bag. For the patient with a neurogenic bladder, treatment with intermittent catheterization results in earlier return of detrusor reflex activity and a decrease in such complications as penoscrotal abscess, fistula, or diverticulum. The patient, however, must have the manual dexterity to insert the catheter and be able to move to a toilet or commode; otherwise a care partner will have to do the catheterization at the prescribed intervals. It should be emphasized that this is a simple procedure and usually very acceptable to the patient and family.

**Precautions and Principles of Care.** Gentleness should be emphasized to avoid traumatizing the urethra. Intermittent catheterization in the home is not advisable if there is urethral stenosis, false passage, diverticulum, or severe urethritis. The patient's daily fluid intake is restricted to 1500 ml to avoid bladder overdistention. Catheterization is initially done every 6 hours until the patient begins to void spontaneously. Before the catheterization, voiding should be encouraged with various assistive measures such as muscular or manual compression of the lower abdomen. The patient should not be allowed to retain more than 600 ml and in such event the frequency of catheterization should be increased or fluid intake lessened. When spontaneous voiding starts and residual urine decreases, the frequency of catheterization may be reduced to every 8 hours, then every 12 hours, and, later, once every 24 hours. Catheterization may be stopped any time the residual urine is consistently less than 100 ml.

**Technique.** A size French 14 to 16 catheter will usually be appropriate for adults, French 10 for adolescents, and French 8 for pediatric patients. Sterile catheters in sterile packets are commercially obtainable. However, the same catheter can be used several times if flushed with tap water before and after its use and kept in a clean container.

The male patient can be taught to self-catheterize in the sitting or standing position. He first washes his hands thoroughly with soap and water. He then holds the penis with one hand, and retracts the foreskin and cleans the meatus with soap and water or antiseptic solution if preferred. The end of the catheter is lubricated with water-soluble jelly, and the catheter is gently inserted into the urethra and advanced into the bladder. The urine is allowed to drain out until the bladder is emptied.

The female patient also washes her hands thoroughly with soap and water. She can catheterize herself in the recumbent position with her thighs flexed and knees abducted or in a standing position with one leg on the seat of the toilet. In either position, the labia can be spread with one hand and the catheter inserted with the other one. Before catheterization, the surroundings of the meatus are cleansed with soap and water or antiseptic solution. The catheter is lubricated and inserted gently into the urethra and the bladder drained of all urine. A mirror positioned in front may be of considerable help to the patient in locating the meatus.

### Indwelling Catheter

An indwelling catheter may be necessary in the following situations:

1. When the patient cannot self-catheterize and intermittent catheterization by others at the prescribed intervals cannot be done
2. Incontinence persists between intermittent catheterizations
3. Continued deterioration of the upper urinary tract in spite of intermittent catheterization in certain patients with neurogenic bladder

**Precautions and Principles of Care.** When a catheter is left indwelling, urinary infection inevitably follows. The entry of bacteria is through the lumen of the catheter and along the urethral mucosa outside the catheter.

The patient must maintain a fluid intake of 3000 ml daily to benefit from the flushing action of a continuous free flow of urine through the catheter. The free end of the catheter should at all times drain into a closed drainage system with the bag situated below the level of the bladder, and a drain-off tube at the bottom. It is advisable to cleanse the periurethral area with soap and water twice a day to prevent accumulation of pus and dried secretions around the meatus adjacent to the catheter.

Catheter changes are done at intervals of 1 to 4 weeks. Some patients have repeated and frequent blockage problems from encrustations and will require catheter changes at shorter intervals. Other patients can wear a catheter for several weeks and maintain a free flow of urine through the catheter. Sometimes it is necessary to irrigate the catheter with physiologic saline solution once or more often daily when encrustation tendency is severe.

In addition to maintaining a high fluid intake, there may be an advantage to keeping the urine in the acidic range to suppress bacterial growth. This may be accomplished with ascorbic acid, 1 to 4 g daily; methenamine mandelate, 1 g four times a day; or methenamine hippurate, 1 g twice a day. Antibiotics in patients with indwelling catheters and no signs of sepsis serve no useful purpose and may lead to growth of resistant organisms. Long-term indwelling catheter treatment has the risk of squamous cell carcinoma (5%–10%) and, because of this, cystoscopy is indicated when there is bleeding in a patient with long-term indwelling catheter drainage.

**Technique.** The catheter must not be too large (a size French 14–16 is recommended for adult patients), allowing drainage from the periurethral glands around the catheter and minimizing the risk of urethral wall necrosis.

Before insertion wash hands thoroughly with soap and water. In the male, hold the penis with one hand, retract the foreskin, and clean the meatus and glans penis with an antiseptic solution. In the female, separate the labia with one hand and cleanse the area around the meatus with an antiseptic solution. Hold the catheter with the other hand, lubricate the free end, and insert the catheter gently into the urethra. Drain the bladder of all urine.

After inserting the catheter, inflate the balloon with 5 ml of sterile water, anchor the catheter on the thigh, and connect it to the drainage bag , being certain to avoid kinking the tubing.

## PHARMACOLOGIC THERAPY

Pharmacotherapy in combination with intermittent catheterization has played a major role in the management of urinary bladder dysfunctions. The choice of pharmacologic agents can be classified as follows:

1. Drugs that facilitate bladder emptying
   a. By increasing intravesical pressure
   b. By decreasing outlet resistance
2. Drugs that facilitate urine storage
   a. By decreasing intravesical pressure
   b. By increasing outlet resistance

### *Drugs Increasing Intravesical Pressure*

**Bethanechol (Urecholine).** Bethanechol is the most popular cholinergic agent. It acts principally by stimulation of muscarinic cholinergic receptors, thereby increasing detrusor tone and decreasing bladder capacity. The indications for its use are nonobstructive urinary retention and acontractile bladder (detrusor areflexia) with increased residual urine volume. The contraindications are mechanical obstruction of the lower urinary tract and gastrointestinal tract, pregnancy, peptic ulcer, asthma, hyperthyroidism, coronary artery disease, epilepsy, and Parkinson's disease. The side-effects include gastrointestinal symptoms such as abdominal cramps, vomiting, and defecation, and cardiovascular symptoms such as bradycardia with subsequent hypotension.

The drug may be administered orally, 50 mg to 200 mg in divided doses, and subcutaneously in 5-mg doses.

**Carbachol.** Carbachol is widely used in Europe. It has properties similar to those of bethanechol but has stronger nicotine-like effects.

The oral dose is 2 mg to 4 mg three times daily.

## Drugs Decreasing Outlet Resistance

**Phenoxybenzamine (Dibenzyline).** Phenoxybenzamine is an alpha-adrenergic blocker that causes relaxation of the urethral smooth muscle resulting in a decrease of urethral closure pressure. It is indicated in urinary retention or elevated residual urine. Although acting on smooth muscle, phenoxybenzamine may reduce residual urine in detrusor–sphincter dyssynergia. Side-effects include postural hypotension, tachycardia, and diaphoresis. Prolonged administration is not advisable because there is experimental evidence of mutagenic effects.

The dosage is 10 mg to 40 mg daily in divided doses.

**Diazepam (Valium).** Diazepam relaxes the striated external sphincter because of its polysynaptic inhibitory action. It is indicated when incomplete bladder emptying is the result of detrusor–sphincter dyssynergia.

The oral dose is 5 mg to 10 mg three or four times a day, being careful that sedation does not, in itself, cause incontinence.

**Baclofen (Lioresal).** Baclofen inhibits both monosynaptic and polysynaptic reflexes and is utilized for skeletal muscle spasticity and detrusor–sphincter dyssynergia. The side-effects include muscular weakness and sometimes stress incontinence.

Baclofen is given orally in divided doses of 10 mg with gradual increments to 80 mg to 100 mg per day.

## Drugs Decreasing Intravesical Pressure

**Oxybutynin (Ditropan).** Oxybutynin has a potent direct effect on the smooth muscle and also inhibits the muscarinic action of acetylcholine on smooth muscle. It diminishes detrusor reflex contractions and increases bladder capacity. It is indicated for hyperreflexic and poorly compliant bladders associated with incontinence or urgency. Contraindications include glaucoma, gastrointestinal and lower urinary tract obstruction, megacolon, myasthenia gravis, and pregnancy.

Side-effects are dryness of the mouth and blurring of vision.

The dosage is 5 mg orally two to four times a day.

**Propantheline (Pro-Banthine).** Propantheline inhibits the action of acetylcholine at the muscarinic receptors and suppresses detrusor reflex contractions in the hyperreflexic bladder. Contraindications are glaucoma and gastrointestinal or lower urinary tract obstruction. The side-effects include decreased salivation and visual blurring. There may be gastrointestinal bloating, constipation, and tachycardia.

The dosage may be as high as 150 mg per day in divided doses for control of hyperreflexic bladder contractions.

**Imipramine (Tofranil).** Imipramine has an alpha- and beta-adrenergic action. It enhances resting intraurethral pressure through its alpha-adrenergic stimulation and inhibits abnormal detrusor reflex activity through its beta-adrenergic effect on the body of the bladder. The drug is, however, more frequently used to treat childhood enuresis. The side-effects are dryness of the mouth, epigastric distress, myocardial infarction, Parkinson's syndrome, delusion, and generalized seizures.

The dosage for children 6 years or older is 25 mg orally at bedtime, and may be increased to 75 mg. For adults, the dosage is 100 mg to 200 mg daily in divided doses.

### Drugs Increasing Outlet Resistance

**Ephedrine.** Ephedrine has predominantly alpha-adrenergic effects but also causes beta-adrenergic stimulation. The effect is increased urethral pressure. It is indicated in stress urinary incontinence, enuresis, and postprostatectomy incontinence. The contraindications are hypertension, angina pectoris, hyperthyroidism, and bladder outlet obstruction. Side-effects are increased irritability, loss of appetite, restlessness, and insomnia. In addition there may be elevation of blood pressure and leg cramps in elderly patients.

The dosage is 25 mg three or four times per day orally.

**Phenylpropanolamine (Ornade).** Phenylpropanolamine has the same mode of action as ephedrine but there is also an increase in the urethral pressure. It is indicated in stress urinary incontinence and postprostatectomy incontinence.

Side-effects are urinary retention and hypertension.

The dosage is one Ornade spansule twice daily.

## INCONTINENCE APPLIANCES AND ABSORBENT UNDERGARMENTS OR PADS

The use of catheters or pharmacologic treatment, or both, may not adequately control urinary incontinence or such modalities may not be feasible for some patients. Another alternative is the use of incontinence appliances or absorbent undergarments and pads. This modality is far from ideal, in large part because the patient continues to be uncomfortable and constantly reminded of his deficit. On the other hand, they can offer a degree of freedom with none of the problems associated with medications or indwelling devices.

### Incontinence Appliances

The condom or Texas catheter is the most widely accepted type of incontinence appliance. There are other commercially available urinary appliances, generally in the shape of a rubber cone pulled over the penis and kept in place by straps around the waist. These are often rejected by the patient because of their bulky nature, complicated arrangement, and unreliability in preventing urine spillage.

The condom catheter consists of a condom fitted over the penis and connected to a rubber tube that drains the urine into a collecting bag. The condom catheter can be home-made or obtained commercially.

**Assembling the Condom Catheter.** The illustrations in Figure 13-1 demonstrate how to assemble a condom catheter that is not only cost-effective, but has also met with high patient satisfaction.

**Application and Care of the Condom Catheter.** To begin, wash the genital area, retract the prepuce, and cleanse any accumulation of secretions around the glans. Be sure to shorten the pubic hair to prevent it from sticking to the skin cement. Paint the skin of the penis with tincture of benzoin and allow it to dry, and then place a paper towel around the penis with a central hole to prevent the skin cement from spilling to the pubic hair. Apply a thin layer of skin bond cement circumferentially around the shaft of the penis (do not apply cement on the glans), and then allow it to dry. Then roll the condom upward until the entire penis is covered. The tip of the penis should be at least 2 inches from the rubber tube to prevent it

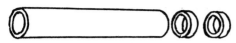

Cut two thin rubber rings from piece of rubber tubing.

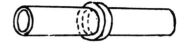

Place one rubber ring over the rubber tubing about 1½" from the end.

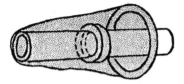

Place the condom over the end of the tubing so that the rolled edge is on the inner side of the condom.

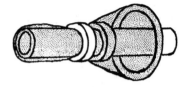

Place the second rubber ring over the end of the condom and down one inch.

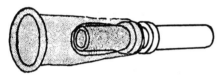

Draw the condom over the second rubber ring so that the condom has the rolled edge on the outside.

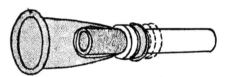

Lift the first rubber ring over the second rubber ring to secure the condom to the tubing.

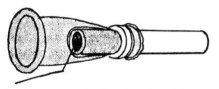

Puncture an opening the size of the tube. The condom is now ready for application.

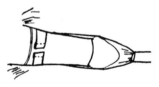

When needed, method used to apply tape around condom.

**Figure 13-1** *Assembling a condom catheter.*

from rubbing. If the penis is small, a strip of adhesive tape is wrapped around the condom and the adhesive surfaces of the ends brought together, thus allowing room for expansion if erection occurs. The drainage tube is then connected to the urinal. When the patient is out of bed, the urinal is strapped to the leg and when the patient is in bed, the drainage tube is connected to a collecting urinal bag, which hangs from the patient's bed. The condom is checked at intervals during the day and night to ensure that it is not twisted and has free drainage. The condom catheter is changed every 24 to 48 hours.

There are commercially available condom catheters, which differ in the way they are kept securely attached to the penis, varying from elastic double-sided adhesive strips to adhesive inner surfaces.

### Absorbent Undergarments and Pads

Unfortunately there are no effective incontinence appliances for women as there are for men. Consequently, when incontinence is unrelieved by other modalities, the female patient has to use absorbent undergarments and pads. One-piece disposable undergarments that drain the urine from the skin through a stay-dry liner and absorbent inner layers are commercially obtainable. They are kept in place with reusable elastic straps. One can also obtain extra-absorbent pads or shields with waterproof backing, which are kept in place with adhesive tabs that stick to the inner surface of close-fitting underwear.

## URINARY DIVERSION

The flow of urine through the bladder can be diverted surgically at the vesical or supravesical level. These operative procedures include

1. Suprapubic cystostomy
2. Nephrostomy
3. Intestinal urinary conduit

### Suprapubic Cystostomy

Suprapubic cystostomy is indicated in urinary retention in patients with an impassable urethral stricture or patients with vesical outlet obstruction whose general condition prevents immediate surgical correction of the obstruction. It is also advocated in patients with severe posterior urethral trauma. Its use as a long-term diversion in the spinal cord injured patient is being supplanted by intermittent catheterization and pharmacologic therapy.

**Care of the Suprapubic Cystostomy Tube.** The tube used is usually a Foley catheter varying in size from French 18 to French 28. Larger tubes are usually preferred because urine flow is less impeded. The objectives of care are prevention of infection and maintenance of unobstructed flow through the tube. Once or twice daily, the tube should be cleansed at its point of insertion with hydrogen peroxide followed by Betadine solution. A $4 \times 4$ gauze dressing is then applied at the site of insertion. The catheter should be taped to the abdomen to prevent tension and to hold it in place while the end of the tube is connected to a drainage bag that should never be higher than the bladder. The bag should be emptied regularly to avoid back flow or back pressure and it should be replaced once a week. Cystostomy tubes are generally changed once a month. Fluid intake should be encouraged to facilitate drainage, prevent tube blockage from clots or sediments, and formation of stones.

### Nephrostomy

Nephrostomy is an operative procedure in which a catheter is inserted through the renal parenchyma into the pelvis and left indwelling. It may be temporary or permanent. Temporary nephrostomy is done to allow recovery of renal function prior to a definitive operative procedure. For example, a bladder cancer may involve both ureters and cause uremia and sepsis. A possible course of management begins with nephrostomy drainage, then proceeds to subsequent cystectomy and intestinal urinary diversion when the renal status and general condition improve. Permanent nephrostomy is indicated where there is irreparable damage to the ureter and other operative procedures such as ileal conduit are not advisable based on the patient's general condition or extent of the disease.

Percutaneous nephrostomy is a relatively new procedure whereby a plastic catheter is inserted into the renal pelvis under fluoroscopic or sonographic guidance. Percutaneous nephrostomy has been gradually but surely replacing operative nephrostomy done solely for supravesical drainage. Percutaneous nephrostomy can be used for various purposes other than drainage, including conversion to a permanent nephrostomy, dissolution of urinary calculi, and extraction of urinary tract calculi.

Care of the nephrostomy tube is the same as that of a cystostomy tube.

### Intestinal Urinary Conduit

Intestinal urinary conduit may be an ileal or colonic conduit. The procedure is performed when the urinary bladder is removed by surgical operation or its functional capacity is destroyed. Severe fibrotic contractures associated with bacterial infection, irradiation cystitis, and bladder cancers are examples of lesions that would require urinary diversion.

**Application of Ileostomy Bag and Care of the Stoma.** The objectives are to apply the ileostomy bag in such a manner that it will remain in place for 4 to 10 days and keep the skin and stoma in good condition. There are many different kinds of ileostomy appliances and the specific instructions of the manufacturer should be followed. In general, the paper on the faceplate is first removed and adhesive spray is applied to the faceplate. The ileal bag is removed and then a 4 × 4 gauze dressing is rolled to form a wick that is placed into the stoma to absorb urine. Next, wash the skin with soap and water and dry and apply the bag over the stoma, gently pushing around the faceplate to help the bag adhere to the skin.

## ARTIFICIAL SPHINCTER

The artificial urinary sphincter has been implanted in patients with incontinence due to incompetence of the urethral sphincters. The conditions that have required implantation of the artificial sphincter are listed in decreasing order of frequency:

1. Myelomeningocele
2. Radical prostatectomy
3. Simple prostatectomy
4. Spinal cord injury
5. Neurogenic bladder
6. Stress incontinence
7. Pelvic trauma
8. Bladder exstrophy
9. Epispadias
10. Sacral agenesis

The AMS Sphincter 800 is the newest generation of artificial sphincters (Fig. 13-2). It has three components: control pump, occlusive cuff, and pressure-regulating balloon. All these components are filled with a contrast-fluid media that is isotonic to minimize fluid transfer across the silicone, which is a semipermeable membrane.

When implanted, the prosthesis simulates normal sphincter function by opening and closing the urethra (vesical neck or bulbous urethra) under the patient's control. To urinate, the patient squeezes the deflate bulb (soft part) of the control pump in the scrotum or labia until if feels empty of fluid. This causes the fluid that pressurizes the cuff to move from the cuff to the pressure-regulating balloon. With the cuff empty, urine passes through the urethra. As soon as the patient stops squeezing the pump, the fluid in the balloon that has been transferred from the pump and cuff begins to return slowly to those components. After a few minutes, the cuff is again sufficiently refilled to occlude the urethra or bladder neck.

The control pump is implanted in the scrotum or labium. The upper part of the control

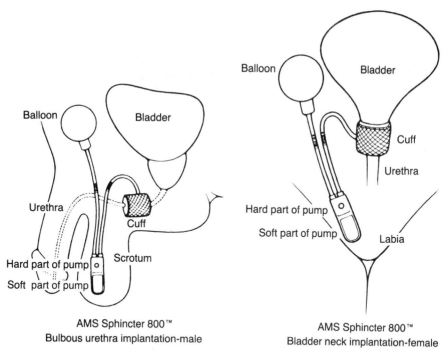

**Figure 13-2** *The AMS Sphincter 800, an artificial urinary sphincter. Illustration courtesy of American Medical Systems, Inc., Minnetonka, MN.*

pump contains the resistor and valves needed to transfer fluid to and from the cuff and a deactivation button connected to a deactivation valve. The bottom half of the control pump is a deflate bulb that the patient squeezes to transfer fluid within the system. To deactivate the device, the cuff is first deflated by squeezing the deflate bulb. The deflate bulb is then allowed to refill, and, when full, the deactivation button located in the hard part of the pump is pressed, causing a block in the fluid pathway from the balloon to the cuff and *vice versa.* To activate, the deflate bulb is squeezed quickly and forcefully; this should unseat the deflate valve and reopen the fluid pathway.

The occlusive cuff is implanted either at the bladder neck (male or female) or the bulbous urethra (male). The cuff occludes the urethra by applying pressure circumferentially. The pressure-regulating balloon is implanted in the prevesical space and controls the amount of pressure exerted by the occlusive cuff.

Complications that can develop after hospital discharge include mechanical failure and infection.

The artificial sphincter is a man-made mechanical device and as such is susceptible to mechanical failure. Leakage of fluid is the most common mechanical problem and can occur in the cuff, pump, balloon, or tubing, but usually involves the cuff. Leakage in the system is recognized by the loss of resistance when applying pressure to the deflate bulb, and is confirmed by x-rays of the prosthesis. A kink in the tubing can occur after hospital discharge and cause blockage of the fluid flow in the system, evidenced by increased resistance in deflating the bulb or complete inability to squeeze the bulb. Mechanical defects can be recognized by x-ray films (that include oblique views) and these failures can be corrected surgically.

Infection can develop from a primary wound infection shortly after discharge or may be a slow process that may become evident up to one year after implantation. Slow infection with bacteria of low virulence should be suspected if tenderness, redness, and induration of the tissue overlying the prosthesis develop. It is easy to detect when the process occurs in the scrotum or labia. However, an infection in one place means infection of the entire prosthetic space. Erosion at the cuff site also occurs and is detected by cystoscopic examination. When infection of the prosthesis is suspected, intensive antibiotic treatment should be instituted, but when skin perforation occurs, immediate and complete removal of the prosthesis is advisable. After removal, a four-month delay is desirable before reimplantation.

## CONCLUSION

The goal in treating incontinent patients is to allow them comfort, freedom of movement, dignity, and a decrease in medical complications. The spectrum of techniques and products discussed here should enable the primary-care physician to accomplish that goal for the majority of his patients. These procedures, like many others in home care, are dependent on patient acceptability and care partner cooperation. As the primary-care physician involved in the care of incontinent patients, you will be called upon, in some instances, to instruct the patient and family in specific procedures, and in others, to arrange for referral after discussing the treatment options. This chapter will facilitate your being able to do both.

### PARTIAL LIST OF MANUFACTURERS OF URINARY APPLIANCES AND CATHETERS

#### Intermittent Catheterization and Indwelling Catheter

1. Red-Nel Catheter
   Argyle
   Division of Sherwood Medical
   St Louis, MO

2. Self-Cath (female, pediatric, adolescent, and long)
   Menthor Corporation
   1499 West River Road N
   Minneapolis, MN

3. Intermittent Female Catheter
   Bard Urological Division
   C.R. Bard, Inc.
   Murray Hill, NJ

4. Foley Catheters
   C.R. Bard, Inc.
   Murray Hill, NJ

   Porges Catheter Corporation
   250 West 56th Street
   New York, NY

   Rusch, Inc.
   53 W 23rd Street
   New York, NY

#### External Catheters or Condom Catheter

1. Trojan Condoms
   Youngs Drug Products Corporation
   Trenton, NJ

2. Self-Adhesive Urinary External Catheter
   Hollister, Inc.
   2000 Hollister Drive
   Libertyville, IL

3. Uri Drain
   Chesebrough Ponds, Inc.
   Hospital Products Division
   Greenwich, CT

4. Freedom Cath
   Mentor Corporation
   Health Care Products
   2700 Freeway Boulevard
   Minneapolis, MN

5. External Catheter for Children
   The Perma-Type Company
   PO Box 175
   Farmington, CT

**Leg Bags and Urine Collection Bags**

1. Dispoz-a-Bag
   Bard Home Health Division
   C.R. Bard, Inc.
   Berkeley Heights, NJ

2. Closed System Urine Collection Bag
   Condor Laboratories, Inc.
   Keene, NH

3. Uri-Meter Drainage Bag
   Davol, Inc.
   Subsidiary of C.R. Bard, Inc.
   100 Sockansseti
   Cranston, RI

**Urostomy Appliances and Accessories**

1. Marlen Manufacturing and
   Development Co.
   5150 Richmond Road
   Bedford, OH

2. Hollister, Inc.
   2000 Hollister Drive
   Libertyville, IL

3. Cook Urological
   1100 West Morgan Street
   Spencer, IN

**Absorbent Undergarments and Pads**

1. Depend Shields and Undergarments
   Kimberly-Clark Corporation
   Neenah, WI

2. ConvaTec
   ConvaTec Pavilion
   Princeton, NJ

# 14

# Ostomy and Bowel Management

ELIZABETH A. PURCELL
THOMAS H. GOUGE

Rehabilitation has been defined as the "dynamic process that restores an individual to the highest possible level of functioning."[1] Rehabilitation and home management of the stoma patient aim to at least return the patient to his preexisting life-style, and in many cases to a better one. Unfortunately, the word *rehabilitation* also connotes disability. In our experience, a stoma is neither a disability nor a handicap. The patient is encouraged to regard himself as a person who happens to have an altered pattern of elimination.[2] In general, unsuccessful adjustment is a failure of proper rehabilitation.[3] Home management is a life-long cooperative process among patient, family, physician, and enterostomal therapist.

A central figure in both rehabilitation and ongoing care is the enterostomal therapist. This therapist is a registered nurse who has specialized training and has been certified in the care of individuals who have stomas. He or she provides direct patient care, teaching, and counseling; acts as consultant and educator; implements discharge planning; and provides outpatient follow-up and ongoing teaching and support of family and patient. The enterostomal therapist is part of a multidisciplinary health-care team and collaborates closely with the surgeon, physician, and ancillary services and coordinates their activities.

The enterostomal therapist's interactions with the patient begin as soon as the decision for stoma surgery has been made. The therapist has two primary goals: to establish rapport and trust and to assess and evaluate both patient and family support systems. Careful assessment of the patient and his support systems leads to a plan of care that will provide proper management of the stoma at home.

A primary concern for patients of any age or sex is body image. How an individual will respond to the alterations in his body will depend on the strength of his ego before surgery.[4] The other major factor is the support of significant others. Significant others may include spouse, other family members, or friends. The enterostomal therapist interviews and assesses these individuals, especially the spouse or other major care partner. The nature and quality of family care are determined by the nature and quality of the preoperative relationship. The operation and its residuals merely introduce new factors that must be integrated into a continuum of existing relationships.[5] If the preexisting relationship is strong, it will withstand the crisis of stoma surgery, and the necessary psychological and physical support will be provided. Likewise, poor relationships impede rehabilitation. The enterostomal therapist and the health-care team must be alert to possible negative dynamics and be prepared to intervene when necessary.

Every patient and care partner should at least understand that the stoma will not prevent or curtail normal activities; that there will be no embarrassing odors; that the presence of the stoma will not be apparent; that teaching and practice in management of the stoma will take place *prior* to discharge; and that neither patient nor family will be abandoned. Continuity and long-term follow-up will be provided by the surgeon and enterostomal therapist together.

Preoperative patient and family teaching and assessment are always geared toward discharge planning and home care. While an important part of this assessment includes anticipation of emotional response to the stoma, it also includes an evaluation of who will assume responsibility for the actual care of the stoma at home. Ideally, the patient himself should learn self-care and independence. However, this may not always be possible or desirable. Obvious contraindications to independence include quadraplegia, mental confusion, crippling arthritis, and Parkinson's disease.

When these disabilities are not present, however, there still may be other considerations related to who will care for the stoma at home. If the patient is extremely physically debilitated, he may very well need the help of his spouse or care partner—at least initially. If the spouse is unwilling or unable to participate in the stoma care, referral to an outside agency such as the Visiting Nurse Service must be made to carry on teaching and supervision until the patient can be independent. This type of referral is especially important if there is no spouse or care partner for the patient. Perhaps the most subtle consideration of all, however, involves the patient and spouse whose mutual dependence, under any circumstances, is extremely high. The need to share and support and be involved is overwhelming. Therefore, although our professional instincts or desires dictate patient independence in stoma care, that may not be an appropriate goal in certain situations.

Thus, there may be any number of extenuating or individual circumstances to be considered in teaching stoma care prior to discharge. The decision should be a collaborative effort on the part of the enterostomal therapist, the nursing staff, and the patient and spouse and/or family.

As recovery from surgery permits, the enterostomal therapist and nursing staff begin detailed instruction on a daily basis (irrigation for the colostomy; appliance change for the ileostomy). There is no specific time frame for completion of this instruction. Teaching is always individualized, as is methodology. Certainly, instruction with demonstration, followed by return demonstration, is necessary. Valuable teaching adjuncts may include written instructions, diagrams, pamphlets, booklets, or audiovisual aids. Virtually all patients prefer to have some printed information to take to the home care setting, "just in case" they need to check on a point of information.

The decision for discharge is based on the following criteria: the patient demonstrates independent ability to care for his stoma at home; the patient and/or spouse demonstrates ability to care for the stoma alone or together; or the patient cannot adequately care for the stoma, but an appropriate referral to an outside agency has been made for home care supervision. Moreover, this decision is based on the availability of continued support, instruction, and follow-up after discharge on the part of the surgeon and the enterostomal therapist. Both the physician and the therapist will see the patient on routine check-ups and remain available by telephone should a problem or question arise.

If possible, patients should leave the hospital with a one-month to two-month supply of equipment and with information about the purchase of supplies once home. Equipment is not particularly cheap. Medicare (for patients 65 years old or older) and major medical (for patients 64 years old or younger) provide 80% reimbursement. Patients with additional medical coverage (*e.g.,* special union plans) should be alerted to phrases such as "prosthetic devices" or "surgical equipment" in their insurance plans, since stoma supplies are included in these categories and costs should be reimbursable. The enterostomal therapist will be aware of sources for discounted equipment that offer the same "name" ostomy supplies at significantly reduced prices. The equipment is available by mail order and can be charged to credit cards. Realistic plans must be made for storing, ordering, and maintaining a sufficient stock of supplies.

Initial home management should be evaluated by the physician and enterostomal therapist together. The stoma may need to be remeasured, equipment changed, or procedures altered, and counseling may need to be continued. Although most patients cope well, they need considerable support and continuous care.[6] Although the primary-care physician will be the one principally interacting with the patient, contact with the surgeon and enterostomal therapist should be maintained because of the late problems that may arise. If the patient has not been seen by an enterostomal therapist in the hospital, the surgeon should try to provide the name of one who can provide follow-up on stoma management in the home. If you do not know of any enterostomal therapists in your area, you can contact the International Association for Enterostomal Therapy, Inc., 5000 Birch Street, PO Box 2690, Suite 175, Newport Beach, California 92660; or the United Ostomy Association, 20001 W. Beverly Boulevard, Los Angeles, California, 90057, for assistance. The International Association for Enterostomal Therapy maintains a list of enterostomal therapists across the country who provide outpatient services either in a clinic or home setting. The United Ostomy Association has a list of ostomy clubs (self-help groups) across the nation, whose advisors are enterostomal therapists and physicians.

Stomal problems that may arise may simply be minor and worrisome, such as granulomas and stomal bleeding, which require no treatment other than modification of technique and which can be managed at home. Other problems may be more serious and require consultation with a specialist or hospitalization. Some complications, such as parastomal abscess, parastomal hernia and stomal prolapse, require prompt treatment to avoid more serious sequelae. Others, such as recurrent disease and intestinal obstruction, may be serious or even life-threatening in themselves. All need to be correctly diagnosed so appropriate level of treatment can be given.

Problems common to all stomas are granulomas and superficial bleeding. Bleeding from the stoma itself is trivial, usually caused by mucosal irritation or superficial laceration. It can usually be stopped by application of simple pressure with a gauze pad for a few minutes. The stoma equipment should be checked carefully to be sure that it is not cutting the stoma. More profuse bleeding will be seen with stomal varices and with bleeding through the stoma. Both require thorough investigation of the underlying cause. Bleeding from the surface will be visible on inspection. Bleeding from within has the same significance as gastrointestinal bleeding in any patient and may be caused by recurrent or new problems.

Stomal granulomas are small pea-sized polyps that most commonly develop on permanent ileostomies. They are innocuous and require no specific treatment. On a colostomy they must be differentiated from inflammatory or adenomatous polyps by biopsy.

Prolapse of the stoma is seen most often with loop colostomy, but may occur with any stoma. The prolapse appears as a pink or purple protrusion of the stoma. The patient will describe that the stoma has lengthened or grown. If the intestine is viable, the color will be normal pink. The treatment is immediate reduction by gentle manipulation. Analgesics and sedatives are usually not required but the patient will require reassurance. If the intestine is ischemic, as indicated by edema and a purple or black color, or if it is not immediately reducible, emergent hospitalization is necessary.

Any patient with stomal prolapse should be referred to a specialist for evaluation. Prolapse is associated with parastomal hernia. Patients with parastomal hernias describe a bulging of the skin around the stoma when they strain. Any such hernias that are symptomatic or increasing in size should be evaluated for repair like any other hernia to prevent the complications of prolapse, obstruction, and strangulation.

# ILEOSTOMY

An ileostomy requires constant wearing of a pouch or collecting device. In a Brooke permanent ileostomy the mucosal surface of the ileum is exposed. The intestine extends outward beyond the skin surface at least 1.5 cm to 2 cm (Fig. 14-1). This protrusion carries irritating small bowel contents away from the skin and allows it to fall into the pouch. A temporary loop ileostomy has a similar but lesser degree of protrusion for the same reason and requires the same care.

Proper management of an ileostomy requires maintenance of the appliance and protection of the skin. Immediately postoperatively, an appropriate skin barrier such as Stomahesive or Hollihesive should always be used, with the opening cut to fit the stoma exactly so that no peristomal skin is exposed. A clear plastic temporary pouch is then applied over this barrier and stoma visibility is ensured. The enterostomal therapist will choose the equipment to be used, based on the individual patient's needs. As long as the pouch is secure, odorproof, waterproof, and comfortable, the brand name is unimportant. The appliance may be one-piece or two-piece, disposable or reusable, clear or opaque. If the patient wishes to switch to a different system, he should first check with the enterostomal therapist or physician for approval. For long-term ileostomy management, we currently recommend one of the two-piece snap-on systems (manufactured by Hollister and Squibb) that work very much like Tupperware. A plastic flange is attached to either a Stomahesive or Hollihesive wafer and the pouch snaps onto the flange (Fig. 14-2). The equipment is secure, unobtrusive, lightweight, easy to apply, and comfortable to wear.

The entire appliance should be changed approximately every 5 to 7 days. Since the stoma is most active shortly after eating, bathing and changing the appliance are best done several hours after a meal. For most patients, changing the appliance is most convenient in the morning before breakfast. As soon as the old pouch is removed, the patient washes

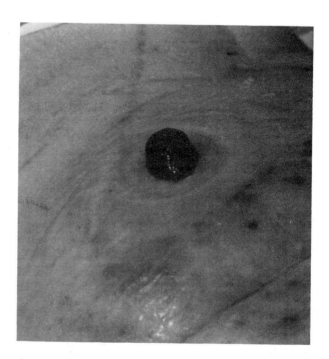

***Figure 14-1*** *Ileostomy stoma.*

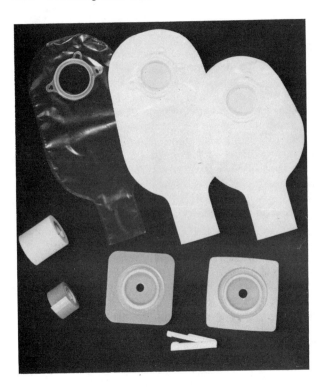

**Figure 14-2** *Snap-on pouches. (Clockwise from top left) Squibb clear and opaque drainable Sur-Fit pouches; Stomahesive wafers (flexible and standard) with Sur-Fit flange; clamp closure; 2-inch micropore and 1-inch dermiclear tape.*

thoroughly in the tub or shower, using mild soap and a washcloth. The skin is then dried thoroughly. A hair dryer on low or cool setting is a useful adjunct. As soon as the skin is completely dry, a protector such as United Skin Prep, Hollister Skin Gel, or Bard Protective Barrier Film is applied. When that coating is dry, the skin barrier or wafer is applied and the pouch is then snapped into place. Finally, four strips of microporous adhesive tape should be applied, covering all edges of the wafer like the frame of a picture. For convenience, some wafers are now manufactured with tape already attached.

Although this procedure is fairly easy and can be managed by most patients, not all ileostomies can be managed so simply. The physician, surgeon, or enterostomal therapist will often be called upon to act as problem-solver and "trouble-shooter" for stomas that are flush with the skin or otherwise poorly constructed, stomas that are poorly placed, and stomas surrounded by irregular skin surfaces. Under these circumstances, ileal contents have a tendency to go sideways and get underneath the skin barrier rather than into the pouch, creating leakage and skin irritation. Some of these problems will be difficult, others will be straightforward, but none should be insurmountable with proper use of available stoma care products. Skin barriers in paste form can be used to level irregular surfaces immediately around the ileostomy. Small convex inserts, which can be snapped into the flange, will also help prevent leakage under the wafer. Ileostomies that are flush with the skin may require a special faceplate, and attachment of a belt may be of further help in maintaining a difficult stoma. No universal solution exists for problem stomas. The available materials far exceed the few items mentioned. The enterostomal therapist is an essential resource who should be consulted early for recommendations in managing a difficult stoma.

## SKIN CARE

Despite meticulous care of the stoma, every patient with an ileostomy faces the possibility of skin irritation due to the caustic nature of the small bowel contents. Skin irritation may be due to leakage, fungal infection, folliculitis, or allergic reactions. The severity of the irritation is related to both the nature and duration of the problem, so prompt diagnosis and treatment are important and can keep minor problems minor. Careful inspection of the skin will exclude the more serious problems of fistula or abscess as a cause of the irritation.

Exposure of the peristomal skin to proteolytic digestive enzymes present in small bowel effluent from ileostomies can cause erythema in less than an hour and erosion in several hours.[7] Excoriation due to leakage is both the most serious skin problem and the most difficult to treat. The red, wet, weeping skin severely impedes or prevents adherence of the appliance and may exacerbate the problem by causing further leakage. Leakage is commonly caused by change in size or configuration of the stoma or by improper techniques. Whatever the cause, the skin needs immediate treatment. Skin sealants are discontinued immediately if the patient describes skin irritation. The alcohol content of these preparations causes burning pain and may further irritate the skin. Immediate treatment of the skin includes application of a steroid aerosol (triamcinolone acetonide 0.1%, betamethasone dipropionate, or dexamethasone) for its anti-inflammatory effect and nystatin powder for its drying and antifungal action. Stomahesive powder is also frequently helpful because it will absorb exudate from weeping skin and still allow a skin barrier or faceplate to adhere properly.

Fungal infections of the peristomal skin are particularly common in the summer months and in humid climates. The faceplate creates a warm, wet environment, which enhances fungal growth. *Candida* is most common. *Candida* infections are characterized by pruritic erythematous patches with red or white papules. The fungal infection should be treated by removing the appliance and faceplate, drying the skin, and rubbing nystatin powder into the involved areas. All excess powder must then be removed to allow proper adherence of the appliance.

More often seen in men, folliculitis is a skin condition characterized by punctate, red, inflamed hair follicles around the stomal area.[8] Peristomal hairs become embedded in the faceplate. If the faceplate is removed without the help of an adhesive or pectin solvent, the hairs are pulled from the skin, and inflammation in the follicles ensues. Treatment includes application of nystatin powder and removal of skin hairs either by clipping with scissors or by shaving with an electric razor. Depilatories are not recommended.

Allergic reactions are uncommon with today's ileostomy equipment. If an allergy develops, the skin will be raised and reddened, with a distinct outline of the causative agent. Treatment must include elimination of the allergen, application of new equipment, and treatment with steroid aerosol spray and nystatin powder. The faceplate should be reapplied without skin prep as already described. Tincture of benzoin, zinc oxide, and aluminum paste have no place in management. More frequent or even daily changes of the appliance may also be necessary until the irritation is resolved.

## CLOTHING

Patients do not need to change their mode of dress, including the wearing of tight-fitting garments and girdles. They should be reassured that nothing can be seen, smelled, or heard when wearing normal attire. If the patient resumes wearing his own clothes at an early stage of recuperation, his process of rehabilitation will probably be accelerated. Clothing has a psychological effect on body image and can promote both self-respect and socialization.[9]

The early hyperactivity of the stoma, with its large volume of effluent and constant filling of the pouch, resolves in the early postoperative period. Ultimately, the ileostomy pouch needs to be emptied about four to six times during a day. Greatest activity generally occurs after meals.

## TRAVEL

Travel need not be restricted because of the ileostomy. Even travel to remote lands is feasible. However, observing some basic guidelines will help avoid problems. On any trip that involves travel by airplane, ileostomy equipment should always be carried as hand luggage. If the patient is separated from checked baggage, toilet articles and clothing are more easily replaced than ileostomy supplies. To be safe, more ileostomy supplies than are usually needed at home should always be taken, especially when traveling to a warmer climate where the pouch may need to be changed more frequently. Since there is always a possibility of traveler's diarrhea, the patient should carry antidiarrheal medication such as loperamide or diphenoxylate hydrochloride with atropine sulfate on all trips and should be instructed to take it if the volume of stool increases significantly.

## GENERAL ACTIVITY

Patients should resume their usual work and leisure activities as soon as possible. There are few restrictions on physical activities. Walking or swimming and active sports such as tennis are encouraged if the patient's general condition permits. With proper protection of the stoma, even contact sports such as football and karate may be permissible. Only prolonged heavy lifting should be avoided because it can predispose to prolapse of the stoma and to development of parastomal hernia.

## DIET

An ileostomy dictates prudence in dietary habits but no absolute dietary restrictions. The two most common problems are dehydration and food blockage. Patients with ileostomies adapt by becoming chronically slightly dehydrated with mild deficits in both sodium and water. They must compensate by adjusting fluid intake. High-fiber foods may cause blockage of the stoma. Common offenders include the pulp of citrus fruits, popcorn, corn, nuts, Chinese vegetables, mushrooms, coconut, artichokes, asparagus, and celery. These foods are not adequately digested by the small intestine. In sufficient quantity they leave residue too large to pass through the stoma.

Food blockage of the ileostomy will usually resolve spontaneously. Severe cramping abdominal pain is followed by passage of the obstructing material, and then by resumption of normal ileostomy function. The patient should be told to notify the physician or enterostomal therapist for any cramping associated with cessation of ileostomy function. When food blockage occurs, the appliance must be removed immediately, since the stoma will swell and the faceplate can become a constriction. If the blockage persists, a physician or enterostomal therapist familiar with the stoma may carefully examine the stoma digitally. If digital examination does not relieve the blockage, a size 16 or 18 French Foley catheter is lubricated and passed through the ileostomy. The resistance of the blockage can readily be felt and the catheter can then be carefully advanced a short distance and a lavage carried out with normal saline in 30-ml to 60-ml increments, using a bulb syringe. Each bolus of fluid must return before further lavage is done. An hour or more of lavage will often be needed before the blockage is relieved, so persistence is required. If lavage is unsuccessful, the patient must be hospitalized and treated for intestinal obstruction. Even if function resumes, the episode of food blockage may actually represent intestinal obstruction, recurrent disease, or other mechanical problems. A careful search should be made for the cause and the patient should be thoroughly evaluated following resolution of the episode.

Dietary instruction should educate patients about food blockage, but not instill a sense of fear about eating. Both the quality and quantity of the food need emphasis. Excess ingestion of nondigestible residue will have the predicted result. Moreover, chewing foods thoroughly is of paramount importance to prevent food blockage and therefore the state of patients' dentition will influence what they can eat.

Depending on food and fluid intake, the ileostomy drainage will vary in consistency from thick and pasty to liquid. Average volume is 500 ml to 700 ml. If high-volume liquid output develops from excess intake, viral gastroenteritis, traveller's diarrhea, or any other reason, large amounts of sodium and potassium may be lost, and the patient can become clinically dehydrated. Dietary instruction must include education in ways to replace these electrolytes. Sodium is easily replaced by eating salty food and broth. Potassium sources include orange juice, bananas, tomato juice, peanut butter, cantaloupe, and watermelon. Commercial beverages such as Gatorade, which are extracellular fluid replacements, are available and the World Health Organization's water rehydration formula is simple and effective. It is made by combining 3.5 g of sodium chloride, 2.5 g of sodium bicarbonate, 5 g of potassium chloride, and 20 g of glucose in 1000 ml of water.

## SEX AND SEXUALITY

Much of the ostomy-related literature addresses the topic of sex and sexuality in terms of patients who have a preexisting relationship, usually with a spouse. Colitis often necessitates surgery at an age when the patient has no spouse or significant other, so the prospect of meeting someone new and becoming physically intimate may generate significant anxiety. The ileostomy presents very real concerns about desirability to the patient, compounded by fear of negative reactions from the potential partner. These concerns can only be addressed by proper counseling and guidance. Without proper guidance, the ileostomy can easily become a scapegoat and a convenient way to avoid healthy socialization.

Both patient and partner need to understand that the stoma will not be harmed in any way during intercourse. The pouch will not fall off if it has been properly applied and emptied. If there has been no nerve damage at the time of surgery, men should be able to achieve and maintain an erection and to have orgasm and ejaculation. Women can and do become pregnant. They can expect a normal pregnancy and delivery with no more complications with than without a stoma.[10] Complications specifically related to pregnancy are stoma prolapse and small bowel obstruction, which may occur as the fetus enlarges.

## PERMANENT SIGMOID COLOSTOMY

### STOMA SITE

The site for a permanent sigmoid colostomy may be different than for an ileostomy. The stoma may be placed in the iliac region or in the abdominal incision. The colostomy will have little or no protrusion. Less protrusion is necessary because the formed stool from the colostomy is potentially less irritating to the skin. The stoma is usually 2 cm to 3 cm in diameter and protrudes 1 mm to 2 mm (Figs. 14-3 and 14-4).

A secondary consideration in colostomy siting is colostomy irrigation. The surgeon will have positioned the colostomy so that it is readily visible and accessible for the irrigation procedure.

### COLOSTOMY IRRIGATION

Physicians and nurses are frequently confused about colostomy management. Colostomy irrigation is used only for permanent sigmoid colostomy. Colostomy irrigation offers the patient the opportunity for control and regulation of his bowel movements, but it is an

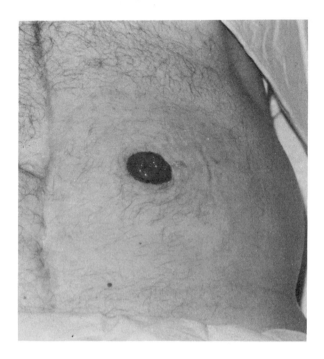

**Figure 14-3** Colostomy stoma located in iliac region.

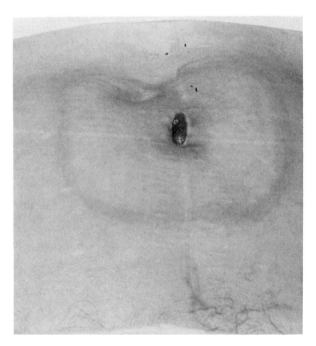

**Figure 14-4** Colostomy stoma located in the incision.

option, not a necessity. The stoma can also be managed simply by use of an odorproof pouch that is changed and emptied at intervals. The decision to have a patient irrigate is based on careful assessment of the capabilities of the patient and his care partner and other resources. Patients who cannot use their hands because of crippling arthritis, paresis, or Parkinson's disease are not candidates for irrigation. Patients with other physical problems, such as blindness or paraplegia, are perfectly acceptable candidates who can be taught to irrigate their own colostomies.

It is our philosophy that the patient with a permanent colostomy should be taught to irrigate. Gaining control of excretions and competence in management of self-care contributes measurably to the reduction of feelings of inadequacy, loss of control, and helplessness.[11] Bowel regulation by irrigation is a goal achieved by 90% of our patients. These patients need wear only a small, protective covering over the stoma. In a study of our patients managed with spontaneous colostomy activity, only 38% achieved an acceptable one or two bowel movements per day managed by spontaneous evacuation, and 32% had more than five colostomy actions per day or had continuous drainage.[12]

This is a time of considerable stress for the patient. Since the colostomy is now functioning, the patient may feel depressed and angry. He may think that he is repulsive to those around him. Moreover, the prospect of actually learning how to care for the colostomy is very frightening. The approach to teaching should be supportive, understanding, and encouraging, with assurances that the irrigation procedure is not painful. We describe and demonstrate it as a simple enema. A high anxiety level impedes learning the procedure so repetition of information and instruction is essential.

We prefer the cone-tip method of irrigation because it is safe and efficient (Fig. 14-5). The cone prevents perforation of the intestine and acts as a dam to retain the water. The irrigation apparatus is otherwise a traditional enema set-up, with a clamp to control the flow rate of the water. One quart of lukewarm tap water is used for the irrigation, although the amount will be adjusted according to individual response. The appropriate volume is the amount that prevents a bowel movement for 24 to 48 hours.

In the beginning the irrigation is done on a daily basis to provide adequate practice and to foster confidence. Later on, frequency of irrigation will also be partly based on previous bowel habits. Patients who usually had infrequent bowel movements (every two to three days) may eventually respond to irrigation every second or third day. However, any such change in irrigating schedule should only be done after control and regularity have been established on a daily basis. To help establish regularity of the colostomy, irrigations should be done at approximately the same time every day. The ideal time is in the morning after breakfast, when the stimulus of the gastrocolic reflex coincides with the irrigation. However, since the procedure can take 45 to 60 minutes, there may be other factors to consider. In the home, the patient must consider not only his routines, but the routines of the other household members as well. The number of bathrooms in the home is significant. The patient should know that he need not sit and wait over the toilet for complete evacuation to occur. In fact, it is desirable for the patient to get up and move around, since physical activity enhances complete evacuation, encourages relaxation, and can be a significant time-saver. Patients may shower, shave, put on make-up, read the newspaper, or the like while waiting for evacuation to be complete. The patient should be counseled to adapt the colostomy irrigation to his routine, not the other way around.

Some patients have significant discomfort when sitting on hard surfaces, even after the perineal incision is healed. For them, colostomy irrigations are more easily done sitting on a chair with some padding until they can comfortably sit on the toilet seat. A painful perineal incision or one that is not completely healed can be helped by sitz baths at frequent intervals.

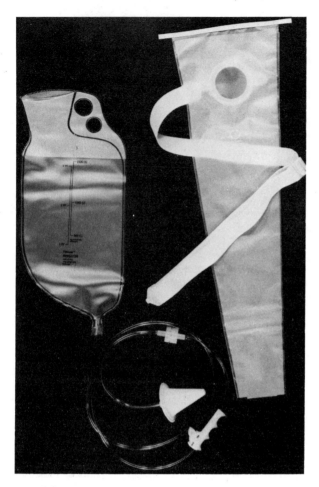

**Figure 14-5** Hollister cone-tip irrigation bag, irrigator drain, and belt.

## DIET

The proper diet for normal colostomy function is one moderately high in residue with 6 to 8 glasses of water daily. The bulk promotes both regularity and a soft, formed bowel movement. Salads, fresh fruits, and vegetables are encouraged. Furthermore, it is important to encourage the patient to return to previous eating habits, because this is what his system is used to. Stress the fact that the patient's gastrointestinal tract has been rerouted, rather than shortened. The patient's spouse, especially, needs to understand that special meals do not have to be prepared at home and that they can go out to dinner. Only those foods for which the patient has a known intolerance should be prohibited. Foods about which the patient is uncertain should be introduced individually on a trial basis. The use of bran or methyl cellulose is also helpful. The amount of bran is adjusted to individual tolerance. The usual dose is three to four tablespoons of unprocessed bran per day. Some patients find commercial methyl cellulose products easier to tolerate.

## SPILLAGE

The most common problem patients have to deal with is spillage (bowel elimination between irrigations). The cause may be diet-related or mechanical. Careful investigation will usually reveal the source. Important considerations about spillage include (1) when it occurs; (2) how often it occurs; (3) the consistency of the stool; and (4) the patient's previous bowel habits. If persistent spillage is diarrheal (loose and watery) the cause is usually dietary. The treatment is careful adherence to the high-residue diet, addition of antidiarrheal food, and more bran. If the spillage is formed or solid stool, a mechanical cause is more likely. A careful review of the patient's irrigating technique will usually reveal the cause of spillage. Many patients lose some irrigating water because they are afraid to hold the cone gently but firmly in place in the stoma. This low-volume irrigation results in an incomplete bowel evacuation. Additional bowel movements then occur later in the day. If no irrigating fluid is being lost, the amount of water used for irrigation should be increased in order to achieve a more complete evacuation. If spillage persists even after dietary and mechanical adjustment, irrigation may be less convenient than spontaneous evacuation. Such patients should be managed by allowing spontaneous evacuation and periodically emptying the pouch. Disposable pouches are convenient for these patients.

## DIARRHEA

Diarrhea is usually episodic. The cause must be identified if appropriate treatment is to be given. Common causes include diet, illness, medication, and other forms of therapy. Foods or fluids that frequently cause loose stools include foods in the cabbage family (cabbage, cole slaw, sauerkraut), broccoli, spinach, beans, fresh fruits, and milk products. Alcohol and fried, spicy, or rich foods are also frequent offenders. Drugs that may cause diarrhea include antibiotics, antihypertensive drugs, and magnesium-containing antacids. Chemotherapy and radiation therapy may also cause diarrhea.

While assessing the cause, recommendations for treatment can be made. Regardless of the cause, food should be eaten that will minimize the diarrhea, such as potatoes, rice, pasta, cheese, and peanut butter. If the cause is dietary, the problem food or fluid should be identified and eliminated. A change or reduction in the amount of medication should be considered when possible. If the cause of the diarrhea is one that cannot be eliminated, such as chemotherapy or radiation therapy, the patient should be instructed to stop colostomy irrigations temporarily, make appropriate dietary adjustments, and take antidiarrheal medication (codeine, Lomotil, or Imodium) in adequate doses to control the diarrhea. A pouch should be worn constantly and emptied frequently until the diarrhea has subsided.

## CONSTIPATION

Constipation is almost always related to diet, and careful questioning usually reveals lack of sufficient intake of both fiber and fluids. Treatment includes an adequate intake of fluid (particularly fruit juices) and increasing the amount of vegetables and cooked or stewed fruits in the diet. Although dietary adjustment is preferable, a mild laxative such as milk of magnesia may be indicated if diet alone does not correct the constipation. Patients must be told to call the physician or enterostomal therapist prior to using laxatives. The difference between constipation (hard stools, which are often difficult to pass) and obstipation or obstruction (an absence of stool passage) must be ascertained.

Patients who have had problems with constipation before colostomy surgery will frequently have problems postoperatively. Whatever measures the patient had previously found effective should be reinstituted if constipation becomes a problem after the surgery. Bulk stool softeners, increased fluids, and dietary adjustment will be effective for nearly all patients.

Constipation can lead to fecal impaction. If stool can not be passed by irrigation, further evaluation will be needed. Digital examination of the stoma usually confirms the presence of impaction, which should be treated by digital relief and by special irrigation. An experienced physician or enterostomal therapist should insert a number 16 or number 18 French

Foley catheter its entire length or until resistance is met. Irrigation through this catheter is then performed with one liter of water, 500 ml of vegetable oil, and approximately 60 ml of dishwashing detergent. More detergent is added if needed to emulsify the mixture. This combination oil enema has been very effective in softening and breaking up an impaction to allow evacuation. The irrigation is usually done by instilling the solution until the patient has cramping pain and then waiting for the fluid to return. If no fluid returns and no stool is evacuated, the procedure should be halted. The patient should then be further evaluated in an emergency room or hospital for possible mechanical obstruction. If fluid returns, the irrigation is repeated until the impaction is relieved.

Medication is frequently the cause of constipation when diet can be excluded. The most common offenders are narcotic analgesics, iron, tranquilizers, and diuretics. Since these drugs are usually necessary, regular use of a stool softener or methyl cellulose may be helpful in controlling constipation.

## GAS AND ODOR

Gas and associated odor are common complaints. Many foods seem to create excess gas. The most common offenders are beans, cabbage, onions, cucumbers, fish, and carbonated beverages. Milk products may also cause excessive gas, particularly in those patients with lactose intolerance, which is common with inflammatory bowel disease and in the elderly. Patients should be told that gas-producing foods are never a source of danger, but they could be a source of embarrassment.

With the sophisticated colostomy equipment available, odor should not be a problem, but many agents for odor control are available. External deodorizers come in liquid, pill, or powder form and should be placed directly in the pouch, but not in contact with the stoma itself. Although aspirin is an effective external deodorant, it is not recommended because stomal ulceration can occur from contact with the aspirin tablets. Internal deodorants for gas include charcoal and chlorophyll (Derifil), which have virtually no side-effects. Bismuth subgallate is a very effective internal deodorant, but it is contraindicated in patients who are anticoagulated with warfarin (Coumadin) and in renal disease. Prolonged use has been associated with heavy metal toxicity.[13]

## SKIN CARE

Although the stool from a sigmoid colostomy is usually formed, peristomal skin irritation can still be a problem. Folliculitis, fungal infections, and allergies may also occur and are treated as described for ileostomy skin care.

## GENERAL ACTIVITY, CLOTHING, AND TRAVEL

The procedures described for a patient with an ileostomy related to activity, clothing, and travel apply equally well to the patient with a colostomy. It is important that the patient and spouse understand that the patient will not be an invalid upon return home. Physical activity is encouraged, including going up and down stairs, taking walks, or even driving a car if appropriate. Common sense should dictate what the patient can tolerate.

Colostomy irrigation requires special consideration if the patient travels to another country or a different time zone. Flight departure and destination must be considered and then the time of the irrigation can be adjusted accordingly. We encourage all patients to wear a security pouch during plane travel until they have settled into a regular schedule, especially in a new time zone. They should irrigate as usual but should exercise care in the water they use. Whatever water is safe to drink is safe to use for irrigation. Water that is unsafe to drink should not be used for irrigation.

# CONCLUSION

Generally speaking, from a psychological and physical point of view, it is easier to manage an ileostomy than a colostomy. Ileostomy surgery often presents an answer to long-term, painful, and debilitating illness. In many cases it is curative treatment, and the disease is benign. Patients frequently are more receptive to the need for surgery. From a practical standpoint, very little time is spent caring for the ileostomy (the pouch is changed approximately once a week and emptied as needed). With a well-constructed, well-placed stoma, there are relatively few management problems.

Managing a colostomy, however, is completely different. A relatively "healthy" individual rather suddenly faces drastic surgery, which may or may not be curative. It may be very difficult for this patient to accept the need for surgery. Considerable time is spent in caring for a colostomy; irrigation takes up to an hour and is done either every day or every other day. Even after irrigation is mastered, there still may be problems to contend with, such as spillage, gas, odor, diarrhea, or constipation. The daily care management problems serve as a constant reminder of the stoma itself and in some cases of the diagnosis of cancer.

The enterostomal therapist, surgeon, or other health-care provider must always consider both psychological and physical concerns in managing the patient with a colostomy or ileostomy. Patient's questions, concerns, and fears may seem to be never-ending, but must be treated with the utmost care, patience, and encouragement. This kind of support can be as important as the surgery itself.

# REFERENCES

1. Johnson JB: Symposium on rehabilitation nursing. Nurs Clin North Am 15:221–223, 1980
2. Watson PG: Applying rehabilitation concepts in the care of persons with ostomies. J Assoc Rehab Nurs 1:99–104, 1976
3. Liss JL: Psychiatric issues in ostomy management. In Broadwell DC, Jackson BS (eds): Principles of Ostomy Care, pp 431–437. St Louis, CV Mosby, 1982
4. Boarini JH: Preoperative considerations. In Broadwell DC, Jackson BS (eds): Principles of Ostomy Care, pp 321–328. St Louis, CV Mosby, 1982
5. Dyk RB, Sutherland A: Adaptation of the spouse and other family members to the colostomy patient. Cancer 9:123–138, 1956
6. Hurney C, Holland J: Psychological sequelae of ostomies in cancer patients. CA 35:170–183, 1985
7. Watt R: Pathophysiology of peristomal skin. In Broadwell DC, Jackson BS (eds): Principles of Ostomy Care, pp 241–253. St Louis, CV Mosby, 1982
8. Esposito Y: Readmission needs of ostomy patients. In Broadwell DC, Jackson BS (eds): Principles of Ostomy Care, pp 399–408. St Louis, CV Mosby, 1982
9. Watson PG, Wood RY, Wechsler NL, Christensen L: Comprehensive care of the ileostomy patient. Nurs Clin North Am 11:427–444, 1976
10. Grubb RD, Blake R: Emotional trauma in ostomy patients. AORN J 23:52–55, 1976
11. Nurses Section, Education Commission (NA): Colostomy, Ileostomy and Ureterostomy Care, pp 6-14. Cleveland Cuyahoga Unit, Ohio Division, American Cancer Society, 1970
12. Grier WR, Postel AH, Syarse A, Localio SA: An evaluation of colonic stoma management without irrigations. Surg Gynecol Obstet 118:1234–1237, 1964
13. Dudas S: Postoperative considerations. In Broadwell DC, Jackson BS (eds): Principles of Ostomy Care, pp 340–368. St. Louis, CV Mosby, 1982

# 15
# The Neurologic Patient

## ABRAHAM N. LIEBERMAN

The physician caring for homebound patients with chronic neurologic diseases will encounter Parkinson's disease (PD), multiple sclerosis (MS), and brain tumors, among other diseases. Principles learned from managing patients with these diseases can be applied to managing most patients with neurologic diseases.

Parkinson's disease is a common disease of the central nervous system (CNS), having a prevalence of 200 cases per 100,000 of population. It is a disease most commonly seen in the elderly, the peak onset occurring after the age of 50 years. PD is progressive, with many patients becoming disabled within 5 to 10 years after its onset. The physician who sees patients at home will see patients with advanced PD, including patients with marked disturbances in gait and balance. One third of patients with advanced PD are demented and this complicates their treatment. Thus, drugs that alleviate the motor symptoms of PD often aggravate the dementia. This feature of the treatment can become burdensome to the family if it is not explained in advance. Depression occurs in more than half of PD patients. The appearance of mental changes, especially dementia, often precipitates a crisis. Thus, a family able to care for a patient with advanced motor disease is unable to care for a patient with both motor disease and mental changes. Another frequent problem among patients with advanced PD is that their response to medication fluctuates during the day and they experience daily oscillations in performance.

To manage PD patients at home, the physician must understand the disease and the drugs used to treat the disease. In addition, since most PD patients are elderly, they often also have heart disease, hypertension, gastrointestinal problems, and diabetes. Such patients are often on several medications in addition to their antiparkinsonian drugs. Thus, the physician will have to know how these other conditions, and the drugs used to treat them, interact with PD and the patients' antiparkinsonian drugs.

Aside from the effects on the patient, PD's greatest effect is on the patient's spouse. The spouse usually behaves as if the disease had struck the couple as a team, which is true. While most spouses can be relied on for support, the physician has to deal with the effects of the disease on both the patient and the spouse.

Multiple sclerosis, like PD, is a common neurologic disease. The prevalence of MS is estimated at 60 cases per 100,000 of population. MS is a disease of the young; the peak onset occurs between the ages of 20 and 40 years. It is unusual for MS to start after the age of 50 years. Although MS is characterized by periods of exacerbations and remissions, the remissions become shorter and the patient's course becomes progressive. The physician who sees patients at home will see patients with advanced disease who are immobile as well as patients who are able to come to the office. Homebound patients with MS are more likely to have bowel and bladder problems than are homebound patients with PD. Of major importance to their management is the fact that homebound MS patients are less likely to be demented than homebound PD patients. To manage the MS patient at home the physician has to understand the disease and has to be able to distinguish an acute exacerbation of the disease from an intercurrent illness (such as an infection) that may bring out previous neurologic symptoms. Additionally, many homebound MS patients receive steroids or immunosuppressive drugs in an attempt to prevent MS exacerbations. The physician must know about these drugs and their associated complications.

Since MS patients are younger than PD patients, their marriages will be shorter and less stable than the marriages of PD patients. MS patients are more likely to have intramarital problems as one member of a recent marriage faces the long-term disability of the other. The home situation of the young MS patient may also be complicated because the spouse is likely to be away from home working and there are likely to be young children to take care of at home. Managing MS patients is truly managing the family.

Patients with brain tumors, although not as common as patients with PD or MS, are likely to require home visits. The physician seeing a patient with a brain tumor will have to know whether the tumor is a primary brain tumor or a metastatic one. The physician will have to deal not only with the complications of the brain tumor or the spinal cord tumor but with the impact the patient's fatal condition has on the patient and the family. The physician who sees brain tumor or spinal cord tumor patients at home sees patients who have had surgery and usually radiation and chemotherapy. Most such patients have increased intracranial pressure and are on steroids. Many of them develop complications of chronic steroid treatment, including bacterial and fungal infections, myopathies, gastrointestinal bleeding, diabetes, and aseptic bone necrosis. Most patients with brain tumors have seizures and are on anticonvulsant drugs. The physician treating a homebound patient with a brain tumor or a spinal cord tumor has to know how to use steroids and anticonvulsant drugs. The physician who can manage a patient with a brain tumor or spinal cord tumor at home can manage any neurologic disease at home.

## PARKINSON'S DISEASE

Parkinson's disease develops because of damage to the extrapyramidal nervous system, that part of the central nervous system (CNS) that controls movement, posture, balance, and walking. This damage results in the primary symptoms of PD: rigidity, tremor, slowness and poverty of movement, difficulty with balance, and difficulty in walking.

Secondary symptoms of PD may include depression, dementia, postural deformity, and difficulty in speaking. PD can also impair the autonomic nervous system, and may result in orthostatic hypotension, seborrhea, blepharospasm, difficulty in voiding, impotence, and constipation.

The cause of PD is unknown. In a few patients, the disease may result from an encephalitis that damages the extrapyramidal nervous system. Many such cases of PD occurred during a worldwide epidemic between 1918 and 1932. In some patients, the parkinsonism occurred at the time of the infection, whereas in others it occurred shortly after the infection (post-encephalitic PD). The majority of these sufferers were young people whose disease often differed from those of today's PD patients.

Recently, parkinsonian symptoms have developed in several young people after they used an illegal drug N-methyl-4-phenyl 1,2,3,6 tetrahydropyridine (abbreviated MPTP) related to the narcotic meperidine. MPTP selectively damages the extrapyramidal nervous system. Based on this, it is thought by some that idiopathic PD might result from damage to the extrapyramidal nervous system from either an exogenous MPTP-like substance or even from an endogenous MPTP-like substance (a substance inadvertently produced in the brain of PD patients).

PD is associated with two areas of the brain: the substantia nigra and the striatum. Neurons in the substantia nigra contain neuromelanin, a pigment that resembles melanin. The neurons in the substantia nigra synapse with neurons in the striatum. The striatum controls movement, balance, and walking. Messages pass between the substantia nigra neurons and the striatal neurons through the aid of dopamine, one of several neurotransmitters in the CNS and the most important one governing the activity of the substantia nigra and the striatum.

In PD, many of the damaged neurons in the substantia nigra contain pink-staining spheres called Lewy bodies, the Lewy body being a marker for PD. Why the Lewy body appears, and how it is involved in damaging the nigral neurons, is not known. Paralleling the degree of neuronal loss in the substantia nigra is a loss of dopamine in the striatum. Loss of approximately 80% of the pigmented neurons in the substantia nigra and 80% of the dopamine in the striatum results in the appearance of PD symptoms.

The pigmented neurons in the substantia nigra synapse with two different types of dopamine receptors in the striatum. One type of receptor (called D1) is found on the body of the striatal neurons and is linked to the enzyme adenyl cyclase. The other type of receptor (D2) is found on axons of neurons that originate in the cerebral cortex and then pass through the striatum (this receptor is not linked to adenyl cyclase). Some antiparkinsonian drugs stimulate one type of receptor and some drugs stimulate both types of receptors. At present most dopamine agonists stimulate the D2 receptor. The exact role of each receptor in Parkinson's disease is not now known.

Another important neurotransmitter in the striatum is acetylcholine, its content being normal in PD patients. However, in order for the striatum to function, a balance between dopamine and acetylcholine is necessary. Because there is a dopamine deficiency in PD, the dopamine–acetylcholine balance is also disturbed. This dopamine–acetylcholine imbalance further aggravates the symptoms of the disease. The use of drugs (anticholinergics) that block the actions of acetylcholine as well as drugs (Sinemet, bromocriptine) that increase dopamine activity restores the balance.

## PRIMARY SYMPTOMS

Rigidity, an increased tone in the muscles, is present when the limbs are still and increases when the limbs are moving. Rigidity is related to an overactivity of gamma motor neurons in the spinal cord, which regulate muscle tone, but it is not known why the gamma motor neurons are overactive in PD. Rigidity is often confused with spasticity, another condition of increased muscle tone. Spasticity, which does not occur in PD and differs from rigidity in several ways, is related to pyramidal tract dysfunction. Spasticity increases during movement of the limbs and then suddenly gives way. Spasticity, not rigidity, follows the paralysis of a stroke. It is associated with increased deep tendon reflexes and a Babinski sign, and is present in MS patients where there is pyramidal tract dysfunction. Rigidity is, by itself, not disabling. However, rigidity is often incorrectly used to describe bradykinesia (slowness and poverty of movement), another primary symptom that is disabling.

Tremor, absent in up to 25% of patients, appears in the hands—and sometimes the feet. The tremor, which may be worse on one side of the body than on the other, may also involve the head, neck, face, and jaw. The tremor usually decreases when the hands are stretched out in front of the patient or when the hands are moving, but in some patients the tremor may increase when the hands are stretched out (sustention or postural tremor). In other patients, the tremor may increase when the hands are moving (action tremor). The resting tumor usually responds to antiparkinsonian drugs, while the sustention or the action tremor usually does not.

Bradykinesia, one of the more disabling PD symptoms, is characterized by a delay in starting movement, slowness and poverty of movement, and arrest of ongoing movement. Bradykinesia may contribute to some of the other parkinsonian symptoms, such as difficulty with balance and walking. Difficulty with balance refers to the inability to maintain equilibrium or to react to abrupt changes in position. This problem contributes to the falls that many patients suffer—falls that may result in injuries. Difficulty in walking includes problems in starting to walk; a decrease in the natural arm swing; short, shuffling steps (festination); difficulty in turning; and sudden, abrupt freezing spells. The difficulty in walking may be complicated by bradykinesia and difficulty with balance.

Scales rating the severity of PD are based on an evaluation of the primary symptoms, and assign a weighted numerical value to each symptom. The scales differ according to which symptoms are evaluated and the weighted value assigned to each symptom. Among the scales are the NYU Parkinson Disease Disability Scale and the Hoehn and Yahr Scale. In the Hoehn and Yahr Scale, the disease is divided into five stages:

Stage 0 = no visible disease

Stage I = disease that involves only one side of the body

Stage II = disease that involves both sides of the body, but does not impair balance or walking

Stage III = disease that impairs balance or walking

Stage IV = disease that markedly impairs balance or walking

Stage V = disease that results in complete immobility

Stages 0 to II are mild disease; stage III is moderate disease; stages IV and V are marked or advanced disease. Homebound patients are usually stage IV or V.

The NYU Parkinson Disability Scale (revised in 1986) is included in the Appendix. A score of 0 indicates no disability. A score of 100 indicates maximum disability. Homebound PD patients usually score at least 40 points.

Complementing the rating scales are functional disability scales that rate the patient's ability to perform activities of daily living. These scales assign a weighted value to a particular activity, such as walking, eating, dressing, hygiene, and speaking, and then grade the patient's degree of disability.

The NYU Functional Disability Scale (also revised in 1986) is also included in the Appendix. The Functional Disability Scale usually gives a better overall picture of the patient's disability than the office examination, and is particularly relevant to the home management of the patient. The office examination evaluates the patient at one moment in time, while the functional disability scale evaluates the patient over the entire day. The physician should ask both the patient and the patient's spouse about the patient's ability to perform the various activities of daily living. These activities include speaking, swallowing, writing, feeding, dressing, personal hygiene, turning in bed, walking, and getting in and out of a chair. There may be a discrepancy between what the patient says and what the spouse says. The patient may claim that he can perform most of the activities of daily living and minimize his difficulties, while the spouse may claim that the patient cannot perform any of the activities of daily living. A major discrepancy such as this indicates a tense home situation. The physician should not pass over this, but rather should deal with it. In the home with a markedly disabled patient, the spouse's assessment is more likely to be correct, and the patient may not see his disabilities the way the person who cares for him sees them. The patient is thus unrealistic. This is a sign that the patient is not dealing with his disability and with how his disability is affecting those with whom he lives. However, the fact that the spouse openly contradicts what the patient says is a sign that the spouse is becoming increasingly resentful of having to care for the patient. Such resentment must be recognized early and responded to. At times the spouse will need to be dealt with as a patient in his or her own right with regularly scheduled appointments. The reasons for the resentment vary, particularly if the resentment has to do with previous unresolved marital problems, reversal of dependency positions in the family, or fatigue and depression in the healthy spouse. However, the physician should remember that if the marriage has lasted a long time, there are many strengths to draw on.

Most spouses can be relied on for support. Patients and their spouses should be encouraged to do as many things together as possible, such as participating in the doctor's home visits and reporting on the patient's progress, difficulties, and needs. A spouse can also ask the doctor for tips on helping the patient at home. If a patient is embarrassed about his disability, there are methods to minimize his psychological distress. This can be a critically important issue in allowing the patient to remain in the flow of his or her usual activities. For example, when expected for a social engagement, the patient can arrive early and leave late; in a restaurant, a waiter can be asked to prepare the patient's food specially before the patient is served so that the patient can eat it easily. When necessary, the family should obtain help in caring for the patient's physical needs. This help, if necessary, can ease the burden on the spouse and, at the same time, minimize the patient's guilt about being a source of distress.

The physician should encourage the patient and his spouse to go to PD support groups, but if the patient cannot go or will not go, the spouse should go alone. The growth of patient self-help support groups is an important factor in alleviating patient's and spouse's adjustment problems. These support groups, consisting of patients, spouses, other family members, and friends, have sprung up throughout the country, usually meeting monthly at some designated place, such as the auditorium of a local school or hospital. The support groups conduct "rap" sessions at which members air problems usually not discussed in the physician's office or at home. Such problems may include the difficulty that PD families have in coping with the illness; the effects of the illness on other family members; or the difficulty patients have in sleeping, driving, working, eating, or sex. At the rap sessions, patients and spouses speak freely with each other about the care they receive, their doctors, and the effects of their therapy. They express their worst fears, those about becoming immobile or senile, and are reassured by others who have overcome similar anxieties. Patients and spouses share their hopes, find friends, and come to terms with the illness.

The largest organization that serves patients with Parkinson's disease is the American Parkinson Disease Association (APDA). Since its founding in 1961, the APDA has been committed to "ease the burden and find the cure" for PD. Although the APDA does not treat patients, it focuses its energies toward patient services and research. APDA sponsors numerous national information and referral centers, each staffed by a nurse coordinator and a supervising physician. These centers provide patient assistance, such as referrals, literature, and trained personnel; they work with area support groups to locate and effectively utilize available community and medical resources. The centers also keep the community informed about developments and issues concerning PD. The APDA provides extensive information through the distribution of manuals, publications, and newsletters. All of the organization's services are free to the public and are funded entirely through private support. Through its research efforts and patient services, the APDA not only enhances the lives of those afflicted with PD, but also promotes efforts toward finding a cure.*

Many patients experience oscillations in their daily performance. For patients who experience such oscillations, the physician should be aware of whether he is seeing the patient on a good or "on" period or in a bad or "off" period. The physician should assess the number of hours each day the patient spends in his "on" periods and the number of hours the patient spends in his "off" periods. Such a determination may be made by

*Further information is available by contacting the toll-free number 1-800-223-APDA; in New York, call (212) 732-9550.

instructing the patient with such daily oscillations to keep a diary at least for one day a week of the number of hours he is "on" during the day and the number of hours he is "off." Through such a diary, the physician can gain a better understanding of the patient's overall performance and can be more helpful in planning the patient's drug treatment. By pointing out these fluctuations, the physician can help the patient plan the day to maximize the periods of better functioning.

The following are the secondary symptoms likely to be encountered in the homebound patient. Depression, which occurs in as many as one half of all patients with early PD, is almost universal in homebound patients with advanced disease. Although depression is usually considered to be an appropriate reaction to a disabling illness, patients with PD experience depression more than patients with other similarly disabling diseases. There is some evidence that PD and depression are linked by a similar reduction in certain catecholamines and indoleamine neurotransmitters. In some patients, the depression may be associated with anxiety and agitation ("agitated depression"). In a few patients, the depression may become so severe that treatment of the depression may become more important than the treatment of PD. Treatment of the depression requires counseling and may require drugs or, when severe, even electric shock. The choice of an antidepressant is individualized to each patient. Thus, among PD patients who are depressed and who are also having difficulty sleeping, the tricyclic antidepressants amitriptyline (Elavil) or imipramine (Tofranil) may be especially useful because both drugs have sedative properties. Patients require between 25 mg to 75 mg of amitriptyline or imipramine given as a single bedtime dose for two to three weeks to achieve an antidepressant effect. Unlike nonparkinsonian depressed patients, few depressed PD patients can tolerate more than 75 mg/day of amitriptyline or imipramine. At higher doses, depressed PD patients, especially those patients who have an underlying dementia, become agitated, confused, or delirious. Among depressed PD patients who are drowsy and sleep during the day, an alternate tricyclic antidepressant is protriptyline (Vivactil) in a dose of 5 mg to 20 mg/day. Amitriptyline, imipramine, and protriptyline all have anticholinergic effects, which may be desirable in depressed PD patients with tremor (where the anticholinergic activity may lessen the tremor), but such anticholinergic effects may not be desirable in depressed PD patients who have difficulty voiding. The tricyclic antidepressants may have an atropine-like effect on the heart and should be used cautiously in patients with underlying heart disease and arrhythmias. Among depressed PD patients who cannot tolerate the anticholinergic effects of the tricyclic antidepressants, a suitable alternative is trazodone (Desyrel), a nontricyclic antidepressant without anticholinergic activity. The dose of trazodone in depressed PD patients is 50 mg to 100 mg given as a single bedtime dose.

Sleep disturbances are a common complaint of PD patients. The disturbances include an inability to fall asleep or an inability to remain asleep, with frequent nighttime awakenings, with the patient and spouse being exhausted in the morning. Some patients experience a reversal of their sleep patterns; they sleep during the day, taking several naps, and are awake all night. Patients may also have vivid dreams and, rarely, nightmares. Bed partners often report that the patients speak in their sleep and have jerking, involuntary movements of their limbs (myoclonus). For some patients, difficulty in sleeping is related to their depression, and the sleep disturbances may respond to antidepressants. Some sleep disturbances such as vivid dreaming or myoclonus may be related to the antiparkinsonian medication, and readjustment of the dose or elimination of the evening dose (if possible) may improve the patient's sleep. On the other hand, some patients require their antiparkinsonian drugs to sleep because a lack of their medications may make them so rigid that they cannot turn in bed and therefore cannot sleep. Standard sleeping drugs are occasionally helpful, especially the benzodiazepines such as flurazepam (Dalmane) or temazepam (Restoril), which usually do not interact with the patient's other antiparkinsonian drugs. However, all hypnotics must be used with caution, particularly in depressed patients. Trying to resolve the sleep difficulties takes on a special significance when you consider that loss of sleep is one of the major problems reported by spouses of disabled patients.

Dementia consists of difficulty with memory, recognition, abstraction, and calculation. Dementia may also be associated with confusion and disorientation, and, when present, usually occurs in elderly patients with advanced PD. If you care for homebound PD patients, you are likely to encounter dementia. However, it is erroneous to assume that dementia is an inevitable outcome of PD. Furthermore, in cases of PD with dementia, the dementia ranges from mild to marked. The dementia of PD resembles Alzheimer's disease. The antiparkinsonian drugs, especially the anticholinergics (Artane, Cogentin, Kemadrin, Akineton) and amantadine (Symmetrel), may, in some elderly demented patients, inadvertently result in increased confusion. The increased confusion is temporary and responds to withdrawal of the drugs.

Speech problems occur in PD. Frequently, the speech impairment is mild and consists of a change in voice volume, phonation, or articulation. Generally, the volume change is the first speech symptom and the patient speaks "more softly." Usually the patient's voice is loud at the beginning of a sentence and then fades. In addition to the decrease in volume, the voice may also become monotonous, lacking variation and feeling, and may sound breathy, tremulous, high pitched, hoarse, or strident. Words may become slurred and indistinct; word endings may be omitted; final consonant sounds, such as the "k" in the word *look,* may be unclear; syllables and words may be crowded and run together; words may be accelerated toward the end of a sentence. Specific measures such as speech therapy, amplification devices, and antiparkinsonian drugs, such as levodopa, may occasionally be helpful.

Sialorrhea usually results from the patient's inability to swallow saliva, leading to its accumulation in the throat, a problem that is evident only at night when patients are reclining and lose gravity's assistance in swallowing their saliva. In a few patients, drooling may result from an overproduction of saliva, but it usually improves with the use of medications, especially the anticholinergic drugs or amantadine, which decrease the production of saliva.

Dysphagia is another common symptom in patients with advanced PD. Patients experience difficulty with both solid and liquid foods. In some patients, the dysphagia arises from an inability to force the food down the throat and an inability of the voluntary muscles of the throat and esophagus to contract. This results in pooling of food in the throat, and these patients may complain of food getting stuck in their throat. To alleviate this problem, the patient should place small portions of food in his mouth and chew and swallow his food slowly and carefully. The patient should always completely swallow one morsel of food before putting another morsel of food into his mouth. In some patients, pooling of food in the throat may cause the food to be aspirated into the lungs. If this occurs chronically, it may present with a recurrent cough or as recurrent pneumonia. The physician must be aware of this and be prepared to treat the patient when it occurs. Likewise, some patients are unable to swallow their pills, a problem that may not be reported by the patient and that only becomes apparent after the patient's PD symptoms worsen. Rarely, the swallowing difficulty becomes so severe or the bouts of the pneumonia so frequent that intravenous feeding or feeding through a nasogastric tube is required. Occasionally levodopa or the anticholinergic drugs may improve the swallowing.

A weight loss of between 10 to 30 pounds is another symptom of PD. The weight loss may be related to the difficulty in swallowing; the large amount of energy used up by the violent tremors or involuntary dyskinetic movements; or the disease's effect on the hypothalamus.

Constipation is frequent among PD patients. It may result from the effect of PD on the autonomic nervous system and may be worsened by some of the antiparkinsonian drugs, especially the anticholinergic drugs or levodopa. After an evaluation, including a rectal examination, blood tests, stool analysis, and, if necessary, a sigmoidoscopy of the lower bowel, has ruled out other causes of constipation, there are several measures the patient can take to ease his bowel movements. The patient should drink at least three 8-ounce glasses of water each day. He should add a cup of unprocessed bran cereal (20 g of fiber) to his diet or take two tablespoons of coarse bran at each meal. When moving his bowels, he should sit comfortably on a low commode with his knees drawn up to help the abdominal muscles pass the stool. If these measures are not helpful, then glycerin suppositories, small doses of senna laxatives, or careful use of Fleet's or saline enemas may be tried.

Breathing problems or shortness of breath after minimal physical activity may occur and should first be evaluated to rule out heart or lung disease. If the results are negative, shortness of breath may be due to rigidity or bradykinesia of the chest wall muscles, which prevents the patient's lungs from expanding. Some patients on levodopa, without rigid chest wall muscles or heart or lung disease, may experience shortness of breath and abnormal grunting respirations because levodopa has the potential to cause uncoordinated involuntary dyskinetic movements of the diaphragm, chest wall muscles, and upper pharyngeal muscles, which cannot be visualized. When shortness of breath arises from rigidity or bradykinesia of the chest wall muscles, increasing the patient's antiparkinsonian medications may improve his breathing. If the shortness of breath is a result of levodopa, decreasing the patient's levodopa may improve his breathing. Distinguishing whether the patient's breathing problem results from too little or not enough medication may be difficult. The simplest solution is to decrease the medication and see if the breathing improves.

Difficulty in voiding is a problem that may consist of urgency, frequency, hesitancy in starting to void, difficulty in completing voiding, and incomplete voiding with dribbling. Rarely, a patient may be unable to void altogether. This difficulty in voiding results from the muscles of the bladder becoming rigid and bradykinetic, thus decreasing the ability of the bladder to contract and expel urine. Some antiparkinsonian drugs, such as the anticholinergics and amantadine, may increase the voiding difficulty by inhibiting the cholinergic nerves that promote urination. In men, this difficulty may suggest prostatism. Indeed, this difficulty may be exaggerated in men with enlarged prostates. All men should have a rectal examination and the physician should estimate the size of the prostate before beginning treatment with an anticholinergic drug. In women, difficulty voiding may suggest laxness of the vagina or uterus, with secondary pressure on the bladder. Patients who experience difficulty in voiding should be checked for these conditions, as well as for infections and diabetes.

Orthostatic hypotension may occur as a symptom of PD itself or may occur in some patients because of the antiparkinsonian drugs (levodopa and the dopamine agonists). Orthostatic hypotension related to the effects of levodopa or the dopamine agonists usually disappears once the body has adjusted to the drugs. It may also be caused by some of the other drugs that some patients take for their other medical conditions such as hypertension, heart disease, and depression. Orthostatic hypotension may also result from dehydration, malnutrition, diabetes, or other intercurrent illnesses. The physician will have to decide which drug or drugs are responsible for the orthostatic hypotension and which may be safely eliminated or reduced.

Dependent lower extremity edema, a common problem for these patients, usually occurs toward the end of the day after a patient has been standing and disappears when the patient lies down. It is important that these patients be evaluated for other causes of dependent edema, including heart failure. The dependent edema in PD patients usually results from the inability of the rigid PD leg muscles to massage fluid from the feet back to the heart. Such fluid accumulates in the feet during the day through the effects of gravity. Rarely, drugs such as amantadine may aggravate the dependent edema. This edema may not require any treatment. However, if the edema becomes very pronounced, a number of measures may be used, including elevating the feet during the day, wearing elastic support stockings, and occasionally diuretics. Rarely, if the edema is pronounced and the patient is immobile, skin breakdown may occur.

Sexual problems between patients and their partners are seldom discussed. For that reason the physician should ask about them. A decrease in the desire for sex may result from the nonspecific effects of a chronic illness such as PD, a fear of being unable to perform satisfactorily, depression, and, occasionally, medications. Some men complain of an inability to achieve or maintain an erection, an effect of the disease on the autonomic nervous system. If this occurs, the patient should have a thorough examination to determine if there are other causes, such as diabetes or primary urologic conditions.

The choice of antiparkinsonian drugs is customized to the patient and to the disease's severity. Levodopa is the single most effective antiparkinsonian drug, crossing into the brain where it is changed into dopamine, thus compensating for the dopamine deficiency in PD. Most PD patients initially respond to levodopa, with the usual period of maximum response (the "levodopa honeymoon") being 2 to 5 years, although this varies from patient to patient. There may be some complications associated with long-term levodopa treatment (involuntary dyskinetic movements, diurnal oscillations in performance) that may be related to the amount and duration of levodopa treatment. It is thought by some physicians that the duration of the "levodopa honeymoon" may, in some patients, be similar regardless of the severity of their disease. Thus, levodopa is reserved by these physicians for patients with at least moderate disease, but many physicians do not believe this and use levodopa very early in PD. Today, levodopa alone is rarely used as a treatment for PD. Rather, levodopa is combined with a dopa decarboxylase inhibitor such as is present in Sinemet. Decarboxylase inhibitors are drugs that block the conversion of levodopa to dopamine outside the brain, while not affecting this conversion inside the brain. About 90% of levodopa (when used alone) is changed outside the brain to dopamine, a substance that cannot cross from the blood into the brain. When dopamine is produced outside the brain, it cannot compensate for the dopamine deficiency in the brain of PD patients. However, the dopamine produced outside the brain may cause nausea, vomiting, and decreased appetite. Since only 10% of the administered levodopa reaches the brain (where it is changed into dopamine), it is desirable to block the conversion of levodopa outside the brain—the function of the inhibitor.

When levodopa is combined with such an inhibitor, only one-fifth the dose of levodopa is required to achieve an antiparkinsonian effect. More than 90% of all PD patients initially respond to Sinemet, with the majority of these patients improving markedly. These inhibitors produce antiparkinsonian effects sooner and the effects are more striking than those produced with levodopa alone, while symptoms such as nausea and vomiting are decreased.

Bromocriptine (Parlodel), a dopamine agonist, can be used at any stage of PD. Dopamine agonists bypass the degenerating cells in the substantia nigra, stimulate the dopamine receptors directly, and are useful in treating all of the primary symptoms of the disease. Bromocriptine may be used alone but is usually combined with other antiparkinsonian medications. When used alone, bromocriptine does not induce the dyskinesias or the oscillations in performance that are associated with chronic levodopa treatment. In mild to moderately affected patients, dosages of less than 20 mg per day of bromocriptine, alone or combined with Sinemet, are usually sufficient. The dosage of bromocriptine should be increased gradually, starting at 1.25 mg (half a tablet) or 2.5 mg (one tablet) with the evening meal. The daily dosage is then increased by half or one tablet each week until symptom control is noted. By using a combination of Sinemet and bromocriptine in mildly to moderately impaired patients, good symptom control can be achieved at a lower dose of each drug. Specific patient problems, such as early morning rigidity, bradykinesia, or leg cramping, may be helped with bromocriptine. The adverse effects of bromocriptine (nausea and orthostatic hypotension) are similar to levodopa, are usually temporary, and may be minimized by gradually building up to a therapeutic dose and taking bromocriptine with meals. Bromocriptine can also be used in patients with advanced PD. In these patients, bromocriptine in low doses, when added to levodopa, may have a good antiparkinsonian effect, but bromocriptine in higher doses may have to be used. These higher doses of bromocriptine may result in more adverse effects, including mental changes. The adverse effects disappear when the dose of bromocriptine is decreased.

Amantadine (Symmetrel) acts by releasing dopamine from the cells in the substantia nigra and is effective in up to 50% of PD patients. Side-effects include livedo reticularis, which may be accompanied by dependent edema, and, rarely, confusion, delusions, and hallucinations. All of the side-effects are temporary and clear within a few days of drug withdrawal.

Anticholinergic drugs, which may be added or substituted if the patient's response to amantadine decreases or side-effects develop, are effective against rigidity and tremor but not against bradykinesia or difficulty in balance or gait. Side-effects include dryness of the mouth, blurred vision, mental changes, or difficulty voiding.

Although the role of diet in PD has been the subject of much debate, no single diet is recommended. However, patients often complain that certain foods cause a change in their symptoms or an undesirable side-effect. Other patients find that milk, meat, meat products, and other foods rich in protein make them stiffer and slower, and usually notice that bland or vegetarian diets cause fewer symptoms. When levodopa is taken with a meal rich in protein, the drug's absorption is delayed and the levels of levodopa in the blood are reduced because some amino acids present in milk and meat may block the absorption of levodopa from the gut or block the entry of levodopa into the brain.

Patients with PD, especially those with mild or moderate disease, benefit from physical therapy. Physical therapy does not reverse or delay the symptoms of PD; however, it does help patients make full use of their potential and may prevent complications, such as contractures of the rigid, poorly moving limbs. Physical therapy is a modality that should be introduced early in the disease. Since PD is a chronic illness that may eventually result in immobility, patients should engage in a daily exercise routine with the same regularity as they take their medication. They should understand both the benefits and limitations of physical therapy and should be encouraged to adhere to their program. For the mild or moderately affected patients who do not become rapidly exhausted, a routine of walking a prescribed distance, simple calisthenics, and active range-of-motion exercises for all the major joints (shoulders, elbows, wrists, hips, knees, ankles) once or twice a day is recommended. However, the routine should not be carried out to the point of fatigue. When fatigue sets in, the patient should rest.

It is important to remember that, for patients with daily changes in performance (the "wearing off" or "on–off" phenomenon), exercising should be reserved for the "on" or "good" periods. Forcing patients to walk or exercise during their "off" or "bad" periods will not "loosen them up." Such exercises in these "off" periods can be painful as well as dangerous. When patients emerge from an "off" period, most are so relieved that they will start moving about on their own. Encouragement and assistance at this time will motivate them even further, and will enable them to complete their exercise. Special care in exercising should be taken for patients who fall easily. Such patients should exercise under supervision while they are seated in a secure chair or when they are lying down.

PD patients often experience difficulties performing routines of daily living. Some tips that may help overcome some of these problems include making dressing quicker and easier by wearing loose, lightweight clothes and putting on and taking off clothes from the stiffer, slower side first. If balance is affected, the patient should sit over the edge of the bed or in a chair with armrests to dress. Other helpful ideas are to use elastic waistbands or Velcro closures instead of buttons or zippers; wear pullover tops, which eliminate fastening; choose clothing that closes in the front; and use elastic shoelaces or slip-on shoes.

The bathroom, which is usually small with slippery tile and porcelain surfaces, is usually the most dangerous place for anyone with impaired balance or difficulty in walking. Some of the preventive measures that can avoid accidents are placing a non-slip rubber mat or adhesive anti-slip surfaces at the bottom of the tub or shower stall, removing glass doors from the tub, using a tub bench or shower chair, installing a shower head on a flexible hose to enable showering while seated, and attaching soap to a rope, which makes retrieving easier. Bathroom fixtures should not be used as grab railings since they are not very strong, but grab bars can be installed. In addition, a raised toilet seat makes rising easier and arm rails can be attached to the toilet seat for leverage.

Freezing, or feet "stuck" to the floor, often occurs when approaching narrow spaces or a doorway. When in a freezing position, patients are usually in a stooped posture with knees bent and heels off the ground. The more patients try to move, the more off balance they become. To alleviate freezing the patient should not try to take any steps, and should place both heels on the floor, straighten the knees, hips, and trunk, and not lean backward. Next, the patient should gently rock side to side, take some marching steps in place, and start taking steps forward by placing both heels down first, keeping the feet about 8 inches apart.

Many patients have trouble standing after sitting on a low surface, such as a chair. To stand, instruct the patient to always bring the buttocks close to the edge of the chair and keep the feet at least 8 inches apart, with one foot slightly in front of the other. The patient then uses momentum by rocking the trunk quickly back and forth three times and, on the third time, brings both shoulders forward, just past the knees. By then pushing down on both hands and straightening up, rising should be much easier. Only by specifically instructing the patient in these maneuvers will mobility be facilitated.

Patients with PD often have other medical conditions necessitating drugs that influence the treatment of PD. The following are some examples: Glaucoma, for instance, may be exacerbated by anticholinergic drugs; these drugs do not necessarily have to be discontinued, but should be used with care. Patients with glaucoma who must continue on anticholinergic drugs should be carefully monitored.

Patients who have had a recent heart attack or whose heart rhythm is irregular may be sensitive to the side-effects of some antiparkinsonian drugs such as the anticholinergic agents or levodopa. A patient with a history of a recent heart attack may be less tolerant of the slight drop in blood pressure sometimes caused by the antiparkinsonian drugs such as levodopa or the dopamine agonists. These drugs may not have to be discontinued as long as the patient's physician feels the drugs' benefits exceed their risks. At present, there are no known contraindications to using any of the antiparkinsonian drugs with digoxin, the beta blockers, calcium channel blockers, quinidine, or procainamide.

In rare instances, drugs used to treat hypertension may worsen PD symptoms. Occasionally, alpha methyldopa (Aldomet) may result in temporary worsening of PD symptoms, but this effect will disappear if the drug is stopped. The use of alpha methyldopa is not contraindicated in PD, but if another suitable antihypertensive drug is available, it should be used instead. Diuretics may aggravate orthostatic hypotension, but this is more likely to affect PD patients who already suffer from orthostatic hypotension or who are already on drugs such as levodopa or dopamine agonists, which may themselves result in orthostatic changes.

In patients with gastrointestinal diseases there have been some isolated reports relating bleeding duodenal ulcers to levodopa and the dopamine agonists. However, no direct cause-and-effect relationship has been established. Levodopa and the dopamine agonists may dilate the lower esophageal sphincter, resulting in gastric juice flowing backward into the esophagus, causing reflux esophagitis. Such reflux esophagitis results in nausea and vomiting, which in turn results in further gastric reflux with increased esophageal inflammation, a particular problem for patients who have a hiatal hernia because of their vulnerability to reflux esophagitis. Patients who have hiatal hernia and who take antiparkinsonian drugs should follow an appropriate diet and may require antacids or other measures to decrease the esophageal inflammation. Cimetidine (Tagamet) or ranitidine (Zantac) may also be useful. Patients with a history of liver disease, jaundice, or hepatitis should have liver function tests before taking antiparkinsonian drugs, and should have these repeated periodically. Metoclopramide (Reglan) should be avoided in patients with PD. Although the drug is a useful antinauseant, its antinauseant effects result from blockade of peripheral and central dopamine receptors, which may worsen PD.

## MULTIPLE SCLEROSIS

Multiple sclerosis (MS) is a disease of the white matter that involves two or more areas of the CNS, two or more separate 24-hour episodes occurring at least one month apart. Symptoms and signs may include loss of vision, double vision, hemiparesis, quadriparesis, incontinence, ataxia, paresthesias, dysesthesias, or any combination of the above. MS may also run a progressive course. The diagnosis of MS is made on the basis of the history and the neurologic examination. The lumbar puncture reveals the presence of oligoclonal bands, which confirm the diagnosis. Magnetic resonance imaging (MRI) revealing multiple plaques is also confirmatory.

Most of the motor and sensory symptoms of MS arise from lesions disrupting the descending corticospinal tracts, the cerebellar pathways, or the ascending sensory pathways, the lesions occurring at any point throughout the respective courses of these tracts. The legs are affected more often than the arms, and bilateral involvement is more frequent than unilateral involvement. Typically, motor symptoms are described as fatigue, heaviness, stiffness, or weakness, whereas leg involvement may result in complaints of tripping or stumbling. A common complaint of patients with MS, more than of patients with PD, is fatigue and low tolerance for any physical activity. Motor signs elicited during an examination may be present without symptoms. Typical motor signs include hyperreflexia, Babinski's sign, and spasticity. Spasticity may develop gradually. Occasionally, the deep tendon reflexes are hypoactive and there may even be amyotrophy as a result of MS lesions involving the intra-axial portions of nerve roots in the spinal cord and brain stem. Spinal cord lesions may result in painful tonic limb spasms, but these may respond to treatment with baclofen (Lioresal). Cerebellar symptoms occur in more than half of patients with MS and include sustention, action, and intention tremors; truncal instability; impaired balance; and "scanning" monotonous speech.

Sensory symptoms are more common than motor symptoms, with patients often complaining of pins and needles, tingling, numbness, a dead feeling, warmth, a tight band around the body, or merely "funny" or "different" sensations on different parts of the body. The distribution of these symptoms may follow no obvious anatomical distribution. Pain mimicking muscle or joint aches or "rheumatism" is often present, and painful dysesthesias occur in as many as 20% of patients. Sensory signs including loss of light touch and loss of pin sensation often do not correspond to the distribution of the sensory symptoms.

Bladder problems including inability to void are more common than in PD. Many homebound MS patients require an indwelling catheter or intermittent clean catheterization. Constipation occurs in up to half of MS patients, but recommendations for treating it are similar to the recommendations for treating the constipation of PD.

Diplopia, a common symptom of MS, usually results from sixth or third nerve involvement or from involvement of conjugate gaze centers in the brain stem. Facial paresthesia or loss of sensation and even painful trigeminal neuralgia may occur in up to 5% of patients. This troubling symptom results from plaques near the fifth nerve nucleus in the pons and can be very painful, requiring treatment. Although trigeminal neuralgia may respond to carbamazepine (Tegretol) or phenytoin (Dilantin), both of these drugs may aggravate the patient's difficulty in walking or balancing. Baclofen (Lioresal) may also be used to treat trigeminal neuralgia. Vertigo, when present, is often severe and may be associated with nystagmus. Bedrest in a comfortable position is the most useful treatment for severe vertigo, and meclizine (Antivert) may be useful.

Optic or retrobulbar neuritis, which occurs in up to 40% of patients with MS, is usually unilateral but may be bilateral. The visual disturbances accompanying optic neuritis may vary from complete blindness to relatively minor impairments of vision. Because examination may disclose only minor differences in visual acuity, it may be necessary to use specialized visual field examinations to disclose the central scotomata that impair vision or use specialized color plates to disclose the impairment of the optic nerves not appreciated by testing visual acuity. It must be emphasized that the patient's visual complaints and difficulty in seeing may not be appreciated by only testing visual acuity.

Dementia is much less common in MS than in PD; however, in MS mood changes are more common than dementia, with depression being by far the most common feature. Unexpected cheerfulness or occasionally marked euphoria does occur, but usually on a background of depression.

MS is a disease noted for its variability. The most common course is that of multiple relapses and remissions with symptoms developing over several days or weeks. However, in 10% of patients, symptoms steadily increase without remission. When new symptoms occur they probably represent new lesions (*i.e.,* new plaques). However, old symptoms or previously apparent signs may appear during an intercurrent illness, usually an infection with fever. Most studies of MS define a "relapse" as an episode lasting more than 24 hours, while shorter episodes are more likely to represent a temporary conduction block. Remission of symptoms after an exacerbation may be complete, especially early in the course of MS, but with the increase in the number of lesions, irreversible deficits often result. As MS progresses, the course may change to that of chronic progression. The chronic progressive form of MS is more likely to occur with motor or cerebellar signs and is more likely to develop in the older homebound patient.

A number of factors, but especially body temperature, are known to affect the status of MS patients. Common infectious complications in homebound MS patients, including cystitis, decubiti, and pneumonia, may result in fever and can aggravate the clinical picture. The reappearance of such old symptoms or signs may represent a temporary block in demyelinated nerve tracts. Increased temperature alone, such as after a hot bath, may bring out not only previously suppressed clinical features, but also new symptoms and signs that represent previously undetectable subclinical lesions. Treatment of such symptoms involves treating the underlying infection and keeping the body temperature normal.

## TREATMENT OF ACUTE RELAPSE

Steroids and adrenocorticotropic hormone (ACTH) are effective in blunting exacerbations of MS, but not in reversing the disease or preventing its progression. Oral prednisone (up to 100 mg per day) is believed to be as effective as ACTH although no definitive trial has been conducted. Recently, pulses of high doses of intravenous steroids (up to as much as 1000 mg per day of methylprednisolone for three days) have been reported to produce abrupt improvement in symptoms. (These have all been in uncontrolled studies.) For an acute relapse, prednisone, up to 100 mg per day for a week, is usually sufficient. The drug should be tapered over another one to two weeks.

Steroids and ACTH probably exert their immediate effects by reducing the edema around a plaque, thus directly improving nerve tract function. Steroids may also stabilize nerve membranes. In addition to these rapid effects, steroids influence immune function, which may be important in blunting subsequent exacerbations of MS. However modest the short-term benefits of steroids in MS, they must be weighed against their potential toxicities and the chance for spontaneous recovery in MS. Thus, patients should be carefully selected for steroid therapy.

Most therapies to prevent exacerbation or reverse progression have been directed at suppressing or augmenting immune reactivity, which is thought to be responsible in some way for the exacerbations and the progression of MS. An alkylating agent, cyclophosphamide (Cytoxan), has been used both alone and in concert with other therapies in several large "nonblinded" studies and is reported to benefit both relapsing and progressive MS. Short-term side-effects of cyclophosphamide include nausea, alopecia, amenorrhea, cystitis, and a decrease in white blood cells. Other immune therapies include cyclosporine. A long-term complication of these therapies includes increases in certain malignancies. Although not yet reported in MS, these are *potential* severe side-effects. The physician seeing the homebound patient with MS should be prepared to give psychological support to the patient and the family. The physician should check all MS patients for signs of infection (bladder, lungs, decubiti), and treat these when necessary, but the patient who is on steroids or immunosuppressive drugs is even more likely to develop infections and such patients must be checked even more frequently.

## BRAIN TUMORS

There are 385,000 deaths from cancer each year and 50,000 (13%) are associated with CNS involvement. It is estimated that of these 50,000 deaths, 8,500 (17%) are caused by primary brain tumors (usually malignant gliomas).

Patients with brain tumors are encountered in three separate circumstances. In the first, the patient presents with a brain tumor and no history of systemic cancer. Work-up in such an instance will as likely reveal the tumor to be metastatic as primary. In the second instance, the patient presents with a brain tumor and a past history of systemic cancer. Work-up in this setting almost always reveals the tumor to be metastatic. In the third instance, a patient with obvious systemic cancer develops a brain tumor that on work-up is invariably metastatic.

Most classifications of brain tumors emphasize the embryogenesis of the various cellular components of the CNS and attempt to classify the tumors in terms of the different morphologic stages that the cells pass through during oncogenesis. Tumors are classified into those of astroglial, oligodendroglial, ependymal, and neuronal series. The glioblastoma is conceived of as originating *de novo* from a primitive stem cell, the glioblast. Occasionally, it is conceived of as originating from an astrocytoma and is referred to as a secondary glioblastoma. Recently, the tendency has been to downplay the concept of embryogenesis and to emphasize the importance of anaplasia. Glial tumors, like neoplasms elsewhere in the body, undergo increasing anaplasia and their classification has been simplified into astrocytomas, oligodendrogliomas, or ependymomas of varying grades of malignancy.

The diagnosis of a brain tumor depends on the correlation of symptoms and signs with neuroradiologic findings. The most common symptoms of a brain tumor are headache (occurring in 30% of patients); seizures (occurring in 20%); personality changes; and motor and speech disturbances. When focal deficits are progressive for several weeks or months, they are usually indicative of a brain tumor. Symptoms of malignant brain tumors are usually present for less than a year before diagnosis. Similar symptoms of more than a year's duration generally indicate a less malignant tumor. Occasionally (less than 5%) brain tumors may present with an abrupt onset resulting from a hemorrhage into a tumor or an infarct of the surrounding brain. The diagnosis of brain tumor has been markedly facilitated by computed tomography (CT) and magnetic resonance imaging (MRI). Despite the progress in increasing both survival and quality of survival, it is apparent that virtually all patients with malignant gliomas die of their disease because of a failure to eradicate the primary lesion. The surgeon is rarely able to do a complete resection, and conventional radiation or chemotherapy falls short of destroying the tumor.

Metastasis to the brain and spinal cord is the most common neurologic complication of systemic cancer. Autopsy studies suggest as many as 15% of patients who die of cancer harbor brain or spinal cord metastases at autopsy. Of these, two thirds to three fourths will have suffered some neurologic symptoms during life, and many will have been disabled by their neurologic disease, having died as a direct result of this. While metastases may appear anywhere within the brain, their distribution generally parallels the blood supply to the brain, occurring about equally in both hemispheres in the territory of the middle cerebral arteries. About 10% to 15% of metastases occur in the cerebellum. In more than half of the patients with brain metastases, the lesions are multiple, a situation more common with certain tumors, such as carcinoma of the lung and malignant melanoma. Spinal cord compression by a metastatic tumor growing into the epidural space in the vertebral body is relatively common, perhaps affecting about 5% of patients with systemic cancer.

The physician managing homebound patients with cancer will encounter patients with both primary and metastatic cancer. These patients will be suffering from complications of brain and spinal cord compression. The physician will have to evaluate and manage these patients, including the complications resulting from immobility, such as aspiration pneumonia, phlebitis, and decubitus ulcers. Additionally, many patients with brain tumors have seizures, which present their own clinical problems.

A seizure is an abnormal discharge of nerve cells within the brain, with the clinical manifestation depending on the location of the abnormally discharging neurons. When relatively few motor neurons in the cortex discharge, there may be only jerking of a contralateral limb, without loss of consciousness. This is called a simple partial motor seizure. When millions of neurons throughout the brain discharge, the seizure is characterized by a loss of consciousness that is accompanied by a tonic–clonic phase and is followed by postictal confusion (a grand mal seizure). Between these two seizure extremes are many different types of seizures. A frequent type is the complex partial seizure formerly called a *psychomotor* or *temporal lobe seizure*. It is important to remember that seizures occur in patients without brain tumors. Indeed, patients with brain tumors represent only a small minority of patients with seizures. More than two million Americans have suffered two or more seizures, and more than four million have had at least one seizure. More than 200,000 Americans have seizures more than once a month despite treatment with antiepileptic drugs. Even though in most patients the cause of the seizures cannot be determined (idiopathic epilepsy), the majority of seizures can be controlled if the correct seizure diagnosis is made and the correct drug is maintained at a therapeutic serum concentration. The physician who can manage the seizures that occur in a patient with a brain tumor can use these principles to manage all patients with seizures.

The pharmacologic principles for effective oral use of antiepileptic drugs relate to drug absorption, distribution, and elimination. Drug absorption depends on the ability of the gastrointestinal (GI) tract to facilitate entrance of the ingested drug into the blood. This, in turn, is a function of the properties of the drug and its interaction with the cell membranes of the GI tract. All antiepileptic drugs are of small molecular weight and cross lipid membranes with ease, thus allowing almost total absorption in most cases. Exceptionally, a specific absorption defect in some patients may interfere with the bioavailability of a particular drug. Drugs taken when the stomach is empty may be absorbed much more rapidly than those taken directly after a meal. Antiepileptic drugs whose lipid solubility is high are distributed to all body tissues in various proportions. As a result the brain concentration is, in most cases, equal to or greater than that of other body tissues. The blood concentrations can therefore be used as an important guide to therapy. Although a drug may be eliminated by metabolism, storage, or excretion, the major clinical concern is with the rate of disappearance of the drug. This rate is usually expressed as the time required to remove half of the active drug from the body. The half-lives, which have been measured for all antiepileptic drugs, determine the frequency of drug administration: drugs with longer half-lives, such as phenytoin (Dilantin) and phenobarbital, can be administered once or twice daily without large fluctuations in their concentrations in the blood, and drugs such as carbamazepine (Tegretol) and valproic acid, which have shorter half-lives, require more frequent dosing.

Drugs with long half-lives may require many days to reach a steady state, the time needed being approximately five times the half-life of the drug. This means that drugs such as phenobarbital and phenytoin may require 5 to 10 days or longer to reach a steady state, but that drugs such as carbamazepine and valproic acid will reach steady state in 2 to 4 days. Another pharmacologic principle of importance relates to the problems of polypharmacy. Recent studies suggest that single-drug therapy may be superior to multiple-drug regimens in mildly to moderately affected patients, thus strongly reinforcing the recommendation of trying single drugs first. Whenever possible, the sedative medications that interfere with behavioral and functional aspects in both children and adults should be avoided. This is especially true for the barbiturates, particularly in a patient who is already drowsy because of increased intracranial pressure. Generalized tonic–clonic seizures are best treated with phenytoin, carbamazepine, or phenobarbital. In resistant cases, two drugs may be used together. If control is not possible with two drugs, it may be necessary to resort to another combination or even a third drug. The partial motor or complex seizures usually respond to the same drugs used for generalized seizures. Thus, phenytoin and carbamazepine are effective for partial seizures, and neither has a prominent sedative effect.

The physician managing a homebound patient with a brain tumor will have to be able to manage seizures, treat infections, and evaluate the patient for signs of increased intracranial or spinal cord pressure. Most homebound patients with brain or spinal cord tumors will already have had surgery, received radiation therapy, and will have completed chemotherapy. The physician managing such patients will be primarily interested in maintaining the patient comfortably and will have to deal with the stresses of the patient's dying. Patients who are showing signs of increased intracranial pressure will either become drowsy or have a worsening of their focal neurologic symptoms. The neurologic symptoms may respond to increased doses of steroids, which reduce the increased intracranial pressure. The temporary improvement gained from the steroids must be weighed against the complications of chronic high-dose steroids. In some instances the dying patient with an inoperable brain tumor who is becoming increasingly drowsy and stuporous may benefit from less, not more, steroids, thus allowing the patient to lapse into coma and die. Such a decision should be discussed with the patient (when possible) and the family. The family should be prepared for the fact that the patient dying of a brain tumor is not in pain, but that when he goes into a coma he may develop heavy rapid breathing suggesting that he is in pain.

## Appendix

### *NYU Parkinson Disability Scale (revised 1986)*

Facial masking
   0: No facial masking
   2: Facial masking present

Salivation
   0: No drooling during exam
   1: Drooling during exam

Speech
   0: Normal, voice soft but understandable
   2: Minimal impairment
   4: Moderate–marked impairment, difficult to understand patient

Total score = 7

Tremor
   Tremor at rest is rated in the upper limbs.
   0: Absent
   2: Minimally present
   4: Moderate–markedly present
   For the upper limbs only, the patient is asked to take his right or left index finger and touch the examiner's finger and then touch his (the patient's) nose.
   The tremor is rated during these maneuvers.
   0: Absent
   2: Present

Total score = 14

Rigidity
   The resistance to passive movement is rated at each of the four limbs and at the neck
   0: Absent
   1: Present
   2: Marked

Total score = 10

Bradykinesia
   The ability of the patient to perform various maneuvers is then assessed. These maneuvers are individually performed and include tapping first the right thumb and right index finger together and then the left, 10 times. Alternately pronating and supinating the right wrist and then the left, 10 times. Tapping the right foot and then the left, 10 times.
   0: No impairment
   2: Minimal impairment
   4: Moderate–marked impairment
   The patient, while seated, is then asked to open and close both hands while simultaneously tapping his feet, 10 times.
   0: No impairment
   5: Minimal impairment
   8: Marked impairment

Total score = 32

Gait and postural stability
   The patient is asked to get up from and sit down in a chair, 5 times.
   0: No difficulty
   5: Minimal difficulty
 10: Marked difficulty
   The patient's posture is assessed
   0: No impairment
   2: Postural deformity present
   The ability of the patient to withstand an abrupt shove against the sternum is assessed.
   0: No difficulty
   5: Retropulsion, but patient recovers
 10: Patient would fall if not caught

The patient's gait is assessed by having the patient walk back and forth several times.

0: No impairment

5: Minimal impairment, manifested by short steps or difficulty with turns or difficulty doing tandem walking

10: Moderate gait impairment, obvious gait difficulty

15: Marked gait impairment

## NYU Functional Disability Scale (Revised 1986)

### *Activities of Daily Living*

Speech

0: Normal

2: Minimal impairment; loss of expression, diction, and/or volume

5: Moderate; slurred but understandable

10: Marked; difficult to understand

Salivation

0: Normal

2: Minimal; but definite excess of saliva, nighttime drooling

5: Moderate–marked; excess saliva, daytime drooling

Swallowing

0: Normal

2: Minimal impairment; occasional choking

5: Moderate–marked; requires special diet

Handwriting

0: Normal

2: Minimal impairment; slow or small, all words are legible

5: Moderate–marked; most words are not legible

Cutting food and handling utensil

0: Normal

2: Minimal impairment; slow and clumsy, but no help needed

5: Moderate; needs some help

10: Marked; helpless

Dressing

0: Normal

2: Minimal impairment; slow, no help needed

5: Moderate; considerable help required, but can do many things alone

10: Marked, helpless

Hygiene

0: Normal

2: Minimal impairment; slow, but no help needed

5: Moderate; needs help to shower or bathe; very slow in hygienic care

10: Marked; requires assistance for washing, brushing teeth, combing hair, going to bathroom

Turning in bed and adjusting bed clothes

0: Normal

2: Minimal impairment; slow and clumsy, but no help needed

5: Moderate–marked; can initiate, but not turn or adjust sheets alone

Walking

0: Normal

5: Walks slowly, may shuffle with short steps; no assistance

10: Severe disturbance of walking; requiring assistance

Freezing when walking

0: None

5: Sudden transient freezing; only when going through a doorway or into an elevator; no falling; recovers in seconds

10: Severe freezing; occasionally falls

Falling (unrelated to freezing)

0: None

5: Falls less than once daily
10: Falls more than once daily

Tremor
0: Absent
2: Minimal; infrequently present
5: Moderate; bothersome to patient
10: Marked; interferes with most activities

Sensory complaints related to parkinsonism
0: None
2: Occasionally has numbness, tingling, or mild aching
5: Frequent painful sensations

# 16
# Skin Care

JOSEPH AGRIS

Care of the skin is one of the most important aspects of home care of the patient with restricted mobility. The skin is accessible and can be readily visualized, a unique feature of this organ system. Most treatments can be done by the patient and care partner in conjunction with the nurse. And, most important, preventive care is easy and extremely effective; in fact, the prevention of decubiti may well be one of the most effective preventive modalities we have for these patients.

What are some of the factors that lead to an elderly immobilized patient's susceptibility to skin problems? Over a period of years, exposure to ultraviolet rays prematurely ages the skin, particularly in fair-skinned individuals. The exposure to the sun is cumulative and some of the end results are pigmentation changes, telangiectasias, and atrophy. Another result is skin carcinoma on the sun-exposed areas such as the scalp, face, back of the hands, and, in women, the lower extremities. As we all spend more time in the sun and wear lighter clothing (and as sun-tanning facilities proliferate) we will be seeing more premature aging of the skin with the resultant increased predilection to skin breakdown in later years. The burden is on the medical community to care for these people so as to minimize these effects.

## GENERAL PRINCIPLES

Caring for the skin in the immobilized patient is an essential and integral part of overall management. The major role of the physician is educating the patient and family as to the importance of preventive skin inspection and early treatment if problems should arise.

Keeping the skin clean and dry at all times is absolutely essential. Areas where perspiration or body fluids accumulate (perianal, perineal, gluteal, and axillary areas) must be cleansed several times a day with a mild soap—the milder the soap, the better and the fewer ingredients the better (no antiperspirants, coloring agents, or perfumes). The skin in these areas is often quite fragile and sensitive to these extraneous chemicals. Many rashes that develop can be "cured" by removing the offending agents before resorting to topical steroids or other medications. After washing, the skin should be rinsed very well with water and patted dry, not rubbed. Next, a lubricating cream or lotion can be applied and gently rubbed into the skin, being sure to neither rub too hard nor leave any residue on the skin. Residual lotion will lead to sensitization and maceration. The same principles apply to these lotions—the fewer ingredients, the better.

A fine powder may be used in the intertriginous areas. Excess powder is to be avoided because it will produce a coarse abrasive sandpaper-like result, causing fine superficial abrasions, which, over time, will lead to further skin breakdown. Also, the skin must be absolutely dry before applying any powder; otherwise the powder will form a paste and retain moisture against the skin surface. When it comes to powder, more is not better. A small amount applied two or three times a day is more effective than a large amount applied once. The powder should be applied sparingly and gently spread over the skin surface, leaving a fine coating. Any combination of moisture, abrasion, maceration, heat, friction, and pressure must be avoided.

Patients with bladder incontinence present with their own special set of problems. Urethral catheters must be constantly checked for leakage. If leakage occurs, the skin should be gently washed and rinsed well to remove any urine contamination. After patting the skin dry a moisturizing lotion can be applied. The appropriate type of incontinence pad or adult diaper can greatly decrease the incidence of skin problems should incontinence be a problem (see Chap. 13).

Bowel incontinence, being more difficult to control and deal with, presents other problems. Here, the first goal is the primary management of the incontinence. If that is not successful it is important to remove the feces and clean the skin, as with urinary incontinence, as soon as possible. In the buttock and perineal area allowing the skin to dry adequately is of prime importance. It may take up to 30 minutes for full evaporation to occur. In fact, if the skin does become irritated, exposure to the air is still one of the most effective measures. After the skin is meticulously washed and completely dried, powder may be applied.

Plastic undergarments are a mixed blessing. They effectively prevent soiling of the bed linen but also keep the moisture in contact with the skin, creating the potential for problems or worsening the problems that already exist. Once skin breakdown has occurred, plastic garments are to be avoided and air circulation maximized. If plastic is used, frequent changes and washings are essential. Many of the newer incontinence products can avoid some of these problems. They are available from a variety of manufacturers in both disposable and reusable forms.

Clothing and bedding should be as wrinkle free as possible. Clothing should be of a porous absorbent material to allow for air circulation and avoid the accumulation of perspiration. Care should be taken to choose clothing without multiple pleats, heavy overlapping seams or closures, clips, buttons, or snaps that could lead to localized areas of pressure. Tight-fitting garments or constrictive elastic bands can also be detrimental by causing skin irritation and obstruction of the venous circulation.

## POSITIONING THE PATIENT

Friction and shearing forces are potentially detrimental to the skin, particularly if chronically present. This is relevant for (1) the patient with flexion contractures where there is constant rubbing of the knees against a bed rail; (2) the patient who is constantly sliding down in bed or in the chair, applying very large shearing forces to the skin of the buttocks; and (3) the patient who is dragged up in bed by a well-meaning family instead of being gently lifted. The solution to the last problem includes lifting instead of dragging, or using a draw sheet if necessary. Patients should be positioned as far back in the chair as possible and, if warranted, a restraining device should be used to maintain an upright position. The constant slow forward slipping creates friction and shearing forces between the skin and underlying bone. In combination with incontinence and skin maceration, these forces can quickly lead to skin breakdown. It is the repetitive, chronic nature of this situation that creates the problem. Because of the rather benign appearance of the slipping and the insidious nature of the damage, the problem is often not recognized early. Necrosis, when it does appear, often seems very sudden and may cover a wide area with deep penetration.

Patients with spasms are at risk from the friction, shearing, and direct trauma that result from these movements. Treatment of these patients should be directed at managing the spasms and providing cushioning and appropriate positioning. If repetitive rubbing is particularly troublesome, some of these patients may benefit from surgical release of the contractures, particularly of the lower extremities. Likewise, regional blocks may prevent the movement. As a last resort, cordotomy or rhizotomy may be needed.

## SENSORY LEVEL AND SKIN CARE

Patients with neurologic disorders such as stroke, demyelinating conditions, paraplegia, and quadriplegia have a spectrum of sensory loss ranging from the normal to the insensate. This is usually a gradual progression rather than a sharp demarcation. It is important to identify these areas because the patient will not be aware of the normal pressure sensation, so that skin damage may be occurring without any warning. Diabetic patients are particularly prone to this complication in the feet due to peripheral neuropathy. Management of these patients requires shifting position on a regular frequent, rather rigid, schedule. If the patient is unable to learn to do this himself, because of the primary disease process or dementia, the care partner should be taught to assume responsibility for repositioning the patient. Contributing to skin breakdown, the patient with a sensory deficit may have skin and muscle atrophy so that pressure is being transmitted directly to the underlying bone.

The application of adhesive dressings, tourniquets, prosthetic devices, and straps for leg bags must be carefully thought out in the patient with a sensory loss. A common site for skin breakdown is the lower leg site of attachment of the drainage bag for urinary catheters. The attachments should not be overly snug and the buckle must not be in direct contact with the skin. The sites of the strap attachments should be rotated periodically. It is particularly important to instruct the patient, care partner, and nurse about these issues which are so easily checked and can result in such an enormous problem if a decubitus ulcer results.

## TEMPERATURE CONTROL

Body temperature control is often impaired in patients with central or spinal cord lesions. Reflex changes and blood flow are altered below the level of the lesion in spinal cord patients, impairing the normal sweating and shivering mechanisms. Maintaining a stable, comfortable room temperature and humidity level becomes important in these situations.

A phenomenon called autonomic hyperreflexia occurs in patients with complete spinal cord lesions above the T5–T6 level. Severe hypertension and profuse sweating, initiated by reflex sympathetic and parasympathetic actions, result from a variety of stimuli. This phenomenon can be caused by stimulation of pain receptors, infection, chemical agents, catheterization, bladder or visceral distention, or stimulation of the skin because of breakdown. The patient may complain of a headache and will be acutely hypertensive, as well as having dilated pupils. It is important for the patient and family to recognize this as it is happening. The particular concern, in addition to discomfort, is the profuse sweating and its effects on the skin.

Treatment consists of removing the trigger stimuli, if they can be identified; monitoring the blood pressure; elevating the head of the bed; and checking for either abdominal distention or a plugged catheter. A rectal examination can be performed to check for fecal impaction. If the problem is recurrent and not amenable to these simple measures, phenoxybenzamine may be helpful. This produces a "chemical sympathectomy," stabilizing the problem. The most important feature, in terms of the skin, is to control the environment and take into account the potential effects of profuse sweating on the skin.

## CRITERIA FOR SKIN ASSESSMENT AND RISK FACTORS

Many factors predispose to the breakdown of the skin. These include paralysis, paresis, malnutrition, anemia, shearing forces, pressure, infection, and the changes associated with advanced age. The debilitated, paraplegic, or comatose patient lacks "protective sensation" that alerts him to the normal discomfort produced by prolonged immobility. Because the patient feels *no* discomfort and is medically debilitated (paralysis, paresis, stroke), he cannot change body position. As a result, localized areas of pressure, aggravated by moisture and such other problems as incontinence of bowel or bladder, result in skin breakdown, with secondary infection developing at these sites. The major cause, in all cases, is pressure.

Prolonged periods of even minimal pressure are just as likely to cause injury as intense pressure of short duration. Tissue necrosis and cell death result when external pressures exceed the normal capillary pressure of 32 mm Hg. When this occurs, the blood supply to the area is compromised, followed by an inflammatory process and subsequent vasodilatation. A circumferential reactive hyperemia is seen. Therefore, the first recognizable sign is erythema. This color change is easily recognized. If the pressure is relieved, thereby allowing perfusion of the tissue and removal of toxic by-products, this initial damage may be reversible. However, if the pressure is not relieved, or if the patient has been in the position over a prolonged period of time, irreversible damage may occur. This can happen in as short a period as 30 minutes, depending on the amount of pressure, the condition of the skin, the adequacy of the blood supply, and the overall health and well-being of the patient. Even when the hyperemia and inflammation are recognized early, and treatment immediately instituted, it is still likely that necrosis of the underlying tissue, as well as muscle, may have already occurred.

## PRESSURE RELIEF

A bedridden person will need to be turned on a schedule, usually every two hours, around the clock. For this, several attendants may be necessary. A turning frame or rotary bed might be helpful but is very expensive. Each turn need not be from prone to supine, but should involve sufficient repositioning to relieve the pressure sites at risk. In the home setting, if such frequent positioning is not possible, the patient should be positioned so that the weight of the body is distributed over the *largest possible area*. Localized pressure is minimized by proper body alignment and the careful placement of foam pads, cushions, and pillows. Use of a foam mattress or air-filled or fluid-filled flotation mattress will lessen the risk of pressure defects. Foam cut-outs and rubber rings should *not* be used, because they result in localized pressure and compromise the surrounding venous circulation. In most instances they will do more harm than good.

Most pressure ulcers develop over the bony prominences of the sacrum, ischium, and trochanter. Thus, patients are more vulnerable in the sitting or supine position. Patients who are susceptible to pressure ulcers should be encouraged to sleep prone, unless they have limited respiratory capacity. With the patient in the prone position, body weight is more evenly distributed over the chest, abdomen, and thighs. Even without special equipment and with only the proper placement of four or five pillows (under the chest, pelvis, thigh, and ankle area), the distribution of forces will be such that pressure will be relieved and decubitus prevention maintained. A patient can be taught to maintain the prone position for increasing lengths of time. After a period of approximately two weeks, the patient should be able to spend the entire night on his abdomen, with little or no disturbance of his sleep. In many cases the prone patient will not require turning during the night. This is a great relief to the care partner, whose own loss of sleep is a major burden.

A wheelchair-bound patient must be taught to shift his weight or elevate himself approximately 1 minute out of every 15 minutes. This relieves pressure and allows him to continue sitting for several hours without the risk of developing skin breakdown. The usual sling seat in a wheelchair is designed for only brief periods of sitting. If a wheelchair is used for more prolonged periods, a special, readily available cushion is necessary to relieve the pressure on the trochanters. Initially, weight shifting will require conscientious attention and exercise to strengthen the arms and upper torso. Of some help are electronic devices with flashing lights or a ringing bell that will remind the patient to do the weight shifts.

## RECOGNITION OF EARLY SIGNS OF SKIN BREAKDOWN

The initial signs that may lead to skin damage and breakdown are *erythema, edema,* and *punctate hemorrhages* (see Recognition of Tissue Breakdown). As little as 30 minutes of pressure may produce an area of erythema, but usually 2 to 6 hours are required to produce a significant problem. Incipient difficulty is easily recognized by the pink to bright red, usually circular or elliptical area that results, most commonly over a bony prominence. The affected area is usually warmer than the surrounding skin, when compared by placing the wrist or the back of the hand against the adjacent skin and then touching the involved area. The central portion is often flattened, and the periphery is elevated and edematous. This is the result of central compression by the bony prominence and the peripheral deposition of fluid from dependency and the inflammatory process. If there is significant pressure for a short duration or a prolonged pressure over many hours, punctate hemorrhages may be seen in the central area. This situation may still be reversible, but is more tenuous.

As the vascularity of the skin is compromised, blisters or serum-filled bullae appear. This is an ominous sign and is an indication of irreversible superficial skin loss with possible underlying damage. Eventually the bullae will rupture and the overlying skin will slough. A circumferential erythematous halo (cellulitis) usually develops. In 3 to 5 days a well-circumscribed focus of necrosis results, initially appearing as a reddish-gray area, progressing to a waxy, yellowish-gray eschar. If the area remains dry, a gray-to-black leathery eschar with a concave center remains. This is actually an area of dry, noninfected, localized gangrene.

An eschar such as this can often be maintained for months to years without any further treatment, provided it remains dry. Moisture, as a result of normal body processes (sweating, urinary or bowel incontinence) may cause the eschar to separate from the surrounding tissue. Secondary infection (usually gram-negative) ensues, with a slowly enlarging circumferential, erythematous halo, often quite brightly colored. If it extends for 2 cm beyond the area of skin breakdown, it is considered an active cellulitis, requiring systemic antibiotics. As the cellulitis progresses, bleeding and a serosanguineous discharge may then develop, with putrefaction becoming evident. Bacterial infection enlarges the defect and destruction of the underlying subcutaneous tissue occurs first, followed by muscle destruction. The next step is abscess formation, which will extend along the plane of least resistance. This process, in turn, initiates thrombosis of adjacent and deeper vessels, causing further necrosis and continued extension of the defect.

## RECOGNITION OF TISSUE BREAKDOWN

### Early Signs*

1. Redness of the skin (erythema) that does not disappear within a few minutes of relief of pressure on the area
2. Surrounding edema that does not disappear after relief of pressure
3. Induration
4. Blistering of the skin or bulla formation
5. Abrasion of the epidermal layer (partial-thickness skin loss)
6. Localized area of infection, with abrasion

### Late Signs and Symptoms†

1. Full-thickness skin loss (ulceration of the skin, with exposure of adipose tissue)
2. Eschar formation (wet or dry necrosis)
3. Infection, cellulitis (greater than 2 cm) surrounding the area
4. Active drainage
5. Fever and tachycardia
6. Septicemia and bacteremia
7. Ulceration and destruction of soft tissue resulting in underlying osteomyelitis or septic arthritis

*In most cases, these problems are reversible with immediate and appropriate care.
†All of these problems indicate permanent damage. In most instances, surgical intervention is required.

---

As a protective measure, the margins of the defect thicken and roll inward toward the base, creating a bursa-lined cavity. No topical medication is of any value once a wet eschar (wet gangrene) develops. At this point the only treatment is surgical intervention, with removal of the entire eschar and the underlying devitalized tissue, followed by packing of the open wound.

If the process is allowed to continue, a large, deep area of destruction results, which may evolve into osteomyelitis and septic arthritis. Ultimately, the largest part of the lesion is not at the skin surface, but at the level of the bony prominence. This can be thought of as an iceberg, in which 70% of the defect lies below the surface, and only 30% above. The same is true for the progression of skin breakdown and ulcer formation. The important point to emphasize to the family and patient is that "a little bit of redness" may be of enormous significance (see Criteria for Skin Assessment).

## WOUND MANAGEMENT

Once skin breakdown has occurred, a program of wound management must be established. Nonoperative management of pressure ulcers is directed at establishing a clean wound and improving the patient's overall condition. An often overlooked facet of this is nutrition, which is of great importance if the wound is to heal well, whether the treatment is medical or surgical. The best of techniques will likely fail if the patient's nutrition is poor. Sometimes definitive treatment must await stabilizing the patient's protein balance.

The first line of defense is the removal of all pressure; this will be repeated over and over because it is of such great importance. If the wound is only a superficial abrasion, it should be cleaned with a mild soap and water solution, gently patted dry, and then coated with Mercurochrome or Merthiolate as an antibacterial and drying agent. This should be repeated three times a day and epithelialization of a superficial wound usually occurs in 14 to

## CRITERIA FOR SKIN ASSESSMENT

Color change (erythema)

Temperature change

Moisture (skin maceration)

Changes in texture

Blisters or bullae on skin

Skin rash

Recognition of bony prominences (pressure points)

21 days. Once this has occurred, the patient may be rotated again to this site, paying meticulous attention to the area in the future.

When blisters or bullae occur, they should not be ruptured. If the blisters are maintained closed, the chance of infection is reduced and epithelialization occurs more quickly. The area should be gently washed with a mild soap and water solution, rinsed well, and covered with a fluff dressing. An alternative is to keep the site open to the air, provided this is an acceptable position and the patient's activities are not too severely restricted.

If a bulla ruptures, the devitalized skin should be debrided, the wound again cleansed with a soap and water solution, and a drying antibacterial agent, such as 10% Mercurochrome, applied. Wounds will do best when left exposed to the air and free from further maceration. If the wound must be covered, a dry porous dressing should be applied (such as mesh gauze, which will not stick to the skin) and then covered by a latex type gauze dressing.

Another option is the use of occlusive dressings, which allow the wound to be managed with a minimum of care partner involvement. Some of the newer products need to be changed only once a week; they can be kept on in the shower and do not have to be changed if they get wet. These are distinct advantages compared to the alternatives. Evidence suggests that wounds heal more quickly, and with a decreased incidence of infection, when these products are appropriately used. In the perineum there is the added advantage of the dressing protecting the wound from urinary or fecal contamination. Regardless of the type of dressing used, paper or hypoallergenic tape should be used in place of adhesive tape because of the vulnerability and sensitivity of the elderly skin.

Full-thickness skin losses less than 1 cm² in size should close spontaneously by peripheral epithelialization if meticulous wound care is provided. Full-thickness loss means that the subcutaneous tissue has been exposed, with an important implication. Fat tissue, having a poor blood supply, is an excellent medium for bacterial growth. Careful cleansing with mild soap and water, followed by the application of a topical antibiotic cream and covering with a porous dressing, is the treatment of choice.

These small wounds are probably the only decubitus problems for which there is a role for topical agents, be they enzymes or antibiotics. Large wounds will rarely respond satisfactorily and the eventual definitive treatment is only delayed. We have a false sense of security in using these products for larger wounds in the unrealistic hope of avoiding debridement.

Larger lesions with a dark *dry* eschar can be approached in a variety of ways. Commonly they can be left alone. The area can be maintained for months to years simply by gentle cleaning and drying. These lesions do not, of necessity, need to be debrided if that is undesirable for other reasons.

On the other hand, an eschar that becomes soft, is concave (indicating fluid collection under the eschar), whose margins have elevated, or is draining needs sharp surgical debridement. Debridement should include all devitalized tissue, including subcutaneous tissue and muscle, continuing until the first signs of bleeding are noted along the wound margin and at its base. Once the first sign of bleeding occurs, debridement should be discontinued. In other words, sharp debridement should not produce bleeding that cannot be controlled by pressure alone. This is a technique easily performed at the bedside with scissors and forceps.

After completing the debridement, the wound should be irrigated every 8 hours with a solution of sterile saline, povidone iodine or 0.25% acetic acid. The acetic acid has the advantage of being inexpensive and will reduce the odor produced by gram-negative bacteria. The wound is packed with wide mesh roll gauze (the gauze is first soaked in either saline, povidone, or acetic acid, being sure to wring it out well), repeating this step every 4 to 6 hours, leaving the longer intervals for bedtime. When packing the wound, the gauze is inserted so that it is completely inside the wound. One of the most common errors is to leave the wet dressing partially outside the wound, leading to maceration of the surrounding skin. Once the gauze is well inside the defect, dry packing is placed on top of this, followed by a dry dressing. Benzoin may be used to toughen the skin, and paper tape is the preferred adhesive. The purpose of the wet-to-dry dressing is to allow the gauze to dry slowly so that it adheres to the base and margins of the wound, accomplishing a very effective debridement each time the process is repeated.

Several times a week the wound should be inspected and further sharp debridement carried out as necessary. This is repeated until a clean, granulating wound has been produced. Depending on the patient's overall status it is either maintained in this fashion or surgical intervention is undertaken. A point that is frequently overlooked in our zeal to reach closure on any and all skin lesions is that not all ulcers need to be closed. Often in an elderly, debilitated, nutritionally deficient patient the risks of closing the wound far exceed the potential benefit, recognizing that the daily maintenance of these wounds is not necessarily terribly onerous. If, on the other hand, the care partner is unable to do this, and nursing home placement is the other option, then closure should be attempted.

The goal of pressure ulcer management is to prevent further extension. That can be accomplished by either of the approaches just mentioned, keeping in mind the patient's perspective of what is going to be least risky and most acceptable in the total case management. As mentioned previously, occlusive dressings offer the advantages of ease of application and decreased frequency of changes.

## SYSTEMIC ANTIBIOTICS

Administration of systemic antibiotics does not lead to adequate tissue levels in granulating chronic wounds. Therefore, their use has little or no effect on the bacteria level. Other than in acute sepsis, systemic antibiotics should not be used in the treatment of chronic pressure ulcers. However, in the preoperative, intraoperative, and postoperative periods, when surgical excision and immediate closure are to be undertaken, systemic antibiotics do play a role. New tissue planes are opened during the surgical procedure and, at this time, systemic antibiotics will prevent the establishment of foci of infection beyond the ulcer. As with any potent therapeutic agent, the antibiotic should be introduced at the time when it is most effective. This is just prior to, at the time of, and for several days after the surgical procedure is undertaken. Thus, in the treatment of chronic pressure ulcers, systemic antibiotics are used only as an adjunct to surgical management.

To determine the antibiotic of choice, a punch biopsy of the granulation tissue at the base of the ulcer is taken and sent for culture and sensitivity. This is simple, quick, and easily done, and provides a more accurate determination of the bacterial flora than the use of a cotton swab on the surface of the defect. Generally, chronically contaminated ulcers contain mixed populations of gram-negative organisms.

## TOPICAL ANTIBIOTICS

Topical antibiotics do not penetrate to the depth of the wound nor do they affect bacterial growth in granulation tissue. An exception may be silver sulfadiazine, which has been shown to penetrate burn eschars. There are no conclusive data on the superiority of topical antibiotics over wet-to-dry saline dressings. Chronic use of topical antibiotics may result in the formation of resistant strains of organisms. The overzealous application of topical antibiotics, cream or ointment, may coat the wound and certain organisms may actually flourish in this atmosphere. Topical antibiotics may cause localized tissue sensitivity, resulting in a detrimental effect on wound healing. There is also the possibility of a systemic reaction to the topical antibiotic. Topical antibiotics should be limited to use on abrasions and partial-thickness skin losses. Once the wound has extended below the dermis and a cavity has formed, the basic principles of wound management, including debridement and packing, are indicated.

Most superficial wounds do better with a drying agent, such as Mercurochrome or Merthiolate, rather than a wetting agent, such as a topical antibiotic. Exposure to the air is also helpful. Because deeper wounds require surgical debridement and packing, topical creams and medications play a small role in the management of these lesions.

## ENZYMATIC AGENTS

Enzymatic agents used for debridement of pressure ulcers include collagenase, papain, urea, chlorophyllin, streptokinase, fibrinolysin, and deoxyribonuclease. If properly used, these agents will debride the superficial layers of a superficial ulceration, and will help in removing serum and a gelatinous exudate. However, their ability to penetrate an eschar or to remove gross devitalized tissue is not proven. They have little or no use in the management of these wounds and often give the patient and the person caring for him false security. Indeed, some of these agents may be toxic if applied over large areas. Proper uses of forceps and scissors can accomplish more in a few minutes than the application of this medication does over many weeks. If good debridement is followed by cleansing of the wound with a mild soap and water solution, the same goals can be achieved faster and less expensively. In addition, none of these agents will remove large amounts of devitalized tissue, they will not penetrate an eschar, and they will have *no* effect on a well-established bursa or sinus tract. These agents will not penetrate to the base of a deep wound and some may actually plug the opening and impede drainage. Topical enzymes should never be a substitute for debridement and meticulous wound care.

Summary of Nonsurgical Treatment of Decubiti
1. Pressure relief of the involved area
2. Preservation of the surrounding, uninjured normal skin
3. Debridement of necrotic and devitalized tissue
4. Systematized cleansing and packing of the wound
5. Treatment of cellulitis if present
6. When ready, surgical closure of the wound, if the general condition of the patient permits

## SURGICAL CLOSURE

The patient is ready for surgery when his physical condition is stable, spasms and contractures have been controlled, and the ulcer is clean and free of infection. The surgical procedure for pressure ulcer defect includes excision of the ulcer, removal of any scar tissue, excision of the bursa and any sinus tract that has formed, and ostectomy of the bony prominence followed by closure of the defect. This is an ideal approach and is applicable to younger, healthier individuals. However, the elderly and the severely debilitated may not tolerate such procedures. For the elderly or debilitated patient, often the most effective treatment of a small acute pressure defect is to excise it before it becomes infected and close it primarily. This can often be done at the bedside, using local anesthesia. With people who are insensate, a local anesthetic will not be required. This aggressive approach will stop the progression immediately, bring about a closed wound, and eliminate a secondary infection.

The procedure of choice for all small defects, when possible, is excision, with primary closure. The next modality is the application of a split-thickness skin graft. However, when the wound is large and a significant cavity is present, the rotation or advancement of local tissue is required. This should be designed so that future flaps can be constructed, if needed, and the scars placed in such a manner, when possible, that they will not cross bony prominences or other pressure points. When properly planned and executed, the "burning of bridges" does not occur and adjacent tissue will still be available if future problems arise.

## PATIENT, FAMILY, AND STAFF EDUCATION

Prevention is the *sine qua non* of skin care. This can only be brought about by education of the patient, the family, and the nursing staff. From a rehabilitation perspective, the ultimate responsibility for prevention of skin breakdown lies with the patient, the exceptions being mentally retarded, severely debilitated, and incompetent individuals. Until the patient realizes that prevention is within his personal control, the possibility of skin breakdown is great. For infants and younger children the responsibility lies with the parent. Beginning at adolescence, the necessary degree of responsibility can be taught and integrated into the daily routine. Age, intelligence, and socioeconomic status should be considered, but in themselves these are not major criteria. It is the individual's desire and willingness to learn to regiment himself to a program of prevention and skin care that can make the difference in how well the integrity of the skin is maintained.

General skin-care measures can be taught, including cleanliness, control of dependent edema, treatment of the intertriginous areas, and skin lubrication. The morning and evening inspection of the skin takes but a few minutes and can be the single most important aspect of skin care. All staff members and family who work with patients who are at risk for skin breakdown should be made aware of the modalities available for prevention and treatment when the early signs or symptoms occur. Individual verbal, audiovisual, and group educational experiences for the patient and those who care for the patient with these problems will enhance their awareness of the problems and the modalities for their management.

## EQUIPMENT FOR TREATING AND PREVENTING SKIN BREAKDOWN

Many types of cushioning devices are available for treating and preventing decubiti. They have to be thought of as assistive in nature and not as substitutes for position changes and good skin care. Ideally, these devices should mold to an individual's contours; they should provide flotation to equalize pressure distribution; they should allow passage of body secretions; they should be financially and practically suited to the individual's life-style; and lastly, they should also be durable, long-lasting, and easily maintained. No single piece of equipment will meet all these criteria. Foam cushions and foam mattresses will relieve, though not abolish, pressure areas. Several companies have produced various configurations to enhance the effectiveness of the foam cushion, the most effective being those that have been cut in the shape of blocks or cones, so that pressure can be absorbed collectively. A protective cover should be placed over foam cushions or mattresses, since they will absorb body fluids. Even when properly cared for, most foam cushions available today need to be changed every three to four months, since they will lose their resiliency. A foam cushion needs to be at least 4 to 6 inches in thickness to provide protection. Various foam or "sheepskin" protective devices are available to cover elbows, heels, and ankles. The need for these items must be individually determined and the selection must also be made on an individual basis.

Air-filled devices require that the individual have the ability to maintain them properly or a staff that can do it for him. Even with the simplest of flotation equipment, skin problems can be caused if they are underfilled or overfilled. The cost of purchasing, maintaining, and replacing the device needs to be considered in relationship to the individual, his life-style, and other items on the market.

Gel-filled cushions are also available. They often become deformed after 6 months to 1 year, losing their protectiveness.

## PRURITUS

Pruritus is another common complaint of the elderly bedbound patient. The itch sensation, an entity difficult to quantitate, is generally mediated at the cutaneous level by histamine. But, like many other symptom complexes we deal with in medicine, there is a major influence by the central nervous system. When we are distracted by a large number of external stimuli, the itch sensation is blunted, but when we are supine in bed, with little else to think about, the itching is allowed to become more prominent. For this reason alone it is not surprising that so many of our patients present with this annoying problem.

What are the first, and simple, things to do when the patient says, "I itch!"? First, remove the offending agents. Many elderly use over-the-counter preparations on the skin for any number of reasons. A few of the more notorious agents are the topical antihistamines, anesthetics, lanolin-containing preparations, and neomycin, either alone or as part of a combination product. A week or two away from *all* topical preparations should be adequate to tell if this is a cause of the problem.

Next, check for dry skin. Low levels of humidity in the room, excessive bathing, inadequate rinsing off of soap, and water that is too hot all contribute to dry skin and subsequent itching. The elderly are more susceptible to dry skin because of the diminished sebaceous gland production of skin lubricants. In fact, regardless of the *cause* of the problem, correcting these factors can substantially reduce the severity of the symptoms. Bath oils (with careful attention paid to safety when used in the tub so that the patient does not slip) and skin lubricants are the next modalities to try, remembering to use the product with the least coloring and perfume. Occasionally a patient will require a few days or a week of topical corticosteroid to initiate the treatment.

I have discussed treatment before making the diagnosis because so many of these patients will respond to these measures, regardless of the etiology of the pruritus. How can we identify the other causes of itching? The first task is a careful inspection of the skin to eliminate obvious infestations or rashes that would indicate a primary dermatologic disease. Next to be excluded are the systemic diseases that cause itching. Some of the more prominent of these include cholestasis, chronic renal disease, hyperthyroidism, diabetic neuropathy, hematologic problems (polycythemia vera and Hodgkin's disease), and malignancies. Not to be overlooked is the possibility of a drug side-effect. Another common, although difficult to prove, cause is a psychogenic etiology. A more detailed discussion of all the causes of pruritus is beyond the scope of this chapter.

If no specific intervention resolves the problem, drug treatment may be appropriate. When treating an elderly, bed-confined patient, there are a few things to keep in mind that make treating this patient different from our more ambulatory patients. The mere fact that the patient is confined to bed can make the itch sensation more prominent because of the paucity of external distracting stimuli. Many patients who itch are complaining about loss of sleep as much as the itching *per se*. For this reason an antihistamine can be useful because of both its specific effect on the mediator histamine and its sedative properties. The tricyclic antidepressants can also be effective in treating the problem. Placebo treatment of pruritus has been shown to be very effective. I mention this not as a therapeutic suggestion but rather to emphasize the possible psychological factors in evaluating and treating pruritus.

## SKIN CARE AND COSMETICS

A discussion of the skin would be incomplete if mention were not made of the cosmetic aspects of skin care for our home care patients. The patient who is nicely groomed feels better about himself and generates a more positive response from those who are providing care. Sometimes the patient needs to be told that it is alright to use cosmetics, particularly if we are berating him for using *too many* on the skin. There are any number of hypoallergenic aesthetically pleasant products available.

# 17
# Respiratory Care

STUART M. GARAY

Technological and organizational advances in health care have created a growing population of patients who depend on mechanical breathing devices for improved quality of life and even survival itself. There are important reasons to transfer such patients with severe respiratory ailments from the hospital to the home environment. These include the benefits of familiar surroundings and family, a decrease in nosocomial infections, and increased hospital savings. However, for the patient's physician, a return home produces new problems, often requiring novel solutions with poorly organized help. The first part of this chapter will review those disease processes requiring home respiratory care. It will be followed by a discussion of the treatment modalities available in the home. Finally, it will end with an overview of the supportive measures for the physician and the patient.

## DISEASE PROCESSES REQUIRING HOME RESPIRATORY CARE

### CHRONIC OBSTRUCTIVE PULMONARY DISEASE

Chronic bronchitis is clinically defined as a disorder in which cough productive of sputum is present on most days for at least three months of the year for two or more successive years. Pulmonary emphysema is defined pathologically as a disease in which destruction of the walls of the respiratory bronchioles, alveolar ducts, and distal alveoli has occurred, resulting in overdistention of the proximal or entire acinus (that portion of the lung distal to the terminal bronchiole). Approximately 4% of the adult population has established chronic bronchitis or pulmonary emphysema, collectively referred to as *chronic obstructive pulmonary disease* (COPD). The incidence of COPD is higher in current or former cigarette smokers compared to nonsmokers and in heavy (greater than 30 cigarettes/day) compared to light smokers. Its onset is usually after the age of 40, with a male predominance. COPD accounts for more than 25,000 deaths/year and an estimated 100,000 man-years of lost labor due to illness. Its economic cost is approximately $2 billion in lost earnings, hospital costs, and disability payments. Over 1 million individuals between ages 40 and 65 are currently receiving Social Security payments for disability on the basis of COPD. The home management of the patient with COPD attempts to prevent progression of the disease, prevent the complications leading to acute deterioration, treat potentially reversible components of the disease, and teach each patient how to participate in his or her management as an active partner with the physician. Unfortunately, patients with COPD tend to become victims of "polypharmacy." To avoid this problem the physician should consider the risk and benefit of each therapy (drugs, oxygen, or mechanical devices) before it is instituted. Spirometry quantitates the severity of the disease and reveals a potential response to bronchodilators. Combined with history, physical examination, and radiographic and electrocardiographic data, such knowledge forms a basis for patient management at home.

Although COPD implies irreversible airways obstruction, patients may demonstrate 20% to 25% improvement in airflow after inhalation of beta-agonist drugs. In addition, these drugs enhance mucociliary clearance and thus promote expectoration of retained secretions. Therefore, inhaled bronchodilators (Table 17-1) should be used regularly to maximize airway patency. Sequential inhalation (up to 3 puffs separated by 2 to 5 minutes) and proper inhalation technique (see discussion under Asthma, below) are essential to obtain benefit from these agents. There is growing evidence that inhaled anticholinergic agents are effective in patients with COPD, especially in reducing troublesome cough.[1] One such drug, ipratropium bromide (Atrovent) will soon be available for general use.

While theophylline is not as effective a bronchodilator as properly inhaled aerosols, the oral route ensures compliance. Theophylline offers the added benefit of enhancing diaphragmatic contractility, which may be a significant limiting factor in some patients with advanced COPD. A long-acting theophylline preparation should be given twice a day in a dose that will maintain serum theophylline level between 10 $\mu$g to 20 $\mu$g/ml. Under certain conditions the dose should be adjusted (see Modifications of Theophylline Dosage).[2] Patients with advanced COPD may benefit from judicious use of corticosteroids.[3] Patients with advanced COPD who receive daily or alternate-day corticosteroid treatment are susceptible to a variety of steroid-related complications such as adrenal suppression, osteoporosis, capillary fragility, easy bruisability, cataracts, glucose intolerance, and weight gain. A carefully monitored regimen of oral calcium and vitamin D may limit the degree of osteoporosis. However, long-term studies substantiating the value of such treatment in COPD patients have not been performed. All patients receiving chronic corticosteroid therapy should be given additional medication at times of physiologic stress (major surgery or serious illnesses) to prevent acute adrenal insufficiency.

Most patients with COPD are cigarette smokers. Cessation of smoking may slow the progression of the disease once the patient has overt COPD. Thus, all patients should be counseled to discontinue (or at least reduce) cigarette smoking, utilizing nicotine chewing gum and behavioral modification techniques such as rapid-smoking therapy.[4, 5]

The most common complication in COPD is the development of viral or bacterial pulmonary infection. Prophylactic influenzal and, possibly, pneumococcal vaccination are

**TABLE 17-1. INHALED ADRENERGIC BRONCHODILATORS**

| Drug | Alpha or Beta$_1$ Side-Effects | Onset of Action (min) | Duration of Effect (hr) | Route |
|---|---|---|---|---|
| Epinephrine | + + + + | < 1 | 1 | SC |
| Isoproterenol | + + + + | < 1 | 1–2 | MDI |
| Isoetharine | + + | 1–2 | 1–3 | MDI, N |
| Metaproterenol | + + | 2–5 | 3–4 | MDI, N, O |
| Albuterol | + | 5–10 | 4–5 | MDI, N,* O |
| Terbutaline | + | 5–10 | 4–5 | MDI, O, SC |
| Bitolterol | + | 5–10 | 4–8 | MDI |

( + + + + = significantly; + + = occasional; + = minor; MDI = metered dose inhaler; N = nebulizer; O = oral; SC = subcutaneous)
*Will be available.

## MODIFICATIONS OF THEOPHYLLINE DOSAGE

Increase Maintenance Dosage
  Young age
  Cigarette smoking
  High-protein diet
  Acidosis

Decrease Maintenance Dosage
  Elderly patients with decreased cardiac and hepatic function
  Cirrhosis and hepatic insufficiency
  Heart failure
  Cor pulmonale
  Acute pulmonary edema
  Pneumonia
  Alkalosis
  Patients taking
    Cimetidine
    Macrolide antibiotics (troleandomycin, erythromycin)
    Barbiturates
  Influenza immunization

indicated. The latter still awaits confirmation that it will reduce the incidence of pneumonia in patients with COPD. As effective antiviral agents become available their use in the COPD patient should be considered. With the onset of bacterial infection, antibiotic therapy should be provided.

Exercise training and breathing retraining play an important role in rehabilitation programs for patients with COPD, though data to support such programs are still evolving. Although mechanical lung function is not improved, an increase in maximum oxygen uptake and the ability to perform work can often be documented. Both graded (walking) exercise programs and regimens limited to exercise of the ventilatory muscles have improved exercise performance in selected groups of COPD patients. Whether ventilatory muscle training alone is as efficacious as other forms of exercise is not clear. Breathing retraining includes instruction of personal breathing patterns.

In COPD patients, maximal expiratory flow rate occurs at relatively low pleural pressures. With vigorous effort the pleural pressure is increased and the increased driving pressure in the alveoli is offset by the pleural pressure, which compresses airways so that expiratory flow rates do not increase. During exercise, dyspneic patients make maximal expiratory efforts in a futile attempt to expire more rapidly from the overinflated lung. The increased pleural pressure compresses the airways so as to prevent increase in expiratory flow rate. The effect is to increase the work of breathing, increase ventilatory requirements, and precipitate respiratory distress. Breathing retraining teaches the patient to breathe in rapidly and deeply. The deep inspiration maximizes lung recoil and flow rate during this subsequent expiration. The rapid inspiration allows more time for expiration so that the lung can empty more completely. Expiration should be performed passively with minimal effort. This rapid, maximal inspiration followed by prolonged, passive expiration should be practiced at rest and in exercise until it becomes natural.

Advanced COPD is characterized by severe airflow obstruction as well as severe mismatching of ventilation and perfusion, resulting in a large alveolar–arterial difference in oxygen tension and profound hypoxemia. Despite similar degrees of airflow obstruction, the patient in whom emphysema predominates may be characterized as a "pink puffer," with a high minute ventilation and normal arterial carbon dioxide pressure. If bronchitis predominates, the patient may be classified as a "blue bloater"; less work goes into breathing, resulting in hypercapnia and severe hypoxemia. Differences in respiratory control may determine the ventilatory response of COPD patients who develop severe ventilation–perfusion mismatch. In some patients, hypoxemia causes pulmonary hypertension that progresses to right-sided heart failure.

As with any serious and debilitating illness, chronic obstructive pulmonary disease can produce psychological difficulties. The patient often consults a physician because of an acute episode precipitated by a viral or bacterial infection. Initial diagnosis of COPD may come as a surprise, causing acute emotional distress and even depression. The patient, however, usually has experienced years of disease that has been subclinical or he has denied symptoms of disease (for instance, obvious exertional limitation, frequent respiratory infections, and productive cough). Patients often resort to denial to cope with this problem. Exertional limitations imposed by moderately advanced COPD may lead to early retirement because of physically taxing occupations; feelings of depression, hopelessness, irritability, and anger often develop. These changes often occur without the patient's awareness. In severe COPD, breathlessness, hypoxia, or both may alter psychological adaptation. In the Nocturnal Oxygen Therapy Trials sponsored by the National Heart, Lung and Blood Institute, 43% of a group of patients with an average $pO_2$ of 68 mm Hg showed moderate to severe cognitive impairment.[6] This proportion rose to 65% among patients with an average $pO_2$ of 45 mm Hg. Typical changes included reduced attention span, impaired abstract reasoning, memory loss, reduced motor speed and dexterity, and impaired sensation. These deficits may be improved with oxygen (see Oxygen Therapy, later in this chapter). Thus, the physician should monitor the COPD patient's emotional reactions as part of his home care. Questions about mood, sleep, physical energy level, sadness, or anxiety can help uncover psychological difficulties. Friends and relatives as well as the patient should be consulted periodically. Care should be taken with respect to prescribing medication to cope with these psychological difficulties. Many antidepressants have anticholinergic properties, which adversely affect clearance of bronchial secretions. The benzodiazepine antianxiety agents and various hypnotics can decrease respiratory drive. Hydroxyzine (Vistaril, Atarax) is relatively safe in the usual clinical doses (100 mg–400 mg daily) and may be the antianxiety drug of choice. Haloperidol (Haldol) is an anti-psychotic drug that can be useful as an antianxiety agent in low doses (0.5 mg–5.0 mg daily).

## ASTHMA

There is disagreement on a universal definition of asthma. In part, confusion stems from the tremendous age distribution of asthmatics, ranging from "cradle to grave." In turn, the clinical manifestations and natural history vary greatly between younger and older patients. In 1975 a joint committee of the American Thoracic Society and the American College of Chest Physicians defined asthma as follows:

> Asthma is a disease characterized by an increased responsiveness of the airway to various stimuli and manifested by prolongation of forced expiration which changes in severity either spontaneously or with treatment. The term asthma may be modified by words or phrases indicating its etiology, factors provoking attacks, or its duration. Note: the central feature of this definition is *reversible* airways obstruction.[5]

The following principles should guide treatment of asthmatic patients: (1) understand the *unique* history of the patient's symptoms and needs before altering therapy; (2) quantitate results with symptoms, scores, diaries, or some form of objective pulmonary function testing; and (3) make one change at a time. It is doubtful whether any physician, no matter how skilled, really understands the patient's disease better than the patient himself. One recent study contrasts patients' and physicians' estimates of the severity of asthma to severity as quantitated by peak expiratory flow rates.[7] Physicians were highly inaccurate in predicting peak expiratory flow rates by examining patients. The patients themselves more accurately estimated flow rates and could tell whether a given day's measurement was better or worse than a previous one. Having the patient measure serial peak expiratory flow rates at home will reveal important patterns of airflow obstruction. A peak flow meter is compact, inexpensive, and highly accurate. Testing may document consistent early morning diminution in expiratory flow rates, which suggests the need for long-acting bronchodilators at bedtime. Home monitoring of peak flow rates can also help, when the patient calls the physician complaining of worsening asthma: a severe reduction would prompt immediate assessment in the office or emergency room. The range of predicted peak expiratory flow rates is shown in Table 17-2.[8]

Treatment of asthma (like that of COPD) combines the use of beta-agonists as well as theophylline. The most effective bronchodilators are beta-adrenergic aerosols, which include isoproterenol, metaproterenol, terbutaline, albuterol, bitolterol, and fenoterol (not yet available in the United States). When inhaled properly into the airways, these drugs reduce airway resistance and improve expiratory flow rates better than the same agent administered by other routes. Small doses induce maximal bronchodilatation without systemic effects. To be most effective, single inhalation should be followed by a short pause (2 to 5 minutes), then another inhalation and possibly a third. The newer selective beta$_2$ agents such as albuterol and fenoterol are useful not only because they are selective on the smooth muscle of the airways, but also because they provide longer duration of action (4 to 6 hours as opposed to 30 minutes with isoproterenol and 2 to 4 hours with metaproterenol and terbutaline). Bitolterol may last 6 to 8 hours as shown in preliminary studies. Unfortunately, proper inhalation technique is often lacking in patients.[9] A majority of patients simply do not inhale the drugs into their lungs. Inhalation consists of actuation of the nebulizer at the beginning of a slow, full inspiration. It is advisable to follow this with a short period of breath-holding up to 10 seconds to ensure maximal deposition of the drug in the airwyays.[10] There is some evidence that beta agonists can be better deposited in the airways when the metered dose inhaler is held a short distance from the open mouth (although some patients find it difficult to master this type of inhalation). Some patients cannot learn to inhale these agents, so various devices have been developed to make aerosol treatment more effective.[11] With these devices, the drug is squirted into a bag, chambers, or bellows and then inhaled. Alternatively, one may insert a "spacer" or small cylinder attached to the metered dose inhaler. The use of such devices may be particularly valuable for the delivery of steroid aerosols, which tend to be more irritating upon inhalation. They are also valuable in patients with poor hand–mouth coordination such as children, the elderly, and those with arthritis. When a jet nebulizer is used to deliver bronchodilators and the flow is continuous, 50% to 70% of the drug is never inhaled. Thus, about five times as much medication must be nebulized as is delivered from the metered dose inhaler to produce an equivalent effect. Routine prescription of home nebulizers should be discouraged, since at

**TABLE 17-2. PREDICTED PEAK EXPIRATORY FLOW RATES BY HEIGHT (INCHES), MALE AND FEMALE**

| Age (yr) | 55 in M | 55 in F | 60 in M | 60 in F | 65 in M | 65 in F | 70 in M | 70 in F | 75 in M | 75 in F | 80 in M | 80 in F |
|---|---|---|---|---|---|---|---|---|---|---|---|---|
| 20 | 390 | | 550 | 420 | 600 | 460 | 650 | 500 | 700 | 530 | 740 | |
| 30 | 380 | | 530 | 450 | 580 | 450 | 620 | 480 | 660 | 520 | 710 | |
| 40 | 370 | | 500 | 400 | 550 | 440 | 600 | 470 | 640 | 500 | 680 | |
| 50 | 360 | | 480 | 390 | 530 | 420 | 570 | 460 | 610 | 490 | 650 | |
| 60 | 350 | | 460 | 380 | 500 | 410 | 540 | 450 | 580 | 475 | 620 | |

least one study has suggested that fatalities have occurred due to patients' over-reliance on the effectiveness of their home nebulizers.

## CHEST WALL DISORDERS

Disorders that adversely affect the thoracic spine may cause varying degrees of respiratory compromise. The most common disorders include scoliosis, kyphoscoliosis, and ankylosing spondylitis. Scoliosis is a lateral deviation of the spine; kyphosis is a posterior angulation. The angle of the scoliosis is defined by the converging limbs of the curve and is expressed in degrees. The degree of kyphosis is defined by the angle between the upper limb of the spine and the vertical plane. Respiratory and cardiovascular compromise is noted most often when these deformities coexist in the form of kyphoscoliosis. The etiology of kyphoscoliosis is unknown in about 80% of cases. In the remaining cases, the most common etiologies include neuromuscular disease (poliomyelitis, syringomyelia, and neurofibromatosis), congenital defects of the spine, vertebral disease (tuberculosis, tumor, osteomalacia), and thoracoplasty. Idiopathic deformities are more common in females and are usually not severe. In contrast, the deformity secondary to polio, tuberculosis, and congenital spine defects is often marked. The respiratory manifestations of severe kyphoscoliosis include dyspnea, cyanosis, somnolence, and cor pulmonale.[12] Severity reflects the degree of deformity. Clinical manifestations are unusual when kyphosis is less than 20 degrees and when scoliosis is less than 100 degrees; however, alterations in pulmonary function can be demonstrated with mild disease (lateral curves of 65 degrees). The physiologic hallmarks of severe kyphoscoliosis include reduced lung volumes and a small tidal volume. These patients have an increased work of breathing and respond to this need for greater ventilation by increasing respiratory rate, not tidal volume. Rapid shallow ventilations result in large dead space ventilation. This will lead to marked reduction in alveolar ventilation with consequent hypoxemia and hypercapnia. Patients with severe thoracic deformity may live for many years without developing respiratory insufficiency. Insidious pulmonary hypertension may result as a consequence of chronic alveolar hypoventilation. Patients with kyphoscoliosis have a higher incidence of disordered breathing during sleep, which may contribute to this pulmonary hypertension. If hypoventilation persists, cor pulmonale develops. Patients with severe thoracic deformities are at risk for respiratory decompensation with minor insults such as viral or bacterial infections. Treatment is preventive and supportive in the adult. Appropriate immunizations (as suggested in the COPD section), maintenance of good hydration, prompt attention to respiratory infection, and avoidance of sedatives are crucial. Supplementary oxygen may alleviate the vasoconstrictive element of pulmonary hypertension secondary to hypoventilation and has been used chronically in some patients. In some individuals with persistent respiratory failure, tracheostomy may decrease dead space ventilation; when combined with intermittent positive pressure ventilation, lung compliance may increase, with a decrease in the work of breathing. Alternatively, nocturnal home use of cuirass negative pressure ventilators (when hypoventilation is greatest) may reverse hypoxemia and hypercapnia, allowing severely affected patients to live at home as well as function professionally (see section on Home Mechanical Ventilation, later in this chapter).[13]

## NEUROMUSCULAR DISORDERS

A variety of neuromuscular and spinal cord diseases may affect the respiratory system, leading to ventilatory insufficiency.[14] These include the muscular dystrophies, polymyositis, myotonic dystrophy, polyneuritis, myasthenia gravis, and spinal cord disorders such as amyotrophic lateral sclerosis. The lung itself is not directly affected unless aspiration, atelectasis, or pneumonia complicate the illness. The neuromuscular abnormality affects three interdependent components of the bellows system: the rib cage, the diaphragm, and the abdomen. There may be a generalized loss of muscle strength or weakening of selected muscle groups. The diseases that cause a generalized loss of respiratory muscle strength include the skeletal muscle disorders, such as the muscular dystrophies and myotonic dystrophies, neuromuscular junction disorders such as myasthenia gravis, and the Guillain-Barré syndrome. The most sensitive test of respiratory muscle weakness is the static maximum inspiratory pressure. A maximum inspiratory pressure of 30 cm of water or less and a vital capacity of 800 cc or less suggest impending ventilatory failure. Arterial blood gases are less reliable predictors of hypoventilation, since patients maintain normal arterial $pCO_2$ until their ventilatory capacity begins to approximate their tidal volume. Disorders that selectively weaken muscle groups include high spinal injuries and amyotrophic lateral sclerosis. Acute spinal cord injuries are the most clearly understood examples of this impairment. Lesions below L-1 rarely cause ventilatory insufficiency. Lesions between C-6 and L-1 compromise the abdominal muscles and limit the ability to expire. Complete paralysis of the abdominal muscles results in almost complete loss of the capacity to expire below functional residual capacity. Lesions in the thoracic spine paralyze the external and internal intercostal muscles and further compromise the ability to expire forcibly. These lesions also limit the inspiratory capacity. If the cord lesion is in the cervical region below C-5, the only remaining muscles of respiration are the diaphragm and accessory muscles. The vital capacity may be reduced to 30% or 40% of predicted value and expiration will be entirely passive. Cord lesions in the C-3 to C-5 region may partially or totally denervate the diaphragm. Consequently, there may be lost ability to maintain adequate, spontaneous ventilation. The accessory muscles alone are able to maintain a tidal volume of 50 cc to 100 cc, but this volume is hardly compatible with life. Patients with amyotrophic lateral sclerosis develop progressive weakness of focal muscle groups. Classically, this disease involves the cervical cord and spares the mid and lower thoracic cord. Thus, diaphragmatic function is affected, while intercostal and accessory muscles are spared. Depending on severity, these neuromuscular and spinal cord injuries result in the need for mechanical ventilatory assistance.

## OBSTRUCTIVE SLEEP APNEA

Obstructive sleep apnea is characterized by repetitive cessation of respiration during sleep, sleep arousal, and transient hypoxemia.[15] The etiology of this disorder is unknown. Decreased central drive to breathe, loss of upper airway motor tone, and anatomical obstruction of the upper airway have been implicated in the pathophysiology of sleep apnea. Sleep apnea syndromes are either obstructive, in which oral and nasal air flow ceases while diaphragmatic efforts continue, or central, in which diaphragmatic and intercostal efforts cease in addition to lack of oronasal air flow. Obstructive sleep apnea is most often encountered clinically. Patients with obstructive sleep apnea are more frequently obese, middle-aged men. They present with marked daytime hypersomnolence and nocturnal loud snoring. The latter is punctuated by periodic apneas that are interrupted by snorting and choking spells. Such events occur cyclically, hundreds of times each night. Abnormal motor activity during sleep may be noted by the bed partner. Changes in personality, deteriorating intellectual function, and impotence may lead to loss of employment as well as family discord. Automobile accidents and ventilatory arrests following administration of sedatives have also occurred. There may be clinical evidence of pulmonary hypertension. While history suggests the syndrome, confirmatory evidence usually awaits a sleep study utilizing polysomnography. Treatment varies and has included weight loss, nasal continuous positive airway pressure, tracheostomy, and uvulopalatal pharyngoplasty.

## MODALITIES OF HOME TREATMENT

### OXYGEN THERAPY

Shortly after his discovery of oxygen in 1774, Priestley wrote

> The feeling of it to my lungs was not sensibly different from that of common air; but I fancied that my breast felt peculiarly light and easy for some time afterwards. Who can tell but that, in time, this pure air may become a fashionable article in luxury.[16]

Within four years of Priestley's discovery, Thomas Beddoes described the use of oxygen in his book *The Medicinal Uses of Factitious Airs*. Unfortunately, oxygen therapy lapsed into obscurity until the early 1900s, when Haldane described its use for chlorine gas poisoning in World War I. In the 1920s, Barach designed oxygen rooms for treating hospitalized patients. The modern era of chronic oxygen therapy began in the late 1960s, when Neff and Petty showed that long-term home oxygen could improve survival in patients who suffered from severe hypoxic chronic obstructive lung disease. Of the 9 million people who have COPD in the United States, nearly 500,000 are disabled with advanced disease. Most of these patients use chronic oxygen therapy. Uncontrolled studies published throughout the 1970s suggested that use of oxygen for 15 hours per day could reduce pulmonary hypertension and prevent cor pulmonale. The latter had long been known to carry a grave prognosis in COPD patients. Other published benefits of low-flow oxygen therapy included a decrease in severe polycythemia and improvements in neuropsychological tests, with less depression, hypochondriasis, and social introversion. In some patients, exercise tolerance improved.

Two important controlled trials of oxygen therapy were initiated in the late 1970s and have recently been published. The British Medical Research Council trial asked whether administration of oxygen for 15 hours each day could improve survival of severely hypoxic patients with COPD.[17] In a multicenter study the National Heart, Lung and Blood Institute (NHLBI) asked whether the administration of oxygen for 12 hours versus 24 hours each day (in practice only 19 hours) could improve survival in COPD patients.[6] In both trials, oxygen treatment included the sleeping hours. In the Nocturnal Oxygen Therapy Trial (NOTT) sponsored by the NHLBI, 203 patients from six institutions were randomly assigned to either continuous or 12-hour nocturnal oxygen therapy and followed for a mean of 19 months. All patients had a resting arterial $pO_2$ of less than 55 mm Hg or a $pO_2$ of less than 59 mm Hg plus either edema or hematocrit greater than 55%, a $FEV_1/FVC$ ratio of less than 0.7% after bronchodilator treatment, and a total lung capacity greater than 80% of predicted. Baseline and follow-up data included pulmonary function testing, arterial blood gas determination, exercise testing, sleep studies, neuropsychiatric testing, quality of life assessment, and right heart catheterization. Oxygen was administered by nasal cannula at 1 to 4 liters/minute to maintain a resting $pO_2$ of at least 60 mm Hg. The flow was increased by 1 liter per minute during sleep and exercise. Optimum medical therapy with bronchodilators, diuretics, and antibiotics was continued as necessary. Both nocturnal and continuous oxygen therapy resulted in some fall in hematocrit and pulmonary vascular resistance, as well as improvement in neuropsychiatric function and the patient's perception of quality of life. There was no significant change in $FEV_1$, lung volumes, or arterial blood gas levels. The mortality in the nocturnal oxygen therapy group was nearly twice as high as in the continuous oxygen therapy group.

In the British Medical Research Council study the trial was designed to compare 15 hours per day of oxygen therapy with no oxygen in severe COPD patients: 87 patients were randomized and followed for up to 5 years. In the British trial the mortality was decreased in oxygen-treated patients: 45% of the treated group died as compared to 67% of the control group during the 5-year observation period. In the NOTT trial, those given oxygen

| Name | John Smith |
|---|---|
| Diagnosis | Emphysema |
| ABG (room air): | $pO_2 = 49$ mm Hg     $pCO_2 = 38$ mm Hg     $pH = 7.42$ |
| O$_2$ described: | Nasal cannula 24 hours/day |
| Flow rates: | 1. Awake, at rest: 1 L/min |
| | 2. Asleep: 2 L/min |
| | 3. Exercise: 3 L/min |
| Type of O$_2$: | 1. Oxygen concentrator (at home) |
| | 2. Compressed O$_2$ in portable canister (for travel) |

**Figure 17-1** *Oxygen prescription.*

for 24 hours per day survived longer than those given oxygen for only 12 hours per day. The 24-month mortality in the continuous therapy group was 22.6%, as compared to 41% in the noctural therapy group. In the NOTT trial, patients were older and did not have $CO_2$ retention, whereas most of the British patients had $CO_2$ retention. The severity of hypoxemia was similar in both studies and most patients had modest pulmonary hypertension at the entry of the trial. Combining the results from both studies, only 30% of those treated without oxygen were alive at 5 years. Survival was significantly better in those given oxygen for 15 hours in the day. However, the most important conclusion was that oxygen given for over 19 hours in the 24-hour day (that is, "continuous oxygen") clearly gave a better survival than did oxygen given for shorter periods in the day.

Early expectations that long-term oxygen therapy could consistently lower pulmonary arterial pressure have proved difficult to conclude from these two controlled trials. In the British study, the pulmonary vascular resistance of untreated men increased more than that of men who received oxygen, but the difference was not statistically significant. In the NOTT study, small but significant differences in the hemodynamic effects of nocturnal versus continuous oxygen were seen when patients were evaluated at 6 months. There was an 11% decrease in pulmonary vascular resistance at rest in the group receiving continuous oxygen therapy, whereas the group receiving nocturnal oxygen therapy showed an increase of 6.5%. With exercise, the continuous oxygen patient showed a 15% to 20% decrease in pulmonary vascular resistance, whereas the nocturnal oxygen patient showed no decrease. Only those patients with the least disturbed pulmonary hemodynamics demonstrate any reduction as a result of continuous oxygen therapy. It has recently been suggested that those patients with cor pulmonale due to COPD who show a fall in mean pulmonary arterial pressure of greater than 5 mm Hg when breathing 28% oxygen for 24 hours will have a better 2-year survival than similar patients whose pulmonary arterial pressure did not fall by this amount.[18]

Polycythemia frequently develops in COPD patients as a consequence of hypoxemia. The increased red blood cell mass may cause increases in pulmonary vascular resistance plus reduced cerebral blood flow. It has long been shown that elevated hematocrit and red blood cell volume decrease if oxygen is given for 12 to 24 hours a day; the reduction can be maintained by nocturnal oxygen alone. Polycythemia will recur if oxygen is discontinued. Hematocrit reductions are greatest in patients with values greater than 55% at the outset, but the prognosis appears to be independent of the hematocrit. No significant difference in hematocrit between the two treatment groups was noted in the British study, although the hematocrit tended to fall in the treated group. In contrast, the NOTT study demonstrated that the patient group receiving continuous oxygen treatment had a significantly greater decrease in hematocrit than the group receiving nocturnal oxygen treatment. The difference was significant at both 12 and 18 months. At 18 months, the hematocrit in the continuous oxygen group decreased 9.2% from baseline, while it dropped only 2% in the nocturnal oxygen group.

As part of the NOTT study, neuropsychological and life quality assessments were made before and 6 months after oxygen therapy. Both pretreatment and posttreatment assessments were made while the patients breathed room air. Baseline evaluation revealed neuropsychological deficits suggestive of cerebral dysfunction in 77% of patients. Moderate to severe impairment was observed in 42% of the patients as compared with 14% of a control group of older subjects without chronic lung disease. Deficits were greater in higher cognitive functions such as abstracting ability and complex perceptual motor integration. Simple motor skills were also disturbed, with impairment of speed, strength, and coordination. The degree of neuropsychological dysfunction correlated best with arterial $PO_2$. Patients were more depressed than controls and had severe social adjustment problems that correlated with neuropsychological status and pulmonary function. When nocturnal and continuous treatment groups were compared at 6 months, no difference in neuropsychological function was noted, but after 12 months of therapy, the continuous oxygen group demonstrated significantly greater improvement. Thus, the NOTT study showed that long-term oxygen therapy yielded modest neuropsychological improvement in almost half of the hypoxemic COPD patients, particularly in cognitive functioning. Because there was no control group of hypoxemic COPD patients who did not receive oxygen, the study may have underestimated the benefit of oxygen therapy. Without oxygen, patients would probably have demonstrated deteriorating mental function.

The NOTT study showed that patients receiving continuous oxygen were hospitalized less often and had fewer long hospitalizations than the nocturnal oxygen group, but the difference was not statistically significant. Likewise, in the British study there was no significant difference in the number of days spent in the hospital or the number of work days missed as a result of exacerbations of the patient's pulmonary disease.

Sleep-associated hypoxemia in COPD patients has been intensively studied. Increased hypoxemia during sleep is common in stable hypoxemic COPD patients, but is usually not severe and probably has only limited impact on the clinical and physiologic status of most patients. Patients with severe COPD who are hypoxemic when awake and have evidence of pulmonary arterial hypertension (the blue bloater) usually have episodes of further profound hypoxemia in rapid eye movement (REM) sleep.[19] These hypoxemic episodes are most often associated with irregular breathing and hypoventilation, which appears to be an exaggeration of the pattern seen in normal subjects during REM sleep. These hypoxemic episodes are associated with further increase in pulmonary arterial pressure. This had led to the suggestion that cor pulmonale may arise from repeated hypoxic pulmonary vasoconstriction during REM sleep, particularly when this is repeated each night over many years. Oxygen therapy during sleep may prevent both nocturnal desaturation and pulmonary hypertension in REM sleep. However, patients with COPD occasionally have associated obstructive sleep apnea. In the latter situation oxygen could increase the number of apneic episodes and raise arterial $pCO_2$ during sleep. Fortunately, most patients with COPD do not present with both sleep apnea and COPD, and oxygen can be safely administered. Sleep apnea can be suspected on clinical grounds (see section on Obstructive Sleep Apnea, earlier in this chapter) and, if necessary, documented by polysomnography.

## DISEASES CAUSING SEVERE HYPOXEMIA

Chronic obstructive pulmonary disease is the most common disorder that may warrant home oxygen therapy. However, patients with other irreversible destructive lung diseases may develop chronic hypoxemia that necessitates treatment at home with oxygen. Cystic fibrosis, severe bronchiectasis, and idiopathic pulmonary fibrosis are unusual disorders in which continuous outpatient oxygen therapy may be needed. Patients with neuromuscular disease or kyphoscoliosis may also need such therapy. Lung cancer patients occasionally need home oxygen, but most often their dyspnea is related to their underlying tumor and not hypoxemia; therefore, dyspnea is not relieved by oxygen therapy.

Before prescribing long-term oxygen therapy, the following four conditions should be met: (1) an accurate diagnosis of pulmonary disease must be established; (2) an optimal medical regimen should have been in effect; (3) the patient should have recovered from any exacerbation and should have been stable for approximately 1 month; and (4) oxygen therapy should have been administered and shown to improve hypoxemia. Smoking by patients receiving supplemental oxygen therapy has inherent safety risks and reduces its full physiologic benefits. Consequently, continued smoking by patients receiving oxygen is contraindicated.

Prior to administration of oxygen, symptoms referrable to hypoxemia (cyanosis, plethora, central nervous system dysfunction, or marked intolerance of exercise) as well as evidence of possible pulmonary hypertension or right ventricular failure (jugular venous distention, dependent edema, a loud $P_2$ on auscultation, a right ventricular heave) should be evaluated. The electrocardiogram should be inspected for P-pulmonale, right ventricular hypertrophy, arrhythmias, and ischemia. A chest radiograph may reveal large pulmonary arteries, cardiac enlargement, or a reversible cause of hypoxemia such as pneumonia and congestive failure. A complete blood count provides information about secondary polycythemia. Spirometry demonstrates whether reversible bronchospasm is present. Finally, arterial blood gases must be measured (in the seated position at rest while breathing room air) to assess hypoxemia. Potentially reversible causes of hypoxemia such as respiratory tract infections, retained secretions, bronchospasm, or left-sided congestive heart failure should be treated. After this initial evaluation, bronchodilators, antibiotics, and diuretics should be adjusted *prior* to oxygen administration. Postural drainage and chest percussion may improve clearance of secretions.

Long-term oxygen therapy should be considered only for those patients who have received such an optimal regimen for at least 4 weeks. When a repeat arterial $pO_2$ is still 55 mm Hg or less, hypoxic organ dysfunction may be considered to be present and long-term oxygen therapy is warranted. Patients receiving an optimal medical regimen who have arterial $pO_2$ values greater than 55 mm Hg may still show evidence of hypoxic organ dysfunction such as secondary pulmonary hypertension, cor pulmonale, secondary erythrocytosis, and impaired mentation; in such instances they should also be considered for long-term oxygen therapy. The indications for administering oxygen therapy during exercise are less well defined. Patients who demonstrate arterial $pO_2$ values of 55 mm Hg or less during exercise and in whom oxygen administration significantly improves exercise duration, performance, or capacity, may benefit from oxygen therapy during exercise. Administration of nocturnal oxygen for control of sleep-related hypoxemia is not well established. However, patients should be considered for continuous nocturnal oxygen therapy, if they develop arterial $pO_2$ values of 55 mm Hg or less during sleep as well as a disturbed sleep pattern, cardiac arrhythmias, or pulmonary hypertension. It should be subsequently demonstrated that the hypoxemia is abolished by nocturnal use of oxygen. The above discussion refers to patients at sea level. Effects of altitude on atmospheric, alveolar, and arterial oxygen tensions are presented in Table 17-3.

The NOTT experience showed that a significant number of hypoxemic COPD patients, initially identified as home oxygen candidates, improved their arterial oxygenation substantially with sustained medical supervision. Approximately 45% of the patients who initially met the NOTT criteria for home oxygen were no longer eligible after a 4-week period of outpatient observation. In patients in whom oxygen treatment is initiated at the time of

**TABLE 17-3. EFFECTS OF ALTITUDE ON ATMOSPHERIC, ALVEOLAR, AND ARTERIAL O$_2$ TENSIONS**

| Altitude (feet) | Barometric Pressure (mm Hg) | Atmospheric pO$_2$ (mm Hg) | Alveolar pO$_2$ (mm Hg) | Arterial pO$_2$ (mm Hg) |
|---|---|---|---|---|
| 0 | 760 | 159 | 110 | 96 |
| 1000 | 733 | 153 | 104 | 91 |
| 2000 | 707 | 148 | 99 | 87 |
| 3000 | 687 | 142 | 94 | 83 |
| 4000 | 656 | 137 | 89 | 79 |
| 5000 | 631 | 132 | 85 | 75 |
| 6000 | 604 | 126 | 80 | 71 |

hospital discharge or when the patient is first seen as an outpatient, the need for supplemental oxygen should be reevaluated after the patient has achieved clinical stability. The reason for such caution is that oxygen is among the more expensive drugs administered on a long-term basis. Based on the use and system prescribed, the cost can average from $300 to $900 per month. It should be remembered that many symptoms such as dyspnea at rest, cough, and sputum production are not alleviated by oxygen therapy. Patients receiving chronic oxygen at home should be taught that this therapy alleviates complications of the disease that may not be readily apparent to them. Educating patients about their illness and the expectations from oxygen therapy will promote compliance.

## OXYGEN DELIVERY SYSTEMS

An oxygen delivery system is suitable only if the patient can operate it at home without assistance. Each system must be partially portable so that ambulatory patients can continue oxygen therapy uninterrupted outside the home. Three types of oxygen supply are available and all are expensive: high-pressure compressed gas cylinders, low-pressure liquid oxygen reservoirs, and oxygen concentrators.[20] There are substantial regional differences in cost and availability of equipment. The amount of time the patient spends away from home, cost, and the amount of oxygen used each day are some of the factors that determine which system is the best for a given patient (Tables 17-4 and 17-5). High-pressure cylinders of compressed oxygen have been the conventional source of oxygen. They are available in most communities, but the tanks are large and cumbersome and they require regular home delivery. The most commonly used cylinders are the large H cylinders, which contain almost 7000 liters. Each tank lasts about 4 days, if oxygen is used continuously at 1 liter/minute; it will last approximately 2 days at 2 liters/minute continuous flow. The patient can move freely about the home by using a long (up to 50 feet) tube connecting the breathing apparatus to the H tank. Smaller, lighter, aluminum cylinders with carrying cases are now available. These can be safely refilled by the patient from the large H cylinders if petroleum-based lubricants are avoided. The lightest available model weighs 6½ lb and provides a 2-hour supply at 2 liters/minute when refilled from a full H cylinder. Compressed gas is the least expensive type of gas for use at home, if flow rates are low or periods of use are brief. The cost is usually covered by third-party payers. Unfortunately, frequent tank deliveries may be needed. The high pressure is a potential explosive hazard.

Low-pressure liquid oxygen systems are possible, because at extremely low temperatures oxygen becomes a liquid that occupies less than 1% of the volume that the same amount of oxygen would displace at room air and pressure. Liquid oxygen is stored at −297°F in a thermos-like container. It is vaporized to a gaseous state continuously and passes out of the container as conventional, ready-to-use oxygen at a concentration of 100%.

**TABLE 17-4. ADVANTAGES AND DISADVANTAGES
OF THE HOME OXYGEN SYSTEMS**

| System | Advantages | Disadvantages |
|---|---|---|
| Cylinders | Widely available<br>Most economical<br>Can be stored for long periods without loss of oxygen | Heavy—cannot be carried or moved easily<br>High pressure—potential explosive hazard<br>Requires an expensive pressure regulator |
| Liquid | Portable unit is lightweight<br>Nationwide network of dealers makes traveling easy | Most expensive except for patients on high flow rates<br>Reservoir requires frequent refilling<br>Slow evaporation of $O_2$ (2% per day) |
| Concentrators | Provides constant, inexhaustible home oxygen supply<br>Attractive equipment<br>Most economical for 24 hours/day<br>Negligible fire hazard<br>Casters permit easy movement within the home | Monthly electrical expense not covered by insurance<br>Relatively noisy<br>Requires periodic maintenance by vendor<br>Requires back-up cylinder and regulator in event of electrical failure<br>Alternative system needed for portable use |

Reservoirs for liquid oxygen contain 40 to 90 lb of oxygen that will last approximately 4½ to 10 days when oxygen is administered at 2 liters/minute continuous flow. At this flow rate 3 to 7 refills are required per month. Portable units weigh from 6½ to 11 lb and provide continuous oxygen at 2 liters/minute for 4 to 8 hours. The portable units may be filled from the stationary reservoirs. The advantage of a liquid oxygen system is that the portable system is easiest to carry and longest lasting. While it is the most expensive form of oxygen, it is least expensive for extended or high-flow portable use. Unfortunately, there is slow evaporation of oxygen (approximately 2% per day), even if the system is turned off. The cost for liquid oxygen is not always covered by insurance companies.

**TABLE 17-5. COMPARISON OF OXYGEN DELIVERY SYSTEMS**

| | Reservoir | Duration of Reservior Supply (at 1 liter/min) | Portable System | Duration of Portable Supply (at 1 liter/min) | Cost of $O_2$* 12 hours/day 1 liter/min | 3 liters/min | 24 hours/day 1 liter/min | 3 liters/min |
|---|---|---|---|---|---|---|---|---|
| *Compressed Gas* | 7000 liters | 4 days | Smaller E tank (625 liters) fits on stroller | 10 hours | $163 | $446 | $304 | $871 |
| *Liquid Oxygen†* | 70 lb | 15 days | Small cannister (wheels or shoulder) | 11–15 hours | $126 | $398 | $252 | $796 |
| *Oxygen Concentrator* | | No limit | Small compressed gas tanks (as above) | | | | $164 | $364 |

*Prevailing monthly rates for Medicare (New York City).
†Additional $45/month rental for stationary reservoir.

Oxygen concentrators are the most convenient system of gas supply for homebound patients. These devices extract oxygen from the air by means of a molecular sieve or a semipermeable membrane. The key to this process is a complex inorganic material, sodium aluminum silicate in pellet form (zeolite), which is tightly packed into two cyclindrical containers. When atmospheric gases pass through this sieve material, certain gaseous molecules including nitrogen, carbon dioxide, water vapor, and hydrocarbons will selectively be absorbed onto the sieve material, allowing the remaining, highly concentrated oxygen to pass through the zeolite. Newer models are capable of delivering 85% to 90% oxygen at flow rates of 1 to 4 liters/minute. Proper maintenance of oxygen concentrators, which includes frequent replacement with filters and equipment checks, is essential. When long oxygen tubes are attached to concentrators, increased back pressure may result and a flow meter should be utilized to ensure accurate oxygen flow rates to the patient. The cost of electricity, which may be as much as $30 per month (depending on regional costs), is not reimbursable to the patient. The electricity required is as much as a small room air-conditioning unit, and it is also subject to power failure. Small tanks cannot be filled from the concentrator, so patients require a separate portable system for use outside the home. This portable system acts as a back-up source in case of power failure. In general, an oxygen concentrator is more economical than cylinders for patients who require 2 liters/minute or more of continuous oxygen.

Most patients receiving compressed or liquid oxygen should use a nasal cannula, which is more convenient than a mask because it does not interfere with speech or eating. If the nasal mucosa becomes dry, one of the two openings in the tubing may be occluded. The needed amount of oxygen can then be given through one nostril at a time, alternating sides as desired. A bubble-type humidifier can also be attached to the oxygen source to add moisture to the oxygen. However, routine humidification of oxygen is not necessary at flow rates of 1 to 4 liters/minute, when environmental humidity is adequate. Elimination of unnecessary humidification of oxygen can result in substantial savings.

## FUTURE TRENDS IN OXYGEN DELIVERY

New approaches to oxygen delivery have been recently described. These include trans-tracheal oxygen delivery, a reservoir nasal cannula, and a pulsed dose demand valve.[21-23] They promise to reduce the cost of home oxygen use dramatically.

The transtracheal concept works by inserting a No. 16 Teflon catheter between the second and third tracheal rings.[21] Because oxygen is delivered directly to the tracheo-bronchial tree, bypassing the anatomical dead space of the upper airway, much lower flows of oxygen, as low as 0.25 to 1.5 liters per minute, are possible. Advantages of the trans-tracheal system include (1) elimination of "wasted" oxygen by reduction in anatomical dead space; (2) standard oxygen equipment may be used; and (3) elimination of the nasal cannula-induced nasopharyngeal irritation. Special low flow regulators or flow restrictors may be further savings. In addition, this oxygen-administering device is less conspicuous than a nasal cannula. Disadvantages of the transtracheal oxygen delivery system include surgery for catheter placement and the possibility of complications such as hemoptysis, subcutaneous emphysema, and infection. The manufacturer suggests that the catheter be replaced every 60 to 90 days and be secured with a necklace to prevent its accidental removal. Patients and their families should be trained to handle accidental removal and to carry a standard cannula. The low flow regulator used with the transtracheal device must be capable of providing the higher flows needed with conventional oxygen therapy for contingency purposes.

Storing oxygen in a reservoir placed adjacent to the nose reduces expiratory waste. An oxymizer (Chad Therapeutics, Woodland Hills, CA) is such a device.[22] Oxygen is inhaled in early inspiration to minimize dead space waste. A small amount of oxygen-enriched gas from dead space may reenter the reservoir during early expiration and be recycled. Such a cannula is most efficient at lower flows and may result in a 70% savings in oxygen. At higher flow rates (3 to 4 liters/minute), savings are less but still substantial (approximately 50%). Flow rates must be increased during exercise because a faster respiratory rate shortens the time available to fill the reservoir. The reservoir cannula utilizes conventional oxygen equipment; special low flow regulators or flow restrictors can enhance savings. Unfortunately, the cannula needs to be frequently replaced (each week) in order to avoid failure of an internal membrane that flexes with each breath. In addition, the current apparatus is esthetically displeasing.

Restricting oxygen delivery to the inspiratory portion of a breathing cycle reduces expiratory waste of oxygen. A commercially available demand valve (Demand Oxygen Controller, Cry $O_2$ Corporation, Fort Pierce, FL) is a modified version of a previously described valve that has been incorporated in a portable liquid oxygen reservoir (Pulsair).[23] A fluidic sensor detects the onset of inspiration through a standard nasal cannula, after which a preset volume of oxygen is delivered as a bolus in early inspiration by an electronically governed valve. This minimizes both dead space and expiratory waste of oxygen and avoids a problem with delayed valve closing. Conventional delivery settings are marked on the device. When it is switched to the pulse mode, a dose of oxygen equivalent to that in a conventional flow is delivered with each inspiration. If failure occurs, the patient easily switches to conventional modes. There has been very little clinical experience with the Pulsed Dose Demand Valve, although preliminary studies suggest that it may reduce oxygen utilization by two thirds. The demand valve eliminates the need to adjust oxygen flow when respiratory rate changes. As noted previously, when a patient with COPD exercises and increases his breathing rate, the flow of oxygen must increase in the same proportion. Unfortunately, the demand valve has a high initial cost (approximately $400) and is limited to use with a liquid oxygen system. However, modifications that will interface with other oxygen delivery systems will soon be available.

These three devices suggest new, exciting, and economical ways to provide oxygen. However, the studies to date have been small, under controlled laboratory conditions, and have generally been conducted by the inventor or by the manufacturer.[24] There are no long-term studies of performance, safety, and cost-effectiveness under field conditions. Comparative studies as well as evaluation during sleep and exercise are lacking. Further research within the next few years will be necessary before these new oxygen delivery systems can be enthusiastically recommended.

## HOME MECHANICAL VENTILATION

The worldwide polio epidemic of the late 1940s and early 1950s marked a period of rapid development in respirator technology. Many survivors of the polio epidemic remained dependent on full-time or part-time assisted mechanical ventilation, resulting in a need for home care programs. Thousands of survivors still live at home today, having led full and productive lives despite their need for mechanical respiration. Thus, the experience with home respirators spans over 40 years, but has been limited until recently to large medical centers, where polio patients received their initial care.

In the mid-1980s home mechanical ventilation has become an accepted concept, because of the following: (1) early diagnosis and treatment of debilitating pulmonary disorders have resulted in increased longevity but only because of continued mechanical ventilatory support; (2) socioeconomic pressure placed on the health-care industry has necessitated reductions in cost (such as implementation of reimbursement based on the DRGs); and (3) technological advancements have yielded simple, portable, and safer home respirators. Although the patient population is still small, it will grow as the general medical community and third-party payors realize the benefits offered by this alternative.

## PATIENT POPULATION

Not every patient is a candidate for home mechanical ventilation. Appropriate patients should have no evidence of acute pulmonary dysfunction, significant oxygenation disorders, or multi-organ system failure. Patients receiving home mechanical ventilation fall into several disease categories. Most often they have neuromuscular or thoracic wall disorders. Such patients may be in an early stage of their disease, when spontaneous breathing may be possible during the day, but require nocturnal mechanical ventilatory support to reverse sleep-induced hypoventilation.[13] Patients with early amyotrophic lateral sclerosis, multiple sclerosis, kyphoscoliosis, diaphragmatic paralysis, or myasthenia gravis fit this category. Another group of patients requires continuous mechanical ventilatory support. These patients have high spinal cord injuries, late-stage muscular dystrophy, or severe chronic obstructive pulmonary disease. There is a third category of patients who usually return home at the request of the patient and family. Their long-term prognosis is poor. Examples of these patients are those with lung carcinoma or end-stage chronic obstructive pulmonary disease. The following discussion will be limited to the first two categories of patients.

## RESPIRATOR SELECTION

The selection of a suitable respirator for home use is vital. Unfortunately, most hospital respirators are far too complicated for the home setting. Several simple respirators have been designed for home use (see the Appendix at the end of this chapter). They are compact and not excessively heavy; some are able to fit under a wheelchair when necessary. Most have been designed for ease of operation so that control knobs are few, easy to manipulate, clearly marked, and withstand considerable jarring. These respirators are usually fitted with alarms to indicate power loss and loss of resistance to inspiratory pressure and excessively high pressures. Home respirators must be durable and not require constant service and adjustment. They must be able to run off a dual power source (*i.e.,* off house current, as well as batteries in the event of a power failure). The breathing circuit and humidifier should be simple to assemble and easy to clean.

## EXTERNAL NEGATIVE PRESSURE VENTILATION

Tank or "iron lung" respirators were first designed for artificial ventilation in the last quarter of the 19th century. The first effective tank respirator was developed by Drinker in 1929 but its use became widespread only during the poliomyelitis epidemics of the 1940s and 1950s.[25] The patient is enclosed in a rigid tank up to the neck and a suction pump creates a negative pressure ranging from 10 cm to 30 cm of water inside the chamber by use of a bellows. The negative pressure is transmitted to the thorax, resulting in negative intrathoracic pressure that causes air to flow into the patient's lungs. The tank is a controlled cycled ventilator with a fixed inspiration-to-expiration ratio. The tank respirator is the most effective form of external negative pressure ventilators. It can be used even when the patient fails to coordinate his or her own inspiratory efforts. Tracheostomy is usually not required, and therefore upper airway defenses and humidification are preserved, which reduces the risk of infection. The tank respirator is mechanically sound with little breakdown difficulties. There are a limited number of tank respirators remaining from the poliomyelitis days and new respirators are expensive. Some patients have custom-built their own tank respirators from dismantled parts. Research into smaller units is now in progress. Tank respirators have been effectively used in patients with scoliosis, neuromuscular diseases including poliomyelitis, muscular dystrophy, spinomuscular dystrophy, and central hypoventilation, as well as patients with chronic air-flow obstruction.[13] The initial claustrophobic experience felt by most patients is overcome as they become accustomed to the tank, but occasionally claustrophobia may force cessation of this type of ventilatory support. Rarely, upper airway obstruction may be exacerbated by the tank respirator.[26] Severe scoliosis may pose problems with a neck seal as well as the ability of the patient to lie on the back during use. Swallowing incoordination in the supine position may lead to aspiration, and a patient should not use a respirator for several hours after eating. Nursing care and accessibility to the patient are difficult with patients in a tank respirator but can be provided by placing the arms through the portholes on the side of the respirator. Access to the patient can also be obtained by opening the tank. One major complication of negative pressure ventilation is hypotension, also known as "tank shock." This is caused by a pooling of blood in the abdominal cavity secondary to negative pressure. Tank respirators are large and may not fit into some homes. Power is only from the house current, which requires that a generator be utilized during power failures. Most tanks come without alarms, but these can be added.

## CHEST CUIRASS AND JACKET RESPIRATORS

Cuirass respirators operate on the same principle as the tank respirator; intermittent negative pressure is generated within a rigid shell but with only the thorax and abdomen encased in the shell. The cuirass may be a standard model or it may be individually shaped to fit the patient's body contour. These respirators are less efficient than the tank respirator, since some negative pressure may be lost around the sides of the shell. Optimal sealing of the edge of the cuirass, as well as providing for adequate room for expansion of the chest and abdomen, is best achieved by molding shells individually for each patient.[27] The customized shells are made from a body mold. A loose fit not only causes pressure loss, but can also injure the skin from constant chafing. However, a tight seal is only necessary when negative pressure is applied. Standard shells often cause pressure and discomfort around the iliac crest. Because cuirasses are less efficient than tank respirators, they may cause problems during times of acute decompensation (such as a mild respiratory infection). Cuirasses may not be able to overcome added airway resistance and a more efficient respirator may be necessary during these acute events; a back-up tank respirator or positive pressure ventilator may be necessary.

A jacket or body wrap respirator avoids the problem of sealing the shell by enclosing the patient's trunk in an airtight garment that is tied or zippered around the patient's arm, neck, and waist. A loose grid-like plastic shell is placed over the chest. A plastic wrap is placed around the shell on the entire body except for the head and neck. The wrap is sealed to prevent a pressure loss and negative pressure is then applied. The shell allows room for the chest to rise, producing inspiration. Such a wrap was used in the early 1950s and has been redesigned recently by the Emerson Company (Cambridge, MA) and Lifecare, Inc. (Boulder, CO).

Cuirass and wrap respirators are small, with little unnecessary space inside the shell. They require smaller suction pumps than tank respirators, although the suction pressure that can be achieved may be reduced. The smaller pumps are portable and may permit travel. The disadvantage of such respirators is that they do not produce large tidal volumes. They may be inadequate in patients with restrictive chest wall or pulmonary disease and may be inefficient during acute exacerbations of respiratory failure. Decubitus pressure sores may develop, particularly with cuirasses or wraps that use a back plate or in the presence of a spinal deformity. Swallowing discoordination with upper airway obstruction precludes the use of cuirass and jacket respirators unless a tracheostomy is present. Unfortunately, a tracheostomy breaks the neck seal necessary for wrap respirators but not with cuirass shells. The effect of incoordination of inspiratory effort with the negative pressure phase of the respiratory cycle is greater than in the tank respirator. These respirators are useful in patients with neuromuscular-related respiratory failure, such as poliomyelitis, some of the muscular dystrophies, or motor neuron disease, and in patients with diaphragmatic paralysis as well as chronic airflow obstruction. Patients with scoliosis tolerate molded shells.

## POSITIVE AIRWAY PRESSURE MECHANICAL VENTILATION

Positive pressure ventilation may be applied intermittently to the mouth using a mask or mouthpiece, or via the trachea using a tracheostomy. In this discussion, intermittent oral positive pressure will be referred to as *intermittent positive pressure breathing* (IPPB), while tracheal intermittent positive pressure will be referred to as *intermittent positive pressure ventilation* (IPPV). The choice between IPPB and IPPV will largely be determined by the number of hours during the day that assisted mechanical ventilation is required as well as by the need for nocturnal mechanical ventilation. IPPB is more convenient for the patient. It can be used in virtually any patient regardless of mobility or deformity. The patient inhales air or oxygen that has been filtered and humidified by the upper airways. Patient-triggered ventilation modes ensure coordination of the patient's own inspiratory efforts with the inspiratory phase of the ventilator cycle, thus reducing the work of breathing. These ventilators can also deliver bronchodilator aerosols, though recent studies have shown that IPPB has no advantage over routine nebulizers (see below). The disadvantage of IPPB is that it can be used for only short periods of time (up to about 6 to 8 hours per day), and the beneficial effects on gas exchange usually recede after two hours. IPPB is usually unsuitable for ventilatory support during the night; some patients, however, manage to maintain a seal with a mask or mouthpiece and can use IPPB for nocturnal assistance.[13] Patients with chest wall disorders will tolerate IPPB, while those with neuromuscular disease will not. Shinha and Bergofsky have shown that the use of intermittent positive pressure by mouth for 20 minutes every four hours in scoliotic patients relieves hypoxemia to the same extent as the administration of 45% oxygen without ventilatory assistance, the difference being that carbon dioxide levels fall rather than rise.[28] In addition to improvement of blood gases, there may be improved lung compliance.

The use of a tracheostomy enables IPPV to be used for longer periods of time than with a mouthpiece, and thus nocturnal or continuous use of ventilation is possible. Dead space is reduced during IPPV, and if a tracheostomy tube is used there is no danger of aspiration. However, the potential complications of a tracheostomy are numerous. Mechanical problems due to a tracheostomy include tracheal stenosis, tracheal dilatation if a cuffed tube is used, hemorrhage as a result of erosion into adjacent arteries, and tracheoesophageal fistula formation if posterior erosion occurs. These complications can be minimized by proper support of the ventilator tubing connected to the tracheostomy, but this is often neglected in the patient's home. Infection of the lower respiratory tract may occur as a result of the loss of protective airway filters. Humidification of the inspired air is necessary during IPPV. One major drawback with the use of a tracheostomy and a respirator is difficulty with speech. Recently several devices used in conjunction with the tracheostomy tube such as Venti-Voice and Communi-Trache have been designed to allow speech.

Positive pressure ventilators offer advantages over negative pressure ventilators: ability to ventilate nearly every patient, ability to make precise adjustment of ventilation, and easy access to the patient. The disadvantages of positive pressure ventilators include increased risk of infection, the need for a tracheostomy tube (usually), increased sputum production secondary to the tracheostomy and humidification system, and mandatory cleaning of the respiratory circuits to prevent infection.

Volume-limited ventilators are the most commonly used home ventilators and deliver a preset amount of air with each breath. The pressure needed to deliver the desired volume will vary with the airway resistance. The maximum pressure the ventilator can deliver is usually preset. These ventilators deliver a roughly constant minute ventilation. Since 1978 a number of respirators have been designed and marketed for home use (see Appendix). The most frequently used include Life Products LP3, LP4, and LP5, and Life Care Portable Volume Ventilator (PVV). These are volume-limited, controlled-rate ventilators. More sophisticated versions of these respirators include the IMV (intermittent mandatory ventilation) mode. Controlled-cycle ventilators work well with neuromuscular patients, where minute ventilation needs are relatively constant. Controlled-rate ventilators are less effective in patients with chronic obstructive pulmonary disease, because these patients vary their minute ventilation. Pressure-limited ventilators deliver air until a preset amount of pressure is reached. They will deliver a constant minute ventilation as long as the airway resistance does not change. When the resistance increases, the machine will deliver a lower tidal volume. However, patients with COPD who have altered airway resistance do better on these respirators. The Thompson Bantam-GS and the Life Care RBR are small, portable, pressure-controlled-cycle ventilators.

## INTERMITTENT POSITIVE PRESSURE BREATHING

Over 40 years ago Barach, Swenson, and Motley suggested that intermittent positive pressure breathing (IPPB) could be beneficial in certain medical conditions. IPPB was widely introduced into American medical practice for hospital and home use in patients with COPD. In 1977, a multicentered study sponsored by the National Heart, Lung and Blood Institute investigated the use of intermittent positive pressure breathing in patients with chronic obstructive lung disease.[29] Approximately 1000 patients with COPD who did not have severe hypoxemia or other serious diseases were recruited. Patients underwent baseline testing including lung function and exercise capacity. They were then randomly assigned either to IPPB or treatment with a compressor nebulizer. Both devices supplied the patient with bronchodilator drugs. The difference between the treatments was that IPPB applied positive pressure to the lungs, the compressor nebulizer did not. Both groups of patients were treated with the standard oral bronchodilators given to patients with COPD. Patients were then followed for 3 years. The study found no advantage for IPPB over compressor nebulizer therapy. Over the 3-year follow-up period, the two groups of patients showed similar death rates and similar figures for number and duration of hospitalizations. Changes in life quality did not differ between the two groups. Lung function showed significant but similar deterioration both in the IPPB and the nebulizer groups. Patients were also separated according to degrees of airways obstruction, reversibility of obstruction, sputum production, and the probability of emphysema. In none of these subgroups was IPPB a significantly better treatment than compressor nebulizer.

## TRACHEOSTOMY TUBES

The use of a tracheostomy in long-term ventilation in patients is to provide access for positive pressure ventilation, access for secretion removal, and airway protection for persons subject to aspiration. Tracheostomy also reduces the amount of dead space in the tracheobronchial tree and thus reduces the work of breathing. For home use the high-volume, low-pressure cuffs are important to eliminate the cuff-related necrosis. As discussed above, inability to phonate is one problem associated with tracheostomy tubes. In addition to new devices attached to the tracheostomy tube, this may be overcome by maintaining adequate ventilation through an uncuffed tracheostomy tube. Volume is increased to compensate for leakage. A major problem occurs in patients who sleep with their mouths open (thus increasing the leakage), which may necessitate an increase in volume at night. Some patients require positive pressure ventilation via tracheostomy tube only during the night. Several approaches to daytime maintenance may be pursued, including removal of the tracheostomy tube during the day, with replacement by a tracheal button (such as an Olympic or Kistner button). These plastic tubes maintain the stoma patency and protrude into the trachea only a very short distance. The button allows for suctioning and may even be attached via an adapter to IPPB.

## INTERFACE BETWEEN THE HOME CARE
## TEAM, PATIENT, FAMILY, AND HOME

Successful home management will be achieved only if (1) the patient truly desires to go home; (2) a competent, trainable family is willing to spend the time required for proper training; (3) the family fully understands the patient's diagnosis and prognosis as well as the imposition on their own life-styles; and (4) the family fully understands the financial responsibilities.

Thorough training of a family prior to discharge is necessary to produce a successful home experience. A participatory, hands-on approach to the equipment should be planned. Family members should become familiar with the home respirators as well as tubing circuitry, suction machines and methods of suctioning, tracheostomy tubes, and tracheostomy tube care kits. They should be trained to change the patient's tracheostomy tube when necessary. This will ensure their ability to place a new tube in the event of an airway emergency. Toward the end of the hospital stay, the family should be encouraged to provide around-the-clock care for the patient. This will provide the patient and family with confidence in their newly acquired abilities.

Infection control is crucial for the ventilatory-dependent patient. Aseptic procedural techniques should be taught for caring of the tracheostomy tube and stoma as well as suctioning. In addition, decontamination of the humidification system, ventilator tubing, and the ventilator itself must be performed. Handwashing and use of gloves should be emphasized before any airway manipulation. Sterile, disposable suction catheters are required for use during each suctioning attempt. Sterile conditions are required during tracheostomy tube changing procedures in the home. Inner-cannula cleaning of the tracheostomy tube is performed as a "clean" technique, and the solution used is often 1-to-1 hydrogen peroxide and distilled water, yielding a 50% solution. Distilled water is required as a suction catheter rinse and for use on all humidification devices. Decontamination of all reusable equipment such as circuitry, aerosol tubing, nebulizers, and humidifiers is performed every three days with an initial washing in non-residue-forming household detergent. This is rinsed and followed by soaking in a double or triple quaternary ammonium compound. The exterior surfaces of the ventilator should be kept clean with commercially available broad-spectrum germicide or 70% ethyl alcohol solution. The family is taught to recognize early signs and symptoms of a respiratory tract infection.

Once the patient and family assessment has been completed, evaluation of the home is performed. Electrical facilities must be inspected to determine adequacy for safe operation of all equipment. Electrical circuitry must be adequate to supply the amperage draw at peak use periods. Grounded electrical outlets must be used for all medical devices. The latter should be placed on specifically designated 15-amp to 20-amp circuits with their own fuse box. This will avoid any power overload or outages on that circuit from overuse or faulty household appliances. Observation of the patient's room is necessary to determine ideal placement of electrical outlets, space requirements for equipment and supply storage, and ease of movement of patient and family. Equipment needs will play a major role in determining space requirements. Thus, in addition to the respirator, other equipment such as oxygen cylinders, suction equipment, humidification equipment, and bedside commode need to be placed in perspective. The room should provide adequate ventilation and air-conditioning, if needed during the summer months.

The care of a patient requiring home mechanical ventilation is best managed by a team

## WRITTEN INFORMATION TO BE SUPPLIED TO PATIENT

Operation of ventilator, including proper settings

Diagrams of ventilator controls, tubing, and humidifier

Schedule for
   Cleaning tubing
   Changing humidifier water
   Changing batteries
   Testing back-up equipment

Suctioning procedure

Tracheostomy care and tube change procedure

Postural drainage procedure

Emergency telephone numbers

Respiratory vendor's telephone number

approach. This usually includes a physician, home care nurse, respiratory therapist, and social worker. The physician is largely responsible for planning the patient goals and coordinating the other members' activities. The respiratory therapist is crucial in helping to select the equipment for home use. Equipment and supplies should be brought to the home one or two days prior to patient discharge. This will allow the family to organize the area and devise a scheduled care routine. The therapist will often make contact with the vendor who will supply the patient's home equipment and will help transfer the patient from the hospital ventilator to the home ventilator. Upon discharge, the home care nurse or respiratory therapist, or both, will accompany the patient home. This is necessary to ensure that all of the equipment is functioning and the patient is safe. The primary physician as well as the home care nurse should see the patient shortly after discharge and determine how the family is coordinating the home care. Prior to discharge the patient should be provided with written information outlining all home procedures as well as a list of telephone numbers to call when questions or problems arise (see Written Information to Be Supplied to Patient). There should be a delegation of responsibilities among the members of the team. The family should be told who should be called for different problems, that is, the physician, the home care nurse, or the respiratory therapist. During the first week following discharge, daily telephone checks and several visits may be necessary. Subsequently, monthly visits to the home (usually by the respiratory therapist) are made to assess the patient's ventilatory status and overall physical condition. In addition, the respirator and supplies should be checked on a routine basis.

The appropriate vendor is critical for success. He should be approached early in the discharge planning stages. The vendor should be provided with detailed information regarding the equipment and supply needs, including ventilator settings, tracheostomy tubes, suction catheters, gloves, and dressings. The vendor must be available 24 hours a day to replace equipment, if necessary. Many vendors will provide respiratory therapists and nurses who can coordinate the approach designed by the physician and other members of the team. This respiratory therapist, who is employed by the vendor, must report on a regular basis to the physician in charge.

Financial obligations will play a major role in determining the feasibility of home ventilator management. Regardless of the nature of insurance, it is rare that a third-party payor will cover 100% of the expenses incurred. The family is responsible for a portion of that cost, which can be significant, depending on insurance coverage. Actual figures, reimbursement approximations, and cost commitments from third-party payers and supplies should be obtained and presented to the family prior to any discharge arrangements (Table

**TABLE 17-6. COST OF HOME MECHANICAL VENTILATION**

| | Monthly Rate (Dollars) |
|---|---|
| Respirator | |
| Primary | 1100 |
| Portable (back-up)* | 490 |
| Liquid $O_2$ (4 liters/min or 28%) | 1100 |
| Suction apparatus | 35 |
| Suction catheters | 300[†] |
| Miscellaneous | 300 |
| Tracheostomy care kit | |
| $4'' \times 4''$ gauze | |
| Normal saline | |
| Hydrogen peroxide | |
| Sterile $H_2O$ | |
| Portable suction unit (not reimbursable)[†] | 550 |
| Deep cycle marine battery | 210[†] |
| Battery charger | 210[†] |
| Hospital bed | 173 |
| Wheelchair (adapted for ventilator use)[‡] | 90 |

*Medicare regulations do not provide for routine back-up respirators. Thus, respirators must be ordered as "primary" and portable (back-up) respirators.
[†] Purchase rather than rental.
[‡] Optional to allow for patient mobility outside the home.

17-6). Before the patient is discharged, the local electric company, telephone company, ambulance service, and fire department should be notified. The electric company will appropriate priority service to the patient during power failures. A portable generator may be provided for restoring temporary power.

It is crucial that someone from the home care team be present at discharge, and usually it is the respiratory therapist or the nurse who attends. This person will help the family in the crucial initial hours, knowing that all systems are operational and the patient is safe.

## CONTINUOUS POSITIVE AIRWAY PRESSURE

### NASAL CPAP IN OBSTRUCTIVE SLEEP APNEA

The pathogenetic basis of obstructive sleep apnea appears to involve transient but repetitive occlusion of the upper airway during sleep, leading to recurrent episodes of hypoxemia. This results in frequent arousals and sleep fragmentation. The clinical symptoms are highlighted by loud snoring (which is due to partial obstruction of the upper airway) followed by a complete absence of noise during sleep (the resulting apnea), which is then interrupted by loud snorting sounds. Over the course of time patients develop marked daytime hypersomnolence (secondary to the disrupted sleep pattern), systemic and pulmonary hypertension (due to recurrent and continuous hypoxemia), and even cor pulmonale. Medical and surgical therapies have been designed to correct this problem. The surgical therapy has included tracheostomy and more recently uvulopalatopharyngoplasty. Success with this latter procedure approximates 50%. Unfortunately, medical therapy apparently does not work. However, a mechanical approach that "splints" open the airway has been successfully utilized via nocturnal use of a nasal continuous positive airway pressure (CPAP) mask. In 1981 Sullivan and his colleagues devised a "pneumatic splint" utilizing continuous positive airway pressure delivered through nostril catheters and showed that this can obliterate apneas in hospitalized patients with the syndrome.[30] Since that time various investigators have shown that CPAP can be successfully used not only in the hospital setting but on a chronic basis at home.[31] The basic nasal CPAP design involves the use of a comfortable mask, either custom built or commercially available, which fits snugly over the patient's nose. Airway pressure can be adjusted to the level required to abolish obstructive apneas. Most patients can be successfully treated with CPAP pressures ranging from 4.5 cm to 10 cm of water. Simplification of the original apparatus has been achieved. The entire system is portable and is now commercially available. Dry nasal mucosa, sinusitis, middle ear infections, pneumothorax, and pneumomediastinum are potential problems arising from this therapy but have not been reported. Despite CPAP pressures of 10 cm to 15 cm of water, there has been no reported adverse effect on cardiac output, nor have pneumothoraces been documented.

This form of therapy must be reserved for cooperative and well-motivated patients. Usually a patient is evaluated in a hospital setting and given nasal CPAP to document the obstructive apneas. Nasal CPAP is then applied to assess whether it successfully obliterates the apneas as well as to derive the necessary amount of CPAP needed. Only after this has been documented can it be used on an outpatient basis. The cost is approximately $1500 (Respironics, Inc., Monroeville, PA) to purchase the mask and the supporting equipment, and is usually covered by third-party payers.

## APPENDIX

### VENTILATOR DISTRIBUTORS
### POSITIVE PRESSURE RESPIRATORS

*LP-3, LP-4, LP-5, LP-6:* Life Products, Inc., Boulder, CO
*Thompson Maxivent, Thompson Bantam-GS, THOMPSON M25B, Thompson M3000XA, Companion 2800:* Puritan-Bennett Corporation, Overland Park, KS
*170C, RBL, PVV, PLV-100, PLV-102:* Lifecare, Boulder, CO
*Bear 33:* Bear Medical Systems, Inc., Riverside, CA

### NEGATIVE PRESSURE RESPIRATORS

*Iron lung, Raincoat:* JH Emerson Company, Cambridge, MA
*Pneumosuit with leggings:* New Tech Associates, Inc., Palisades Park, NJ
*Porta-Lung:* Massachusetts Rehabilitation Services, Inc., Brockton, MA
*Chest Cuirass:* Lifecare, Boulder, CO

## REFERENCES

1. Gross NJ, Skorodin MS: Anticholinergic, antimuscarinic bronchodilators. Am Rev Respir Dis 129:856–870, 1984

2. Bukowsky M, Nakatsu K, Mundt PW: Theophylline reassessed. Ann Intern Med 101:63–73, 1984

3. Mendella LA, Manfreda J, Warren CPW, Anthoniesen NR: Steroid response in stable chronic obstructive pulmonary disease. Ann Intern Med 17–21, 1982

4. Russell MAH, Merriman R, Stapleton J, Taylor W: Effect of nicotine chewing gum as an adjunct to general practitioner's advice against smoking. Br Med J 287:1782–1785, 1983

5. Sachs DPL, Hall RG, Hall SM: Effects of rapid smoking: Physiologic evaluation of a smoking cessation therapy. Ann Intern Med 88:639–641, 1978

6. Nocturnal Oxygen Therapy Trials: Continuous or nocturnal oxygen therapy in hypoxemic chronic obstructive lung disease. Ann Intern Med 93:391–398, 1980

7. Shim CS, Williams MH Jr: Evaluation of the severity of asthma: Patients versus physicians. Am J Med 68:11–13, 1980

8. Garay SM: Arterial blood gas analysis and pulmonary function testing. In Goldfrank LR, Flomembaum N (eds). Diagnostic Procedures in the Emergency Department. Topics in Emergency Medicine. Germantown, Aspen Systems, 1984

9. Epstein SW, Manning CPR, Ashley MJ, Corey PN: Survey of the clinical use of pressurized aerosol inhalers. Can Med Assoc J 120:813–816, 1979

10. Newman SP, Pavia D, Clarke SW: How should a pressurized beta-adrenergic bronchodilator be inhaled? Eur J Respir Dis 62:3–20, 1981

11. Newman SP, Woodman G, Clarke SW, Sackner MA: Effect of InspiEase on the deposition of metered-dose aerosols in the human respiratory tract. Chest 89:551–556, 1986

12. Bergofsky EH: Respiratory failure in disorders of the thoracic cage. Am Rev Respir Dis 119:643–669, 1979

13. Garay SM, Turino GM, Goldring RM: Sustained reversal of chronic hypercapnia in patients with alveolar hypoventilation syndromes. Am J Med 70:269–274, 1981

14. Weiner WJ (ed): Respiratory Dysfunction in Neurologic Disease. Mt Kisco, NY, Futura Publishing, 1980

15. Guilleminault C, Dement WC (eds): Sleep Apnea Syndromes. New York, Alan R Liss, 1978

16. Bean JW: Effects of oxygen at increased pressure. Physiol Rev 25:1–147, 1945

17. Stuart-Harris C, Bishop JM, Clark TJH et al: Long-term domiciliary oxygen therapy in chronic hypoxic cor pulmonale complicating chronic bronchitis and emphysema. Report of Medical Council working party. Lancet 1:681–686, 1981

18. Ashutosh K, Mead G, Dunsky M: Early effects of oxygen administration and prognosis in chronic obstructive pulmonary disease and cor pulmonale. Am Rev Respir Dis 127:399–404, 1983

19. Wynne JW, Block AJ, Hemenway J et al: Disordered breathing and oxygen desaturation during sleep in patients with chronic obstructive lung disease. Am J Med 66:573–579, 1979

20. McDonald GJ: Long-term oxygen therapy delivery systems. Respiratory Care 28:898–905, 1983

21. Heimlich HJ: Respiratory rehabilitation with transtracheal oxygen system. Ann Otol Rhinol Laryngol 91:643–647, 1982

22. Soffer M, Tashkin DP, Shapiro BJ et al: Conservation of oxygen supply using a reservoir nasal cannula in hypoxemic patients at rest and during exercise. Chest 88:663–668, 1985

23. Mecikalski M, Shigeoka JW: A demand valve conserves oxygen in subjects with chronic obstructive pulmonary disease. Chest 86:667–670, 1984

24. Shigeoka JW, Bonekat HW: The current status of oxygen-conserving devices. Respiratory Care 30:833–836, 1985

25. Drinker P, Shaw L: An apparatus for the prolonged administration of artificial respiration. J Clin Invest 7:229–237, 1929

26. Sharf S, Feldman N, Goldman MD et al: Vocal cord closure. Am Rev Respir Dis 117:391–397, 1978

27. Powner DJ, Hoffman LG: Bedside construction of a custom cuirass for respiratory failure in kyphoscoliosis. Chest 74:469–471, 1978

28. Shinha R, Bergofsky EH: Prolonged alteration of lung mechanics in kyphoscoliosis by positive pressure hyperinflation. Am Rev Respir Dis 206:47–57, 1972

29. The IPPB Trial Group: Intermittent positive pressure breathing therapy of chronic obstructive pulmonary disease: A clinical trial. Ann Intern Med 99:612–620, 1983

30. Sullivan CE, Berthon-Jones M, Issa FG: Reversal of obstructive sleep apnea by continuous airway pressure applied through the nares. Lancet 1:862–865, 1981

31. Rapoport DM, Sorkin B, Garay SM, Goldring RM: Reversal of the "Pickwickian syndrome" by long-term use of nocturnal airway pressure. N Engl J Med 307:931–933, 1982

# 18
# Infectious Disease

JEFFREY GREENE

Home administration of intravenous antimicrobials is a therapeutic modality not yet widely accepted or available to most practicing physicians. The directions for the near future are clear however. Significant social and economic changes in the practice of medicine provide a driving force to the home therapies movement. Better means of safely delivering intravenous medication have become available. Newer antibiotics with improved pharmacokinetics and therapeutic efficacy have been developed in response to the potentially huge outpatient antimicrobial market. Health insurance companies are carefully exploring the financial implications of home antibiotic programs. Medicolegal specialists are attempting to define the physician's liability exposure to negative outcomes incurred in such programs. Finally, hospital administrators and planning boards are speculating on the role of outpatient antibiotic programs in the context of the new prospective reimbursement schedules and changing patient referral patterns.

The past decade has led us to the threshold of being able to comprehend the proper place of home parenteral antibiotic programs and how they might change the current standards of medical therapy for infectious diseases. The following discussion will review the published experience with prototype programs. General considerations of various issues as they apply to the creation of home antibiotic facilities will then be addressed as well as some specific areas of special importance.

## RECENT EXPERIENCE

The feasibility of administering parenteral antimicrobials at home has been explored only recently. The earliest study was undertaken by Rucker and Harrison in 1974.[1] These investigators safely employed 127 courses of either gentamicin or colistimethate in 62 patients with pulmonary infections complicating cystic fibrosis. The therapy was begun in the hospital setting and continued at home using heparin locks. Forty antibiotic courses were considered unsuccessful and the patients required rehospitalization. Despite the potential toxicities of both antimicrobial agents employed, observed complications of therapy were limited to intravenous site thrombophlebitis. This low rate of complications may be accounted for by the youth of the patients (range 7–27 years) and the relatively short duration of the treatment courses (10–12 days). Since the publication of this pioneering study, at least twelve other trials of home intravenous antibiotic therapy involving nearly 700 patients have been reported (Table 18-1). Critical assessment of these programs is important in determining the applicability of home parenteral antibiosis to widespread use.

All but one of the thirteen cited studies enrolled patients who were already hospitalized, fully diagnosed, and undergoing antibiotic therapy with observed beneficial clinical responses. Patients were not entered into the home therapy programs directly. Most of the patients were hospitalized for several weeks prior to their discharge. The enrollment criteria were not standardized among the different studies. In general, patients had to have stabilized infections without other complicating or unresolved medical problems. Attempts were made to exclude individuals with psychiatric disorders, a history of alcohol or drug abuse, poor venous access, and limited household support systems. Most of the studies were not funded by grants and therefore inadequate insurance reimbursement was another criterion for exclusion.

The structure of the study programs invariably involved a hospital-based facility. Here a team consisting of a physician (usually an infectious disease specialist), a nurse practitioner, and a pharmacist coordinated the operations. Intake assessment was usually the designated responsibility of the physician. The physician also monitored patient progress during periodic visits to the "infusion center" and decided on the need for change in therapy or rehospitalization. In addition the physician generally developed a protocol for monitoring the complications of therapy, using the laboratory, based on the chosen antibiotic regimen.

The nurse practitioner generally served as the major liaison between the patient and the treatment programs. Duties in patient education vis-à-vis vascular access management, drug administration, drug-induced complications, and clinical signs of treatment failure were often assigned to the nurse. The members of the nursing staff were usually responsible for routine changes of the intravenous sites and were on "first-call" for patients with problems or questions.

### TABLE 18-1. SUMMARY OF PUBLISHED SERIES OF HOME ANTIBIOTIC TREATMENT PROGRAMS

| Reference Number | Year | Number of Patients | Osteomyelitis, Septic Arthritis | Cystic Fibrosis | Soft Tissue | Endocarditis | Orthopedic Prosthesis | Pyelonephritis | Otolaryngologic | Gynecologic | Central Nervous System | Fungal, Actinomycosis | Miscellaneous |
|---|---|---|---|---|---|---|---|---|---|---|---|---|---|
| 1 | 1974 | 62 | | 62 | | | | | | | | | |
| 3 | 1978 | 13 | 11 | | | 1 | | | | | | | 1 |
| 4 | 1978 | 23 | 14 | | | 2 | | | | | | 5 | 2 |
| 5 | 1979 | 15 | 12 | | | 2 | | | | | | | 1 |
| 6 | 1981 | 8 | 4 | | | 1 | 2 | | | | 1 | | |
| 7 | 1982 | 150 | 94 | | 18 | 2 | 4 | 10 | 8 | 5 | | | 9 |
| 8 | 1982 | 95 | 45 | 10 | 9 | 14 | | | | | | 8 | 9 |
| 9 | 1983 | 1 | | | | | | | | | 1 | | |
| 10 | 1983 | 48 | 30 | | 10 | 6 | | | | | 2 | | |
| 11 | 1984 | 76 | 76 | | | | | | | | | | |
| 12 | 1984 | 10 | | 10 | | | | | | | | | |
| 13 | 1985 | 135 | 53 | | 21 | 9 | 33 | | | | | | 19 |
| 14 | 1985 | 45 | 28 | | | 6 | | | | | | | 11 |
| Totals | | 681 | 377 | 82 | 58 | 43 | 37 | 12 | 8 | 5 | 3 | 14 | 52 |

The pharmacist's role centered on drug and equipment preparation and dispensing although in several of the studies the pharmacist represented the central figure and was primarily responsible for patient education.

The team approach to home antibiotic therapy has been stressed in several editorials on the subject and would seem critical to the success of these programs.[2] Not every study has been conducted in a large university-affiliated teaching hospital. Most have been in community hospitals that have a large referral base.

The infectious diseases treated in the 13 studies were diverse but heavily weighted in favor of osteomyelitis and septic arthritis (377 of the 681 patients), reflecting the fact that the usual long treatment courses and lack of systemic infections were viewed by the investigators as suitable for inclusion of osteomyelitis in their programs. *Staphylococcus aureus* was the most commonly encountered pathogen although gram-negative (including *Pseudomonas* species) and mixed gram-positive/gram-negative infections were also treated in home programs. Clinical outcomes for patients with osteomyelitis treated at home were difficult to assess or to compare to in-hospital treatment. The various studies lacked suitable control groups, had different periods of follow-up, and lacked consistent therapeutic regimens. In general, three fourths of the skeletal infections treated in home programs were considered "cured."[7, 11, 13]

Other infections that were treated include cystic fibrosis related pulmonary infections, soft-tissue abscesses, infective endocarditis, orthopedic prosthesis infections, pyelonephritis, and various systemic fungal infections, among others. The reported cure rates for these infections were again roughly commensurate with those to be expected in hospitalized patients, but the same caveats in assessing the results apply here.

Success or failure of a home antibiotic program may be measured in many ways.[15] Table 18-2 examines several parameters in eight of the published studies that provide sufficient data to allow analysis. One is the "significant complication rate," which refers to those treatment-associated side-effects considered by the investigators to be severe enough to warrant a change in therapeutic regimen, to stop therapy early, or to rehospitalize the patient. It does not include minor toxicities (mild rash, eosinophilia, intravenous site phlebitis, asymptomatic bacterial colonization of the intravenous catheter) through which the therapy could be maintained. "Patient-initiated drop-out" signifies instances where the family or patient felt they were unable or unwilling to continue home therapy. Only individuals who had already been enrolled in a home therapy program and chose to withdraw are reflected in the figures. The numbers do not reflect patients rejected prior to enrollment because of psychosocial, medical, or financial reasons. "Dollars saved per course" estimates the difference between the estimated charges if the patient had remained

**TABLE 18-2. SUCCESS OF PARENTERAL HOME ANTIBIOTIC PROGRAMS AS MEASURED BY SIGNIFICANT COMPLICATION RATES, PATIENT DROP-OUT, AND DOLLARS SAVED PER PATIENT COURSE**

| Reference Number | Significant Complication Rate* (%) | | Patient-Requested Drop-out* (%) | | Dollars Saved/ Patient/Course* |
|---|---|---|---|---|---|
| 3 | 3/13 | (23%) | 1/13 | (7.7%) | $3,700.00 |
| 4 | 1/23 | (4.4%) | 0/23 | (0.0%) | $2,214.00 |
| 5 | 2/15 | (13%) | 1/15 | (6.7%) | $1,620.00 |
| 6 | 0/8 | (0.0%) | 0/8 | (0.0%) | $2,371.00 |
| 7 | 1/150 | (0.7%) | 0/150 | (0.0%) | $2,885.00 |
| 8 | 0/95 | (0.0%) | 0/95 | (0.0%) | $3,289.00 |
| 10 | 7/48 | (14.5%) | 0/48 | (0.0%) | $5,728.00 |
| 14 | 5/52 | (9.6%) | 0/52 | (0.0%) | $3,324.00 |

*See text for definition of terms.

in the hospital for the entire treatment course and the actual costs incurred by treating the patient at home for part of the course.

The significant complication rates in the eight studies listed ranged from 0% to 23%. The majority of these toxicities involved skin rashes and aminoglycoside-associated vestibular/ auditory toxicity. No secondary sepsis due to infected intravenous sites occurred and there were no deaths resulting directly from home-administered antibiotics. The published reports were often vague as to what measures were employed to monitor side-effects and as to the duration of follow-up.

The most impressive measures of success of the home parenteral antibiotic programs were the low rates of patient-initiated drop-outs. Six of the eight studies had a zero drop-out rate. This certainly is in part due to the selection bias of the program's patient populations. Clearly the more motivated and "home-oriented" patients will have sought and agreed to be included in the studies. Nonetheless, these low rates of drop-out establish that the patients felt adequately prepared for the daily task of self-administration of parenteral antibiotics and that they were secure in the support of the program's base and personnel.

The cost benefit of the published programs is qualitatively apparent but quantitatively difficult to assess fully. Savings were reported in all eight studies ranging from $1600 to $5700 per patient course. The figures listed in Table 18-2 span more than a decade's experience and they are not adjusted for inflation. Furthermore, the cost savings analysis was performed differently in several of the reports, making direct comparisons difficult. While antibiotic and supply expenditures were usually computed, the direct costs of maintaining the home antibiotic program were not. Once a hospital makes a full-scale commitment to maintain a home antibiotic therapy unit (beyond that needed to support an investigational trial) the actual patient expenditures may be greater. This notwithstanding, it is clear that hospitalization for the sole purpose of administering intravenous antibiotics is significantly more costly. Further savings in health-care delivery may be realized by avoidance of additional hospital-related expenses, such as those incurred in the treatment of nosocomial infections. Patients may also be able to assume their avocational activities and therefore generate income that would otherwise be unavailable to them.[16]

## GENERAL CONSIDERATIONS

Political and socioeconomic influences on the medical profession during the past decade have provided an impetus for the creation of home intravenous antibiotic programs. In many areas of the country there is a relative shortage of acute-care hospital beds. Patients who occupy these beds for the sole purpose of receiving parenteral antibiotics underutilize the costly services of inpatient care. Infections requiring 4 to 6 weeks of antimicrobial therapy such as osteomyelitis and bacterial endocarditis became the subjects of clinical trials employing orally administered antibiotics.[17,18] Although some of these studies showed a very acceptable rate of cure, they were often criticized because of their highly selective patient populations, and oral therapies for life-threatening infections never became widely accepted or practiced.

The declining federal subsidy of health care under the Tax Equity and Fiscal Responsibility Act (TEFRA) of 1982 impacted significantly on the home therapy movement. With the application of prospective payment programs (diagnosis related groups [DRGs]) pressure from hospital administrators is being levied to explore alternatives to inpatient care for treatment of serious infections. Faced with allotted lengths of stay for bacterial endocarditis and osteomyelitis of 18.4 days and 12.3 days, respectively, hospitals stand to lose significant sums in the treatment of patients with these infections. An anticipated 1990 market for home antimicrobials has been estimated at $16 billion.[19] In the hope that third-party payers will begin to recognize home therapy of serious infections as appropriate and cost effective, many hospital-based and commercial parenteral antibiotic programs are appearing across the nation.

Along with the financial motivations to explore home therapies come the pressures from patients with their heightened consumerism. Patients present a more sophisticated approach to their own treatment and are more willing to assume an active role in their medical care. The same moods that pervade obstetrics or surgery in requests for natural childbirth or outpatient herniorrhaphies are beginning to influence patients with infectious diseases. Patients may be willing to partake in home parenteral antibiosis so long as they are convinced that the outcomes are not compromised.

The social milieu notwithstanding, expansion of home antibiotic programs would not have proceeded at the current rate had it not been for the extensive clinical experience with related therapies. Feasibility of home intravenous therapy was realized in 1972 with a description of a heparin-lock device for intermittent infusions.[20] Subsequent advances in vascular access, such as arteriovenous fistulas, prosthetic grafts, and subcutaneously tunneled central venous catheters, have provided means of long-term parenteral therapy in patients with poor peripheral venous access.[21] These technical achievements paved the way for central venous hyperalimentation, home-administered chemotherapy, and various blood-product (*e.g.,* Factor VIII) replacement therapies. During the past decade these constitutive therapies have become entrenched in our modern medical armamentarium because of their efficacy and relative safety. The treatment of a dynamic illness such as endocarditis shares the technical requirements of intravenous medication delivery, but has the added need of clinical surveillance of therapeutic response, progression of infection, and complications of therapy throughout the entire treatment course.

Patient selection for entry into a home antibiotic program must take into account many aspects of the individual's psychosocial background. Ideally the patient should be well educated and motivated toward the concept of home therapy. A clean, orderly household is necessary, as is transportation to the treatment center or laboratory. A telephone, good language skills, and adequate support systems are all important. A patient with prior history of substance abuse or medical noncompliance is a particularly poor candidate. In addition, coexistent medical conditions should be fully considered as they may interfere with the administration of intravenous drugs. Neurologic disorders (Parkinson's, cerebrovascular accident with motor deficit), ophthalmologic disease (cataracts, diabetic retinopathy), or rheumatologic conditions (severe osteoarthritis) are but several examples. Consideration must also be given to the possible interactions between the patient's medical regimen and the proposed antibiotic therapy.

Patient evaluation will also address the means by which therapy will be administered. Patients with poor venous access will be identified early and referred for placement of alternative vascular access devices (see below).

Disease selection should address several criteria suggested by published series. Most importantly, home therapy should not be considered until an infection is proven to be under control. Firm objective parameters must be identified (*e.g.,* fever, white blood count, erythrocyte sedimentation rate) as indicators of infection activity, and a clear therapeutic response should be demonstrated. Local infections requiring protracted therapy would seem safer for home therapy than systemic infections. The pathogenesis of the infection should be understood. Sources of bacteremia, deficiencies of host immune defenses, surgical intervention for debridement or drainage of abscesses, and control of underlying predisposing medical conditions (*e.g.,* diabetes) need to be kept in mind prior to sending a patient home for intravenous antibiotic therapy. Furthermore, late suppurative or immunologic sequelae of various infections should be weighed in the decision for treatment in the home. A patient with endocarditis, for example, may suffer a ruptured mycotic aneurysm, hemodynamic decompensation due to a perforated valve leaflet or torn chordae tendineae, or life-threatening conduction disturbances due to intramyocardial abscess well after it appeared that the infection was under good control. Finally, the infectious disease being considered for home therapy should have its microbiology defined. This will allow *in vitro* testing of antibiotic efficacy and help in making rational changes in regimens should it become necessary (see below).

Home antibiotic programs have been reported to reduce the costs of treating some infections by more than 50%. Nonetheless, the daily costs may be $200 to $300 per day. Exactly who is saving money is not always clear, and was the subject of a recent editorial.[22] Third-party insurance companies have not adopted a standard approach to reimbursement. Many major medical policies will pay up to 80% of the costs of home antibiotic administration. This still leaves the patients with a greater out-of-pocket cost as compared to in-hospital treatment in most cases. Thus, ability to pay for therapy is yet another inclusion criterion for home treatment. Medicare does not recognize outpatient parenteral antimicrobial therapy as an accepted standard of medical practice and as such offers no reimbursement for the cost of the drugs but will reimburse for nursing visits.[23] Hospitals faced with the DRG-designated lengths of stay for infections such as osteomyelitis may find it advantageous to subsidize home therapy for Medicare patients rather than assume the greater losses attendant with complete in-hospital courses of therapy.

The medicolegal issues surrounding home antibiotic therapy programs are as yet untested. In an excellent review of the pitfalls of outpatient parenteral therapy Goldenberg points out " . . . that the legal accountability of each member of the ambulatory program team is unknown, and that the medicolegal culpability among pharmacist, physician, hospital, I.V. nurse, administration and patient is still in evolution."[24] It would appear that until such therapy is considered medical standard, patients should be required to sign an informed consent detailing their home therapy as investigational. In this highly litigious society it is probable that patients will seek damages for a variety of negative outcomes including drug-induced complications, failure to eradicate an infection, or delays in diagnosing secondary conditions.

## VASCULAR ACCESS ALTERNATIVES[25]

For relatively short-term antibiotic administration, peripheral vein devices constitute the best means of vascular access. Heparin locks utilizing either steel-needled "butterfly" or short plastic (polyvinylchloride/polytetrafluoroethylene) catheters are most commonly employed. The steel needles have a lower rate of bacterial colonization and clinical infection than the plastic catheters but they are less stable in an ambulatory patient. The successful use of these devices relates to the availability of venous access sites. Elderly or obese patients or individuals with lymphatic insufficiency (*e.g.,* postmastectomy) will have limited access. Furthermore, some individuals with adequate peripheral veins quickly develop chemical phlebitis due to the large doses of various antibiotics administered in small-caliber vessels. Peripherally placed central venous catheters have a high rate of bacterial colonization and secondary thrombophlebitis. They have no role in home parenteral antibiotic therapy.

Surgical creation of an arteriovenous fistula has been the major modality of vascular access for patients on chronic hemodialysis. This is rarely useful for patients requiring home antibiotics. The arteriovenous shunt must mature and cannot be used for several weeks after its placement. In rare patients requiring months of therapy (*e.g.,* amphotericin for disseminated coccidioidomycosis) this means of vascular access may be useful. However, new techniques have essentially supplanted this modality.

Delivery of antibiotics directly into the central venous circulation may be carried out by percutaneously placed central vein catheters. These devices are composed of polyvinyl chloride and are easy to insert. The principal drawbacks of this line are subclavian vein thrombosis and catheter-associated sepsis. The former complication is related to the duration of placement and may be somewhat prevented by frequent heparin flushes. Sepsis occurs because the cutaneous entry site of the catheter is situated close to the vascular puncture site. Use of this type of catheter for more than two weeks is not advisable.

An alternative to the above-mentioned system is the silicone rubber (Silastic) central venous catheters, such as the Hickman or Broviac catheters. These are surgically placed and are then tunneled subcutaneously to a site several inches away where they exit. A polyester cuff in the tunneled portion of the catheter anchors the line and inhibits bacterial movement along the tract. Local exit-wound infections may occur without septicemia, and early treatment may save the line. These Silastic catheters may be kept in place for many months. The published rate of catheter loss due to malfunction or sepsis is 10% to 15%.[26] The generous inside diameter of these lines also affords the ability to sample blood or administer transfusions. At New York University Medical Center we have utilized Hickman catheters in 35 individuals with the acquired immune deficiency syndrome who required chronic amphotericin-B therapy. Despite their severe immune depression, only two lines had to be removed because of septicemia.

While the tunneled Silastic catheters will satisfy the needs of most patients requiring prolonged home antibiotic therapy, a recent advancement, the totally implantable port system, may be a reasonable option for individuals requiring very prolonged therapy or multiple courses of therapy. These devices utilize Silastic catheters attached to a self-sealing subcutaneously implanted port. Percutaneous access to the system is via a small-gauge angled needle that may be left in place for several days. The placement of this device requires the creation of a pouch to accommodate the port.

Many patients enrolled in home antibiotic programs will find it feasible to complete their therapy with heparin locks. In those patients with poor peripheral access, or who suffer chemical phlebitis due to sclerosing antibiotics, a percutaneously placed plastic central venous catheter is plausible. If therapy for more than two weeks is anticipated, a tunneled Silastic catheter is preferred.

## THE ANTIBIOTIC REGIMEN

The choice of an antibiotic regimen for home use may be a difficult one.[27] In addition to usual considerations of drug efficacy against a particular pathogen, tissue penetration, and cost, several other factors must be taken into account. Because the drug is being administered with little supervision, an attempt is made to minimize use of agents that require intensive monitoring of serum levels or renal function. Single drug regimens with infrequent dosing schedules (every 12 hours or every 24 hours) are preferred to allow the patient to resume work or other daily activities. The newer cephalosporins have been developed to satisfy these requirements. Their use may be a compromise favoring drug potency, safety, and long half-life over the lower cost and narrower spectrum of some of the older agents. Any regimen chosen for home use should be started early in the course of treatment to allow for observation of drug-related side-effects and efficacy prior to discharge. If a newer cephalosporin such as ceftriaxone or cefonicid is used for a *Staphylococcus aureus* infection, for example, it would be advisable to assess the serum bactericidal levels prior to discharge since the minimal bactericidal concentrations for these drugs are higher than for the semisynthetic penicillins, such as nafcillin. Peak serum levels of 1 : 8 and trough levels of 1 : 2 have been associated with successful treatment outcomes in patients with osteomyelitis and endocarditis.[28] The microbiology laboratory should be instructed to maintain any clinical isolates by subculture to allow for *in vitro* testing.

Cost considerations are of importance in home care programs as they are in hospital formularies. Interestingly, the cost of the drugs may be exceeded by preparation and handling costs in the pharmacy. This favors a drug that can be infrequently dosed. Older drugs, such as oxacillin, gentamicin, carbenicillin, penicillin, erythromycin, cephalothin, cefazolin, cefoxitin, and cefamandole, may be stored in minibag admixture containers at − 20°C for a month or longer.[29] This allows for storage of large amounts of drug in the home and reduces pharmacy costs. Little information is available for the newer cephalosporins in terms of their storage stability.

The cost of the medications represents a significant fraction of the total expenditures in home antibiotic programs. Table 18-3 summarizes the pharmacokinetics and comparative costs of a number of antibiotics suitable for home use. The daily costs of treatment with the second- and third-generation cephalosporins are roughly equivalent. Overall, prices range from 66¢ for gentamicin to $70 for vancomycin.

*Staphylococcus aureus* has been the most frequently encountered pathogen in infections treated at home. The semisynthetic penicillins (oxacillin and nafcillin) remain the most active drugs. However, because of its long half-life and excellent minimal inhibitory concentration/minimal bactericidal concentration (MIC/MBC) against *Staphylococcus,* cefazolin is a good alternative. The second-generation cephalosporins, cefuroxime, ceftriaxone, cefonicid, and cefamandole, have somewhat lower activity against this pathogen. In patients who are allergic to the cephalosporins, vancomycin or clindamycin are alternative therapies.

Against gram-negative organisms the third-generation cephalosporins have considerable advantage over the aminoglycosides and the penicillin derivatives such as ticarcillin, carbenicillin, and mezlocillin. They have lower minimal inhibitory concentrations, are safer to administer, and have a broader spectrum of activity. It should be kept in mind that the cephalosporins with N-methyl-thio-tetrazole substituent at the 3-position of the beta-lactam ring have been associated with hypoprothrombinemia and hemorrhage as well as a disulfuram reaction after alcohol consumption. Moxalactam, the first completely synthetic cephalosporin, is the most likely to cause bleeding complications and probably has no role in home therapy of infections. Vitamin K administration may decrease the incidence of hemorrhage.

The aminoglycosides are limited by their well-recognized nephrotoxicity, ototoxicity, and vestibular toxicity. These drugs should be reserved for severe infection due to multiply resistant gram-negative rods such as *Pseudomonas aeruginosa* and *Enterobacter clocae.* They are often combined with a semisynthetic penicillin or a cephalosporin. Aminoglycosides are also used for antibiotic synergy against the enterococcus in serious infections such as endocarditis. Careful monitoring of peak and trough aminoglycoside levels is important as is frequent assessment of renal function and periodic audiometry.

Several new non-cephalosporin drugs of extremely broad spectrum and potency have recently been marketed. Ticarcillin–clavulinic acid has a broader spectrum than ticarcillin alone because of the fact that clavulinate is an inhibitor of the beta-lactamases produced by *Staphylococcus aureus,* resistant gram-negative rods, and anaerobes. While it may be useful in certain polymicrobial infections as a single agent, its short half-life is a drawback in the home setting. Another new agent is imipenem-cilastatin. This is the first thienamycin derivative to reach the market. It is a potent inhibitor of cell-wall synthesis and has an incredibly wide range of activity, including against staphylococcus, enterococcus, gram-negative rods including pseudomonas, and anaerobes. Cilastatin, by way of renal dipeptidase inhibition, maintains good urinary levels of the drug. This drug may be used on a schedule of every 6

**TABLE 18-3. COMPARISON OF SELECTED ANTIBIOTICS BY DOSING INTERVAL, DOSE, AND DAILY COSTS**

| Antibiotic | Interval | Dose | | Daily Costs ($)* |
|---|---|---|---|---|
| Gentamicin | q8h | 80 | mg | .66 |
| Tobramycin | q8h | 80 | mg | 14.76 |
| Netilmicin | q12h | 150 | mg | 10.00 |
| Amikacin | q12h | 500 | mg | 37.38 |
| Cefazolin | q8–12h | 1000 | mg | 5.22–7.83 |
| Cefamandole | q6–8h | 2000 | mg | 33.72–44.96 |
| Cefonicid | q24h | 1000 | mg | 13.85 |
| Cefuroxime | q8h | 1500 | mg | 31.44 |
| Cefoxitin | q6–8h | 2000 | mg | 40.77–54.36 |
| Ceftriaxone | q12–24h | 1000 | mg | 23.64–47.28 |
| Cefoperazone | q12h | 2000 | mg | 37.18 |
| Ceftazidime | q8h | 1–2 | g | 34.26–68.52 |
| Ticarcillin | q4–6h | 3 | g | 25.08–37.62 |
| Ticarcillin + clavulinate | q4–6h | 3.1 | g | 37.80–56.70 |
| Mezlocillin | q6–8h | 4 | g | 25.80–34.40 |
| Penicillin G | q4–6h | $2 \times 10^6$ | U | 7.12–10.68 |
| Ampicillin | q4–6h | 2000 | mg | 5.08–7.62 |
| Nafcillin | q4–6h | 2000 | mg | 12.08–18.12 |
| Oxacillin | q4–6h | 2000 | mg | 10.80–16.20 |
| Trimethoprim/ sulfamethoxazole | q6–8h | 10 | ml | 16.74–22.52 |
| Vancomycin | q6–8h | 500 | mg | 45.39–60.52 |
| Clindamycin | q8h | 900 | mg | 44.37 |
| Metronidazole | q6–8h | 500 | mg | 8.52–11.36 |
| Imipenem-Cilastatin | q6h | 500 | mg | 59.80 |

*Costs refer to the price paid by hospital pharmacy but do not include the cost of preparing the drugs, or the costs of infusion apparatus.

hours and there may be a role for it in some serious polymicrobial infections treated at home.

## FUTURE DIRECTIONS

The administration of intravenous antibiotics at home is a concept that is still in evolution, but it will unquestionably assume a niche in the future as an accepted standard of therapy. Before this is realized, however, much more experience is needed. Infections other than osteomyelitis and joint infections must be treated in home therapy programs in numbers large enough to convince investigators that outcomes are comparable to hospital-treated patients. Long-term follow-up is needed and future studies should use a more systematic approach to monitoring for drug-induced side-effects. New antibiotics should be judged not only on their pharmacokinetic characteristics, but also on their therapeutic efficacies. Many years will be necessary to generate enough confidence in a new drug to allow for changes in treatment recommendations for serious infections.

The multidisciplinary approach to home therapy will undoubtedly proceed at its current rate. The future will see a shift of responsibility away from the physician and more to the nurse practitioner and pharmacist. Experience is needed to assess this interplay of professionals in providing optimal patient supervision and care. Critical to the survival of the concept of home parenteral antibiotic therapy is the stance to be taken by the third-party reimbursers. The success of such programs hinges on their being recognized as acceptable alternatives to hospitalization. Commercial enterprises will generally be stymied until they can depend on reimbursement from health insurance carriers. Once commercial outfits enter the marketplace in a major way, there will be an interesting interplay with hospital-based programs. Competition for patient referrals may be significant.

Home intravenous antibiotic therapy is a management approach by which health-care consumers may either benefit or lose. Only by careful analysis and cautious trials will its true niche be defined.

## REFERENCES

1. Rucker RW, Harrison GM: Outpatient intravenous medication in the management of cystic fibrosis. Pediatrics 54:358–360, 1974
2. Smego RA Jr: Home intravenous antibiotic therapy (editorial). Arch Intern Med 145:1001–1002, 1985
3. Antoniskis A, Anderson BC, van Volkinburg EJ et al: Feasibility of outpatient self-administration of parenteral antibiotics. West J Med 128:203–206, 1978
4. Stiver HG, Telford GO, Mossey JM et al: Intravenous antibiotic therapy at home. Ann Intern Med 89:690–693, 1978
5. Kind AC, Williams DN, Persons G et al: Intravenous antibiotic therapy at home. Arch Intern Med 139:413–415, 1979
6. Swenson JP: Training patients to administer intravenous antibiotics at home. Am J Hosp Pharm 38:1480–1483, 1981
7. Poretz DM, Eron LJ, Goldenberg RI et al: Intravenous antibiotic therapy in an outpatient setting. JAMA 248:336–339, 1982
8. Stiver HG, Trosky SK, Cote DD, Oruck JL: Self-administration of intravenous antibiotics: An efficient cost-effective home care program. Can Med Assoc J 127:207–211, 1982
9. Bergstein JM, Kleiman M, Ballantine TV: Long-term outpatient amphotericin-B therapy via a silicone central alimentation catheter. J Pediatr Surg 18:199–200, 1983
10. Rehm SJ, Weinstein AJ: Home intravenous antibiotic therapy: A team approach. Ann Intern Med 99:388–392, 1983
11. Eron LJ, Goldenberg RI, Poretz DM: Combined ceftriaxone and surgical therapy for osteomyelitis in the hospital and outpatient settings. Am J Surg 148(4A):1–4, 1984
12. Winter RJ, George RJ, Deacock SJ et al: Self-administered home intravenous antibiotic therapy in bronchiectasis and adult cystic fibrosis. Lancet 1:1338–1339, 1984
13. Rehm SJ: Home intravenous antibiotic therapy. Cleve Clin Q 52:333–338, 1985
14. Manzella JP, McConville JH, Klaus B, Brenner T: Home intravenous antibiotic therapy. Penn Med 88:52–54, 1985
15. Grizzard MB: Home intravenous antibiotic therapy. A practical management approach for the 1980's. Postgrad Med 78:187–189, 192–195, 1985
16. Poretz DM, Woolard D, Eron LJ et al: Outpatient use of ceftriaxone: A cost-benefit analysis. Am J Med 77(4c):77–83, 1984
17. Dunkle LM, Brock N: Long-term follow-up of ambulatory management of osteomyelitis. Clin Pediatr 21:650–655, 1982
18. Guntheroth WG, Cammarano AA, Kirby WM: Home treatment of infective endocarditis with oral amoxicillin. Am J Cardiol 15:1231–1232, 1985
19. Eron LJ: Intravenous antibiotic administration in outpatient settings. J Infect Dis Jan:4–11, 1984

20. Stern RC, Pittman S, Doershuk CF, Matthews LW: Use of a "heparin lock" in the intermittent administration of intravenous drugs. A technical advance in intravenous therapy. Clin Pediatr 11:521–523, 1972

21. Ogden DA: Comparing vascular access methods. Trans AM Soc Artif Intern Organs 29:782–794, 1983

22. Bosso JA, Stephenson SE, Herbst JJ: Feasibility and cost savings of intravenous administration of aminoglycosides in outpatients with cystic fibrosis. Drug Intell Clin Pharm 19:52–54, 1985

23. Hittel WP: DRG's and Medicare reimbursement for outpatient intravenous antibiotic programs (letter). Am J Hosp Pharm 41:1310, 1312, 1984

24. Goldenberg RI: Pitfalls in the delivery of outpatient intravenous therapy. Drug Intell Clin Pharm 19:293–296, 1985

25. Gyves JW, Ensminger WD: Long-term vascular access, including Hickman catheter and other devices. In Petersdorf et al (eds): *Harrison's Principles of Internal Medicine, Update VII,* pp 133–141. New York, McGraw-Hill, 1985

26. Fuchs PC, Gustafson ME, King JT, Goodall PT: Assessment of catheter-associated infection risk with the Hickman right atrial catheter. Infect Control 5:226–230, 1984

27. Reed MD: Evaluation of antibiotics for home care programs. Drug Intell Clin Pharm 19:288–290, 1985

28. Jordan GW, Kawachi MM: Analysis of serum bactericidal activity in endocarditis, osteomyelitis, and other bacterial infections. Medicine 60:49–61, 1981

29. Dinel BA, Ayotte DC, Behme RJ et al: Stability of antibiotic admixtures frozen in minibags. Drug Intell Clin Pharm 11:542–548, 1977

# 19
# Nutritional Support

PAUL S. KURTIN

Over the past decade there has been increased awareness by physicians of the problems related to malnutrition in hospitalized patients. The enormity of this problem is evidenced by several surveys that have shown that approximately 50% of general medical and surgical patients are malnourished to some degree.[1,2] Malnutrition can adversely affect the prognosis of an individual patient. It can also have broader societal implications in that malnourished patients have been shown to require prolonged hospital stays to recover from their primary illness, which in turn lead to increased costs for hospital care.[3]

Our ability has improved in identifying patients who are already malnourished or who are at risk of developing malnutrition due to their underlying disease or its treatment. So too has our ability improved in providing these patients with specialized nutritional support. While our understanding of the pathophysiology of malnutrition remains incomplete, nearly twenty years of clinical experience in treating these patients has been accumulated. Recently, clinical studies have shown that nutritional support, especially in surgical patients, can significantly decrease patient morbidity and mortality,[4] and this decrease in patient morbidity can lead to significant savings in the cost of patient care.

The nutritional deficiencies of many patients requiring specialized support can be corrected within the course of their hospitalization. However, there are a number of patients who remain hospitalized solely for the purpose of nutritional support. Whether they require this support as a life-sustaining procedure or as an adjuvant to other treatments, or as the primary treatment modality for their illness, this support can now be delivered safely, efficiently, and cost-effectively at home.

Since Shils managed the first parenterally fed patient at home in 1969 over 2000 additional patients have been treated with home parenteral nutrition.[5] Many more patients have been supported at home on enteral tube-feeding programs. The following discussion is intended for physicians who do not have specialized training in clinical nutrition, but who will assume primary responsibility for the long-term, comprehensive care of the patient receiving home nutritional support. Because this review is not intended to be an exhaustive discussion of the theories and practice of total parenteral nutrition (TPN) or enteral nutrition (EN), it is assumed that the primary physician will call upon a physician–clinical nutritionist to act as a consultant in planning and implementing a nutritional support regimen. However, this discussion will familiarize the reader with the basic principles and techniques of TPN and EN to guide the physician in applying these practices in the home care setting. Under optimal conditions, a patient receiving home nutrition will be supported by a team of care providers. In the hospital this team consists of the physician-nutritionist, a nurse, a dietitian, a pharmacist, a social worker, and, if appropriate, a business manager. This multidiscipline approach to patient care is essential to the proper evaluation, preparation, and training of the home care patient. Such teams exist in many but certainly not all medical centers. When a team is not available, the primary physician may call upon a home care company to provide the nursing, social work, and pharmacy expertise that is otherwise unavailable. In either case, the role of the primary physician becomes one of coordinating the activities of the team with the patient. Because the primary physician knows the patient best, he can help the team establish reasonable goals for the patient, and help both the patient and the team by assessing the patient's ability and willingness to accept this form of therapy. In addition, the primary physician can best interact with the family while the patient is still hospitalized and after discharge, and, of course, the physician will be the primary contact between the patient and the team once the patient goes home.

The first issue to be considered is the selection of the patient appropriate for home nutritional support. In the simplest terms, the patient who requires specialized home nutritional support is one who is unable to eat enough to maintain a normal nutritional status. When the primary disease process or its treatment limits the normal ingestion or absorption of adequate nutrients, the patient may require nutritional support for a finite period of time or for the duration of his life. The decision to initiate home enteral nutrition or parenteral nutrition ultimately depends on the level of functioning intestine. Although other variables, discussed below, enter into the decision, any patient who has a sufficiently functioning gastrointestinal tract can and should be managed with enteral feeding. ("If the gut works, use it.")

Patients suitable for long-term enteral support include those who are able to eat but who do not take in enough to prevent progressive weight loss and the development of malnutrition. (See Indications for the Use of Enteral Nutritional Support.) For example, patients who are anorectic due to their disease or its treatment (*e.g.,* chemotherapy) can be evaluated with a 3-day diet history. If they consistently ingest inadequate amounts of protein and calories, a trial with an oral liquid formula is indicated. If this supplemental therapy is not successful, then enteral support is necessary. Other indications for long-term enteral nutritional support include patients with anatomical blockade to normal ingestion. Such patients may have oral or esophageal cancer or may be recovering from the surgery or radiation therapy of their malignancy. Other patients with primary intestinal diseases that lead to malabsorption may require specialized (elemental) diets that are unpalatable and therefore must be infused directly into the stomach or small intestine. However, prior to starting enteral feeding in such a patient, the degree of malabsorption must be evaluated

## INDICATIONS FOR THE USE OF ENTERAL NUTRITIONAL SUPPORT

Anorexia

Malabsorption

Gastrointestinal tract fistulas

Inflammatory bowel disease

Short bowel syndrome

Radiation enteritis

Head and neck surgery

Esophageal carcinoma

Anorexia nervosa

Cerebrovascular disease

to determine the nature and quantity of nutrient losses. Such an evaluation is necessary to decide on the proper mode and composition of nutritional support.

The primary reason for not choosing enteral feeding for the patients described above would be the presence of severe pulmonary disease because of the risk of an aspiration pneumonia, which could severely stress their already limited pulmonary function. However, while aspiration has been reported with nasogastric feeding, it is very unlikely when the feeding tube is passed into, or enters directly, the small intestine.

Patients who require long-term parenteral nutrition simply lack, either anatomically or functionally, adequate intestinal absorptive area. (See Indications for the Use of Parenteral Nutritional Support.) Patients who fall into this category include those with severe Crohn's disease, pseudo-obstruction, radiation enteritis, short bowel syndrome, or severe malabsorption, or those who have had massive intestinal resections. Home parenteral nutrition has also been used as a treatment modality for patients with enterocutaneous fistulas.

For a home care nutrition program to succeed, the physician must assess the motivation of the patient, the patient's ability and willingness to learn about the techniques, and the likelihood that the patient will comply with the therapeutic program. The physician should also discuss the reasons why one modality was chosen over another, what are the potential complications and benefits of the therapy, what role the family will play in assisting with the therapy, and what are the long-term goals of the treatment program. If the patient does not have the ability to master the methodology of his treatment, a family member can be trained. This is commonly done for young children and physically or mentally limited adults.

Entering into a program of home nutritional support often places the patient and his family under great emotional stress, and it is imperative to deal with these issues while the patient is still hospitalized.[6] Some of the issues that need to be considered include the real or perceived financial strain that long-term care will place on the patient and his family. This includes not only the cost of the treatment but also the potential loss of income if the patient is unable to return to work. These costs should be contrasted with the costs of a prolonged hospital stay. With home nutritional support (HNS), however, many patients are able to regain sufficient strength and function so that they can and do return to work.

Eating is such a basic human function that patients in these programs often go through periods of depression and anger as they adjust to new body images as well as a new dependency on a tube, a machine, a bag of nutrients, and the time and care required for the proper infusion of the nutrient solution. Meal time is also often a major time of social interaction for the family, and the patient and his family may have to adjust to new roles and activities at these times. Other basic functions of life can also no longer be taken for granted. For example, patients worry about sleeping while attached to equipment; they worry about sexual relationships; they worry about how they will, or won't, be accepted by their friends.

## INDICATIONS FOR THE USE OF PARENTERAL NUTRITIONAL SUPPORT

Inflammatory bowel disease
Obstruction of gastrointestinal tract
Radiation enteritis
Enterocutaneous fistulas
Short bowel syndrome
Pseudo-obstruction
Chronic diarrhea or malabsorption
Massive intestinal resection

Patients worry about becoming too dependent on their families, and the families are often fearful of allowing the patient to do too much. While the primary physician should encourage a discussion of these issues, recruiting the aid of a home parenteral nutrition nurse or social worker experienced in dealing with these problems is often of great benefit to all involved.

The actual process of initiating home nutritional support begins when the patient's nutritional status and requirements are assessed by a physician trained in clinical nutrition. The physician–clinical nutritionist makes the decisions regarding the nature of the nutritional support and writes the basic prescription in terms of nutrients, electrolytes, and volume.

Table 19-1 illustrates the types of enteral formulations frequently used in this setting. Although it is beyond the scope of this discussion to describe in detail all the variables that go into choosing one product over another, several excellent reviews of this topic have been published.[7,8] However, it can be noted that the products listed in Table 19-1 differ in terms of the amount and types of protein available; the amount and sources of calories per milliliter; osmolality; amount of electrolytes included; and the amount of vitamins and trace elements included. In addition, although many of these products can be purchased ready for use, others involve some amount of preparation by the patient.

In addition to selecting the proper product, the mode of delivery must also be determined. Tables 19-2 to 19-4 list frequently used enteral feeding equipment. The feeding tubes differ in terms of ease of self-intubation and ultimate location in the gastrointestinal tract (*i.e.,* nasogastric, nasojejunal, or percutaneous jejunal tubes). Some patients may want to remove their feeding tubes when not in use, whereas other patients may not want to or may not be able to remove their tubes. For example, patients with esophageal cancer may not be able to intubate themselves easily due to anatomical obstruction, whereas percutaneous jejunal tubes should not be manipulated by the patient.

Once a formula and tube are selected for the patient, he is then stabilized on that regimen for a period of approximately 1 to 2 weeks to ensure adequate nutrient intake and the lack of metabolic complications such as hyperglycemia. The 24-hour feeding regimen (for patients with malabsorption) of this phase of the hospitalization is then gradually reduced to 8 to 12 hours. This will then allow the patient many hours of freedom from the feeding bags and pumps and leads to significant benefits in terms of quality of life. When either anorexia or difficulty in swallowing is the main problem, intermittent "bolus" feeding rather than continuous feeding is indicated. During the several days it will take to shorten the hours of formula delivery, the patient begins instruction in managing his own feeding program. For example, if the patient (or the family) will eventually intubate himself, he is instructed in this procedure. The patient and family will also be instructed in preparing and mixing, if necessary, the formula for delivery. They will also be taught how to operate the infusion pump and aspirate stomach contents, checking for residual formula from previous meals. Although the patient should be metabolically stable before discharge, he will be instructed in monitoring his urine for glucose as well as monitoring his weight for any sudden changes that could represent fluid retention or dehydration. Only when the patient is comfortable with all these procedures and responsibilities is he ready for discharge.

Once at home most patients feed during the night to leave their days free for other activities. In order to minimize trips to the hospital or pharmacy to obtain their formulas and other supplies, some arrangements must be made for the proper storage of these products. A formula, once mixed or emptied from the can, can be safely used only within 24 hours without risking bacterial contamination. Therefore, refrigeration space must be made available, and some patients have purchased separate refrigerators for their formulas.

(*Text continues on page 268*)

# TABLE 19-1. COMPOSITION OF NUTRITIONALLY COMPLETE, LACTOSE-FREE ENTERAL FORMULAS

| Category and Product | Manufacturer* | Kcal/ml | mOsmol/kg water | Price/1000 kcal† | Non-protein kcal/g nitrogen | Protein G | Protein kcal % total | Protein Source | Fat G | Fat kcal % total | Fat Source | Carbohydrate G | Carbohydrate kcal % total | Carbohydrate Source | Na, mg/1000 kcal | K, mEq/1000 kcal | Form | Kcal to meet vitamin RDA | Clinical Studies |
|---|---|---|---|---|---|---|---|---|---|---|---|---|---|---|---|---|---|---|---|
| **1 kcal/ml** | | | | | | | | | | | | | | | | | | | |
| **Standard protein** | | | | | | | | | | | | | | | | | | | |
| **Tube/oral** | | | | | | | | | | | | | | | | | | | |
| Ensure | Ross | 1.06 | 450 | 2.80 | 153 | 37 | 14 | CAS, SOY | 37 | 31.5 | CO | 145 | 54.5 | HCS, SUC | 797 | 38 | READY-TO-USE | 2000 | X |
| Travasorb | Trav | 1 | 450 | 2.20 | 144 | 37 | 15 | CAS, SOY | 37 | 33 | CO, SO | 145 | 58 | SUC, CSS | 736 | 30 | READY | 2000 | |
| Renu | Bio | 1 | 300 | 2.69 | 154 | 35 | 14 | CAS | 40 | 36 | SO | 125 | 50 | MAL, SUC | 500 | 32 | READY | 2000 | X |
| Nutri-Aid | McGaw | 1.1 | 290 | 3.37 | 142 | 37 | 15 | CAS | 35 | 31.5 | CO, M/D GLY | 135 | 54 | CSS, SUC | 690 | 30 | READY | 2075 | |
| **Tube only** | | | | | | | | | | | | | | | | | | | |
| Ensure HN | Ross | 1.06 | 470 | 3.20 | 124 | 44 | 17 | CAS, SOY | 35 | 30 | CO | 139 | 53 | HCS, SUC | 877 | 38 | READY | 1400 | |
| Osmolite | Ross | 1.06 | 300 | 2.96 | 153 | 37 | 14 | CAS, SOY | 38.5 | 31 | MCT, CO, SO | 145 | 55 | HCS | 518 | 25 | READY | 2000 | X |
| Isocal | Mead | 1.06 | 300 | 3.28 | 167 | 34 | 13 | CAS, SOY | 44 | 37 | SO, MCT | 132 | 50 | MAL | 498 | 32 | READY | 2120 | X |
| Osmolite HN | Ross | 1.06 | 310 | 3.28 | 124 | 44 | 17 | CAS, SOY | 37 | 30 | MCT, CO, SO | 141 | 53 | HCS | 877 | 38 | READY | 1400 | X |
| Compleat-modified | Doyle | 1.07 | 300 | 7.16 | 131 | 43 | 16 | BEEF, CAS, VEG | 37 | 31 | BEEF, CO | 140 | 53 | H CER S, FRUIT, VEG | 636 | 34 | READY | 1600 | |
| Vitaneed | Bio | 1 | 375 | 5.16 | 154 | 35 | 14 | BEEF, CAS, VEG | 40 | 36 | SO, BEEF | 125 | 50 | MAL, FRUIT, VEG | 506 | 32 | READY | 2000 | X |
| **Low-fat, Oligomeric** | | | | | | | | | | | | | | | | | | | |
| Travasorb STD | Trav | 1 | 560 | 6.24 | 202 | 30 | 12 | H LAC | 13 | 12 | MCT, SUN O | 190 | 76 | GO | 920 | 30 | POWDER | 2000 | |
| Criticare HN | Mead | 1.06 | 650 | 11.12 | 148 | 38 | 14 | H CAS, AA | 3 | 3 | SAF O | 222 | 83 | MAL, MCS | 598 | 32 | READY | 2120 | X |
| Standard Vivonex | Nor | 1 | 550 | 5.68 | 286 | 22 | 8 | AA | 1 | 1 | SAF O | 231 | 91 | GO | 468 | 30 | POWDER | 1800 | X |
| Vital HN | Ross | 1 | 460 | 8.35 | 125 | 42 | 17 | H WHEY; MEAT, AA | 11 | 9 | SAF O, MCT | 188 | 74 | HCS, SUC | 467 | 34 | POWDER | 1500 | X |
| Travasorb HN | Trav | 1 | 560 | 11.25 | 126 | 45 | 18 | H LAC | 13 | 12 | MCT, SUN O | 175 | 70 | GO | 920 | 30 | POWDER | 2000 | |
| Vivonex HN | Nor | 1 | 810 | 9.87 | 127 | 44 | 18 | AA | 1 | 1 | SAF O | 210 | 81 | GO | 529 | 30 | POWDER | 3000 | X |
| **Fiber-containing** | | | | | | | | | | | | | | | | | | | |
| Enrich | Ross | 1.1 | 480 | 3.22 | 148 | 39 | 15 | CAS, SOY | 37 | 30 | CO | 160 | 55 | HCS, SUC, SP | 773 | 36 | READY | 1530 | X |

| | | | | | | | | | | | | | | | | | | | |
|---|---|---|---|---|---|---|---|---|---|---|---|---|---|---|---|---|---|---|---|
| **High protein** | | | | | | | | | | | | | | | | | | | |
| Sustacal | Mead | 1 | 625 | 3.08 | 79 | 61 | 24 | CAS, SOY | 23 | 21 | SO | 140 | 55 | SUC, CSS | 938 | 53 | READY | 1080 | X |
| Isotein | Doyle | 1.2 | 300 | 12.48 | 86 | 68 | 23 | D LAC, CAS | 34 | 25 | SO, MCT | 156 | 52.5 | MAL, FRUC | 565 | 18 | POWDER | 2100 | |
| **1.5 kcal/ml** | | | | | | | | | | | | | | | | | | | |
| **Standard protein** | | | | | | | | | | | | | | | | | | | |
| Ensure Plus | Ross | 1.5 | 600 | 2.19 | 146 | 55 | 15 | CAS, SOY | 53 | 32 | CO | 200 | 53 | HCS, SUC | 761 | 40 | READY | 3000 | X |
| Sustacal HC | Mead | 1.5 | 650 | 2.42 | 134 | 61 | 16 | CAS | 57.5 | 34 | SO | 190 | 50 | CSS, SUC | 563 | 25 | READY | 1800 | |
| Ensure Plus HN | Ross | 1.5 | 650 | 2.41 | 125 | 63 | 17 | CAS, SOY | 49 | 30 | CO | 197 | 53 | HCS, SUC | 789 | 31 | READY | 1420 | |
| **High-protein** | | | | | | | | | | | | | | | | | | | |
| Traumacal | Mead | 1.5 | 550 | 3.14 | 89 | 83 | 22 | CAS | 68 | 41 | SO, MCT | 143 | 38 | CSS, SUC | 800 | 24 | READY | 3000 | X |
| **2 kcal/ml** | | | | | | | | | | | | | | | | | | | |
| **Standard protein** | | | | | | | | | | | | | | | | | | | |
| Magnacal | Bio | 2 | 590 | 2.07 | 154 | 70 | 14 | CAS | 80 | 36 | SO | 250 | 50 | MAL, SUC | 500 | 16 | READY | 2000 | X |
| Isocal HCN | Mead | 2 | 740 | 2.26 | 145 | 75 | 15 | CAS | 91 | 40 | SO, MCT | 225 | 45 | CSS | 400 | 18 | READY | 3000 | X |

\* American McGaw, Irvine, CA; B, Biosearch Medical Products, Somerville, NJ; Doyle Pharmaceutical Co, Minneapolis, MN; Mead Johnson & Co, Evansville, IN; Norwich-Eaton Pharmaceuticals, Norwich-NY; Ross Laboratories, Columbus, OH; Travenol Laboratories, Inc, Deerfield, IL.

† Institutional list prices, based on minimum reasonable order size and smallest reasonable package, standardized to 1000 kcal. Given for comparison; however, price may decrease as much as 50% when ordered in large quantities; some manufacturers lower prices in competitive bid more than others. Price charged to patient is generally higher than institutional price.

CAS, casein; VEG, vegetables; H LAC, hydrolyzed lactalbumin; AA, amino acids; H WHEY, hydrolyzed whey; D LAC, delactosed lactalbumin; CO, corn oil; SO, soy oil; M/D GLY, mono- and diglycerides; MCT, medium-chain triglycerides; SUN O, sunflower oil; SAF O, safflower oil; HCS, hydrolyzed corn starch; SUC, sucrose; CSS, corn syrup solids; MAL, maltodextrin; H CER S, hydrolyzed cereal solids; VEG, vegetables; GO, glucose oligosaccharides; MCS, modified corn starch; SP, soy polysaccharide (fiber); FRUC, fructose. X indicates studies have been done. Not all studies have been done (some done in-house by manufacturer), but all make some reference to adequate support of nutritional status by the product. Some products not designated by X may have been studied, but if references were not supplied to the authors by the manufacturer, they are not listed.

(Heimburger DC, Weinsler RL: Guidelines for evaluating and categorizing enteral feeding formulas according to therapeutic equivalence. JPEN 9:51–67; copyright © by American Society of Parenteral and Enteral Nutrition, 1985)

**TABLE 19-2. ENTERAL FEEDING EQUIPMENT—CONTAINERS (BAGS)**

| Trademark (Company) | Volume (ml) | Features |
| --- | --- | --- |
| Kangaroo bag (Chesebrough-Pond's) | 500, 1000, 1200 | Tubing attached to bag |
| Vivonix bag (Eaton Lab) | 1000 (?) | Tubing attached with screw clamp |
| Keofeed bag (Health Development Corp) | 500, 1500 | Tubing with liner-slip adaptor |
| Travenol (Travenol) | 1500 | Tubing optimal with universal port |
| Vitafeed (Pharmaseal) | 1200 | Universal port |
| Dobbhoff (Biosearch) | 1000 | Optimal tubing, universal port |
| Ethox-Barron (Ethox Corp) | 1000 | Tubing attached |
| Monitor (Corpak) | 1000 | Tubing not attached |

(Walker WA, Hendricks KM: Manual of Pediatric Nutrition. Philadelphia, WB Saunders, 1985)

**TABLE 19-3. INFUSION PUMPS DESIGNED FOR ENTERAL USE ONLY***

| Trademark | Company | PSI | Flow Rate ml/hr (Increments) | Features |
| --- | --- | --- | --- | --- |
| Kangaroo 200 | Chesebrough-Pond's | 12 | 5–295 (5 ml) | Alarms: low battery (3 hours battery life); rate change; occlusion/empty |
| Flexiflo I | Ross | 15 | 75–200 (25 ml) | No alarm; no battery; (for nonambulatory patients only) |
| Flexiflo II | Ross | 17.5 | 20–60 (20) 75–125 (25) 150–250 (50) | Alarms: empty, low battery, occlusion |
| Biosearch | Biosearch | 6 | 20–250 (10 ml) 125–250 (25 ml) 5–300 (5 ml) | Alarms: low battery (8 hours battery life); occlusion |
| Keofeed 500 (IVAC) | Hedeco | 15 | 1–400 (1 ml) | Alarms: occlusion/ empty; low battery (5 hours battery life); door open |
| Harvard Pump | Harvard Apparatus Company | | | None |
| Barron | Ethox | 28 | 21–140 (20 ml) | Alarms: rate change |
| VTR 300 | Corpale | 12 | 1–299 (1 ml) | Alarms: occlusion/ empty; low battery |

*Compiled by Nancy Hsu, MS, RD, Nutritional Support Unit, Massachusetts General Hospital, Boston, MA.
(Walker WA, Hendricks KM: Manual of Pediatric Nutrition. Philadelphia, WB Saunders, 1985)

## TABLE 19-4. ENTERAL FEEDING TUBES

| Company | Trademark | French Size | Length Inches (cm) | Material | Other Features |
|---|---|---|---|---|---|
| BioSearch Medical Products | Dobbhoff | 8 | 43 (109) | Radiopaque polyurethane with hydrometer | 7 g mercury weight; stainless-steel stylet |
| | Entriflex | 8 | 36 (91) | | 3 g mercury weight; stainless-steel stylet |
| | | 8 | 43 (109) | | |
| | | 8 | 20 (50) | | 3 g stainless-steel weight; nylon stylet |
| | | 6 | 20 (50) | | Nylon stylet |
| Health Development Corp | Keofeed | 5 | 20 (50) | Radiopaque silicone | 0.8 g mercury weight |
| | | 6 | 36 (90) | With Keolube | 3 g mercury weight; nylon stylet |
| | | 7.3 | 30 (75) | | Preassembled into the feeding tube |
| | | | 36 (90) | | |
| | | | 42 (105) | | |
| | | 9.6 | 36 (90) | | |
| | | | 42 (105) | | |
| | | 14.6 | 36 (90) | | |
| | | | 43 (105) | | |
| | | 18.0 | 36 (90) | | |
| | | | 43 (105) | | |
| | Surgifeed | 7.3 | 36 (90) | Silicone | Needle catheter; jejunostomy |
| Sherwood Medical | Duo-Tube | 5 | 40 (102) | Radiopaque silicone | 14 Fr silicone weight |
| | | | | | 15 Fr mercury weight |
| | | 6 | 40 (102) | | 15 Fr silicone weight |
| | | | | | 16 Fr mercury weight |
| | | 8 | 40 (102) | | 16 Fr silicone weight |
| | | | | | 17 Fr silicone weight |
| Health Care Group, Inc | Vitafeed | 5 | 15 (38) | Radiopaque silicone | No mercury weight |
| | | 6 | 42 (105) | | 3 g or 7 g mercury weight |
| | | 8 | 15 (38) | | No mercury weight |
| | | | 42 (105) | | 3 g or 7 g mercury weight |
| | | 10 | 42 (105) | | 3 g or 7 g mercury weight |
| | | 14* | 42 (105) | | 3 g mercury weight |

(Continued on next page)

**TABLE 19-4. ENTERAL FEEDING TUBES—CONTINUED**

| Company | Trademark | French Size | Length Inches (cm) | Material | Other Features |
|---|---|---|---|---|---|
| Norwich-Eaton Pharmaceuticals | Vivonex Jejunostomy Kit | 5 | 36 (90) | Radiopaque polyurethane | Needle catheter |
| Argyle* | Indurell | 5 | 20 | Polyurethane | |
| | | 5 | 36 | | |
| | | 8 | 42 | | |
| | Duotube | 5 | 40 | Silicone | Weighted tip |
| | | 6 | 40 | | |
| | | 8 | 40 | | |

*These tubes are not supplied with preassembled, stainless-steel stylets; all others are.
(Walker WA, Hendricks KM: Manual of Pediatric Nutrition. Philadelphia, WB Saunders, 1985)

In addition, there must be adequate dry storage space for these supplies. The development of home nutrition companies, which often provide weekly deliveries, has helped alleviate some of these storage problems.

Once at home the patient is seen weekly by the physician for the first month, biweekly for another month, and then monthly for the duration of the therapy if the patient is stable. At each visit, in addition to the physical examination and a history looking for any problems, medical, financial, or emotional, the following blood tests are performed: complete blood count, electrolytes, creatinine and blood urea nitrogen, calcium, phosphorus, total protein, albumin, prothrombin time, and liver function tests. Additional blood tests may also be performed periodically. These include Fe/TIBC, copper, zinc, folate, $B_{12}$ levels, urine oxalate, and citrate. These additional tests are particularly important in patients with significant malabsorption.

Complications with home enteral feeding are infrequent and usually minor when they occur (Table 19-5). The risk of aspiration pneumonia with nasogastric feeding was mentioned above. In order to avoid this potentially serious complication, the head of the bed should be raised approximately 30 degrees if the patient feeds while sleeping. Otherwise the patient should be sitting upright during the formula infusion. Also important in avoiding the complication of pneumonia due to aspiration is the checking for residual formula prior to infusing additional formula during the early observation period. This is done by using a large 60-ml syringe and aspirating the stomach contents prior to feeding, at the completion of feeding, and any time the patient feels bloated. If there is less than 100 ml of material, it should be returned and the feeding can be started. If there is more than 100 ml, only 100 ml should be returned and the infusion rate should be lowered for the next two hours when the residual volume is checked again. Finally, at the end of a feeding period the tube should be flushed with water to prevent its clogging with the formula, or if the tube is to be removed, it can be flushed after its removal. Although the most common complication of enteral feeding programs is having the tube fall out, other tube-related problems, though rare, include intestinal obstruction due to knotting of the tube, spillage of the mercury from the tube's bulb, intestinal perforation, and intussusception. Common but minor complications include nasal irritation, epistaxis, mucosal irritation, and sinusitis.

The cost of home enteral nutrition will depend on the amount and type of formula used, but it is obviously much less expensive than home parenteral nutrition or prolonged hospitalization. Excluding the "start-up" costs involved in purchasing the pump, the formula bags, the feeding tube, and other supplies, the cost of this therapy is approximately $700 to $1200/month.

As with enteral nutritional support, the patient who will eventually go home on parenteral nutritional support may or may not be completely stabilized with respect to weight and

**TABLE 19-5. COMPLICATIONS OF ENTERAL HYPERALIMENTATION
AND THEIR MANAGEMENT**

| Type of Complication | Frequency | Therapy |
|---|---|---|
| *Mechanical* | | |
| Tube lumen clogged by solution | Infrequent (<10%) | Flush with water; replace tube if unsuccessful |
| Pulmonary aspiration of stomach contents | Rare (<1%) | Unlikely with head of bed elevated; discontinue if aspiration occurs |
| Esophageal erosion | Rare (<1%) | Discontinue tube |
| *Gastrointestinal* | | |
| Vomiting and bloating | 10%–15% | Reduce flow rate and add peripheral hyperalimentation if needed |
| Diarrhea and cramping | 10%–20% | Reduce flow, dilute solution, consider different type solution, add antidiarrheal drug |
| *Metabolic, Fluid, and Electrolyte Abnormalities* | | |
| Hyperglycemia and glucosuria | 10%–15% | Reduce flow, administer insulin |
| Hyperosmolar coma | Rare (<1%) | Discontinue therapy |
| Edema | 20%–25% | Usually none; may reduce Na content or slow hyperalimentation rate; rarely use diuretics |
| Congestive heart failure | 1%–5% | Slow hyperalimentation, administer diuretics and digoxin |
| Hypernatremia, hypercalcemia | <5% | Adjust electrolyte content of hyperalimentation |
| Essential fatty acid deficiency | Common* | Linoleic acid supplement orally or Intralipid† intravenously |

* If enteral feeding mixture lacks linoleic acid.
† Cutter Laboratories, Berkeley, California.
(Heymsfield SB, Bethel RA, Ansley JD, et al: Enteral hyperalimentation: An alternative to central venous hyperalimentation. Ann Intern Med 90:63–71, 1979)

physiologic and metabolic status prior to discharge from the hospital. Hence, formulas may be, and often are, modified at home as the situation demands. Reviews are available detailing the technical aspects of determining the proper solution for a given patient.[9, 10] Table 19-6 outlines a standard parenteral formula. Of note is the need to add vitamins, trace elements, and fat to the amino acids and glucose to avoid a myriad of depletion syndromes that have been described in patients maintained on inadequate parenteral nutrition. Much of our understanding of the human requirements of trace elements, such as chromium or copper, and vitamins and fatty acids was derived from early experience with this therapeutic technique when the need for these substances was unknown. It has been through clinical studies as well as trial and error that we are now able to devise a program such as the one in Table 19-6.

Once the patient is clinically and metabolically stabilized on his solution, the infusion rate is gradually adjusted over several days such that the total period of infusion is 8 to 12

**TABLE 19-6. ADULT TPN SOLUTION (PER 1000 ML)**

| | |
|---|---|
| Amino acids | 42.5 g |
| Dextrose | 250 g |
| Na | 35 mEq |
| K | 33 mEq |
| Mg | 8 mEq |
| Acetate | 71 mEq |
| Chloride | 49 mEq |
| $PO_4$ | 15 mM |
| Multivitamins (MVI 12) | 4 ml |
| Trace elements | 1 ml |
| Total Kcal | 1020 ml |
| Carbohydrate Kcal | 850 ml |
| Nitrogen Kcal | 170 ml |
| Lipid 20%* | 200 ml |

*Lipid may be added daily to increase delivery of calories or may be given three times a week to avoid essential fatty acid deficiency.

hours. During this period critical factors to follow are the patient's ability to tolerate the fluid, fat, and amino acid loads infused. This is especially true for the diabetic patient who is often intolerant of the large glucose loads involved in parenteral nutrition. The initiation of TPN in a diabetic should be done under the direction of the physician–nutritionist. In brief, a fraction of the patient's insulin requirements is given as regular insulin in the TPN solution. Frequent blood glucose determinations are needed to assess the need for additional subcutaneous insulin, which is then added to subsequent solutions. During this time of adjustment, the patient will be instructed in the care of his indwelling catheter, the preparation of his formula (if necessary), and the operation of his infusion pump.

By far the most common and most serious complications related to home parenteral nutrition are related to the indwelling catheter. A great deal of time must be spent teaching the patient the principles of aseptic technique. Areas to be covered by the training nurse include how to change dressings, how to cleanse the skin, and even how to bathe and swim. Localized skin infections and, more important, bacterial sepsis are the most common complications with this therapy, and a patient (or family) unable or unwilling to follow minimal but essential procedures will not be a candidate for this treatment modality without competent support by someone else.

Another complication with this technique is clotting of the catheter and, less commonly, of the vein into which it is inserted. This can be avoided with the use of heparin after each infusion period. Though various regimens exist, the patient is instructed in the use of a heparin lock so that approximately 1 ml to 2 ml of 10 to 100 unit/ml heparin is injected into the catheter prior to capping it off. Other catheter complications include the inadvertent cutting of the proximal end of the catheter, as well as the catheter becoming dislodged or leaking.

The multitude of metabolic complications that can occur during parenteral nutrition, as listed in Table 19-7, are fortunately rare in home patients once they have been stabilized as hospital inpatients. However, a critical metabolic problem that the primary physician may be called upon to evaluate is glycosuria. If urine testing consistently reveals glycosuria, a 24-hour urine collection for total glucose together with serum glucose levels should be performed during the solution's infusion. If the serum value is greater than 200 mg/dl, regular insulin in a dose of 1 unit per 100 carbohydrate calories can be added to the solution.

## TABLE 19-7. SUMMARY OF PHYSIOLOGIC COMPLICATIONS THAT MAY OCCUR AS THE RESULT OF TOTAL PARENTERAL NUTRITION

| Complication | Probable Cause |
|---|---|
| 1. Hyperglycemia with glycosuria, osmotic diuresis, and dehydration | Diabetes with inadequate insulin coverage; large or rapid glucose infusion prior to adaptation—especially in elderly, septic, or stressed patients |
| 2. Hyperosmolar nonketotic coma | Large or rapid glucose infusion in patients with or without diabetes who are septic and dehydrated with consequent increased insulin needs. |
| 3. Hypernatremia | Inadequate water intake in relation to sodium intake, particularly in face of large fluid losses |
| 4. Hyponatremia | Impaired ability to excrete sodium and water; increased ADH with hypervolemia associated with excessive water administration |
| 5. Hypokalemia | Insufficient potassium intake associated with protein anabolism; metabolic alkalosis |
| 6. Hyperkalemia | Excessive potassium intake especially in presence of renal dysfunction |
| 7. Hypocalcemia | Calcium deficiency in infants; magnesium deficiency ($Ca^+$ related to albumin level) |
| 8. Hypercalcemia | Excessive calcium intake with immobility |
| 9. Hypophosphatemia | Insufficient inorganic phosphate intake, especially when initiating large glucose infusions in malnourished individuals |
| 10. Hypoglycemia | Sudden cessation of infusion |
| 11. Congestive failure | Excessively rapid infusion |
| 12. Hypomagnesemia | Inadequate intake of magnesium |
| 13. Anemia | Failure to replace blood loss; iron deficiency, folic acid and $B_{12}$ deficiency; copper deficiency |
| 14. Increased SGOT and alkaline phosphatase; hepatomegaly | ? Hepatotoxicity due to amino acid imbalance; excessive glycogen or fat deposition in liver |
| 15. Bleeding | Deficiency of vitamin K |
| 16. Demineralization of bone | Inadequate calcium, inorganic phosphate or vitamin D intake; prolonged bedrest |
| 17. Hypervitaminosis A and D | Excessive administration of vitamin mixture |
| 18. Azotemia | Excessive administration of amino acids, particularly in presence of renal dysfunction |

(Adapted from Shils ME: A program for total parenteral nutrition in the home. Am J Clin Nutr 28:1429–1435, 1975)

The most serious and frequent problem that the primary physician will be called upon to evaluate is fever. If a source for the patient's fever not related to the catheter is obvious and is deemed to be of bacterial origin (*e.g.,* cystitis), it should of course be treated and the catheter need not be removed. Even in this instance, blood cultures should be obtained in addition to urine cultures, chest x-ray, and a complete blood count with differential because the discovery of a source of infection does not necessarily mean that the central venous catheter is not colonized. Blood cultures should be obtained both through the catheter and from another peripheral vein. Blood cultures should include cultures for aerobes, anaerobes, and fungi. If the infusion associated with the fever is still available, a sample should be taken and sent for culture since a grossly contaminated solution can cause fevers.

If no obvious source can be found and the patient's fever is $> 102°F$, a microbial cause should be suspected. The subclavian or jugular central catheter should be changed over a sterile guidewire, the removed catheter tip cultured, and the patient started on antibiotics. If all blood and catheter-tip cultures are negative at 48 hours, the antibiotics can be stopped. However, if the blood cultures are positive, the appropriate antibiotics are continued for a full treatment course. It is absolutely essential that the patient or the family be given detailed, written instructions for dealing with a fever and when to notify the doctor. If blood cultures are positive for *Candida,* the central venous catheter must be removed over a sterile guidewire and changed daily. If blood cultures become negative and remain so for 7 days, no further treatment is necessary. If blood cultures remain positive and if the patient is immunocompromised, a course of intravenous antifungal therapy is necessary. Pollack examined the complications related to indwelling catheters in 100 patient-years of home parenteral nutrition in 198 patients.[11] Out of 369 episodes of fever, 20% remained culture negative and resolved without specific therapy. However, 13% (37 episodes) of the fevers were related to the catheter, with 9% of the episodes being documented bacteremias and the remaining due to local cellulitis at the insertion site. Cellulitis can be treated with local and systemic antibiotics without removal of the catheter. Despite the potential seriousness of these problems, it should be realized that it is often possible for a single catheter to remain in place for over a year without complications.

Fluid, electrolytes, and various nutrients may have to be modified as the patient's clinical state dictates. The most common reason for rehospitalization in these patients is the primary disease, with the second most common reason being the catheter complications mentioned above.[12] This means that patients who would otherwise spend a large percentage of their time in the hospital are now able to spend that time at home. Steiger compared the hospitalization rates of patients with similar diseases with and without home nutritional support and found that home nutritional support greatly reduced the total amount of time spent in the hospital by these patients.[13]

Two technical aspects of parenteral nutrition that were mentioned briefly above require more explanation. First is the issue of solution preparation. The necessity of accurate and aseptic preparation cannot be overemphasized. Who should prepare the formula and where it should be mixed are the questions that need to be addressed. Standard solutions that are suitable for most patients are commercially available. However, vitamins, electrolytes, and trace elements often need to be added to these solutions, and each addition theoretically increases the risk of bacterial contamination.

The patient or a family member should master the methods of aseptic technique and learn how to insert the relatively few additives to the solution safely. If this is not possible, then a decision must be made to have help come into the home to prepare the solutions or whether the solutions should be prepared outside the home by a nutrition company and then delivered to the patient.

When ending a parenteral feeding session, the solution cannot be terminated abruptly or else the patient is at risk of developing severe hypoglycemia when the concentrated glucose solution is stopped. Therefore, when an infusion is to be stopped for any reason it should be tapered off in the following way. With 30 minutes remaining in the feeding period the infusion rate should be decreased by 50%. After 15 minutes the rate should again be halved, and then after an additional 15 minutes the infusion can be safely stopped in most patients. However, each patient should be checked regarding his tolerance to this protocol and instructed in the symptoms of hypoglycemia prior to discharge.

Home parenteral nutrition is not inexpensive, although it costs much less than a hospital stay of the same duration. Costs will vary depending on the exact type and amount of formula a patient requires daily, the need for a visiting nurse, and the need for close and continuing medical and other support at home. Start-up costs for this treatment include the infusion pump, catheter filters, dressings, heparin, needles, and syringes. Maintenance costs depend on the formula and, more importantly, on who mixes the formula. These costs can range between $50 to $200/day. These costs, as well as the entire process of home parenteral nutrition, should be thoroughly explained and studied when the decision to institute home care is first entertained.

Malnutrition is not a necessary complication of any disease and should not be an expected one. Depending on the long-term goals of the patient, family, and physician, any patient is a candidate for specialized nutritional support. Because of closer governmental scrutiny of hospital costs, it is no longer practical to provide the long-term nutritional support that many patients require in a hospital setting. Fortunately, the technology now exists that enables this therapy to be delivered at home. Because the early metabolic complications that can be associated with any form of intensive nutritional support program are managed in the hospital prior to discharge, home nutritional therapy is remarkably free of acute medical problems. When this is considered in conjunction with the significant improvements in quality of life gained by allowing the patient to remain at home while maintaining a normal nutritional status, home nutritional support should become a mainstay in the care of chronically ill patients.

## REFERENCES

1. Butterworth CE: The skeleton in the hospital closet. Nutrition Today March/April:4–8, 1974
2. Weinsier RL, Hunker EM, Krumdieck CL, et al: A prospective evaluation of general medical patients during the course of hospitalization. Am J Clin Nutr 32:418–426, 1979
3. Rombeau JL, Barot LR, Williamson CE, et al: Preoperative total parenteral nutrition and surgical outcome in patients with inflammatory bowel disease. Am J Surg 143:139–143, 1982
4. Mullen JL, Buzby GP, Matthews DC, et al: Reduction of operative morbidity and mortality by combined preoperative and postoperative nutritional support. Ann Surg 192:604–613, 1981
5. Shils ME: A program for total parenteral nutrition in the home. Am J Clin Nutr 28:1429–1435, 1975
6. Rabinovitch AE: Home total parenteral nutrition: A psycho-social viewpoint. JPEN 5:522–525, 1981
7. Chernoff RI: Enteral formulas. Nutritional support: Formulas and delivery of enteral feeding. J Am Diet Assoc 79:426–429, 1981
8. Gordon AM: Enteral nutritional support guidelines for feeding product selection. Postgrad Med 71:72–82, 1982
9. Shils ME: Principle of nutritional therapy. Cancer 43:2093–2102, 1979
10. Lokey H, Hitt D, McMahon JJ: A hyperalimentation manual for the small hospital. Surg Clin North Am 59:411–440, 1979
11. Pollack PF, Kadden M, Byrne WJ, et al: 100 patient years' experience with the Broviac silastic catheter for central venous nutrition. JPEN 5:32–36, 1981
12. Byrne WJ, Ament ME, Burke M, et al: Home parenteral nutrition. Surgery, Gynecology and Obstetrics 149:593–599, 1979
13. Steiger E: Morbidity and mortality related to home parenteral nutrition in patients with gut failure. Am J Surg 145:102–105, 1983

# 20

# Cancer Care

DIANE S. BLUM
RONALD H. BLUM

Earlier diagnosis of cancer, longer survival of cancer patients, and changing policies in health-care reimbursement are leading to the home becoming the primary arena for the treatment of the cancer patient. The cancer patient receiving care at home, regardless of diagnosis, must be more informed, more independent, and more aware of community resources than the hospitalized patient. However, patients and families enter the diagnosis of cancer with varying coping abilities and widely different resources for support, and they differ in their abilities to incorporate and apply information appropriately. The attitude and support of the physician are of crucial significance in helping each patient and family deal with the home care situation. The physician who as "captain of the ship" assesses the patient's physical and psychosocial needs and strengths, anticipates the patient's and family's problems at home, and calls on the services of other professionals, optimizes the possibility of the patient coping at home. This chapter will present specific assessments and interventions that the physician can use toward effective home care for the cancer patient. Psychosocial assessments and interventions at various stages will be described first, and then the diagnosis and treatment of the symptoms of cancer by organ system will be discussed.

## THE VALUE OF PSYCHOSOCIAL ASSESSMENT AND INTERVENTION IN HOME CARE

Psychosocial assessment and intervention by the physician have direct benefits for the patient at home, as well as for his or her family, at any stage of cancer. Among other things, patients are allowed to express their concerns about survival, pain, loss of self-esteem, and increasing dependence that affects the equilibrium of the family. Patients also express concern as to what they will derive from the health-care system, specifically the technical quality of care, the degree of continuity of care, the financial burden, and the resources of the system for support for them while at home. The opportunity to express these concerns directly to the physician allows the patient a greater degree of participation, control, and improved self-esteem, all of which enhance the possibility of successful home care.[1]

   The physician derives benefit from increased attention to psychosocial issues as well. By developing the psychosocial database, the physician can make certain predictions about the patient and family that have a direct impact on treatment planning. The physician can look at their competence, potential compliance, resources, and coping styles, and can work with the patient and family to develop a realistic approach to treatment.[2] A treatment plan that will be feasible for the patient and family directly benefits the physician in that the patient and family will be able to function more independently and cope effectively at home.

Psychosocial assessment allows the physician to look at the patient's and family's capabilities realistically so the physician will not set unrealistic goals for himself or herself.[3,4] Stress on the physician is further reduced by early identification of the need for referral to other health-care professionals.[5,6] This is particularly important if the patient has limited resources for support at home. Nurses, social workers, liaison psychiatrists, clergy, rehabilitation specialists, and nutritionists have all developed expertise in the psychosocial treatment of cancer patients. Early referral to other members of the health-care team facilitates the development of relationships with the patient and family that will ease adjustment during the illness, and enables the physician to share the significant responsibility of caring for his or her patients in the home setting.

## STAGE-SPECIFIC ISSUES FOR HOME CARE

The role of the physician changes at each stage of cancer. At different points in the illness, the physician may need to play a greater or lesser role as diagnostician, treater, educator, and source of psychosocial support, and share in the responsibility for both medical and psychosocial decisions. The physician should be willing to assume these various roles and be receptive to the varying expectations of patients and families at the different points in the illness. At each stage, specific interventions on the part of the physician can facilitate the patient's adjustment at home.

## THE INITIAL INTERVIEW

The first meeting may be at the time of the initial symptoms and the diagnosis of cancer, at the point of presentation of metastatic disease, or at the terminal stage. In the context of today's health-care environment, it is clear that even if the patient is hospitalized at the time of the first meeting, the significant physician–patient contact will take place while the patient is living at home. The physician's assessment should begin with the development of a psychosocial database of demographic information, including age, marital status, occupation, and address. The address is particularly important because it has a bearing on the logistics of treatment and also provides initial socioeconomic data. Insurance information is also useful in defining patient resources for the patient functioning at home. Prior to seeing the patient, the physician should use the resources of the referring physician, the chart, and other members of the health-care team in order to learn from previous experience with the patient and family.

A psychosocial history should be part of the initial assessment. This history should include the description of the family constellation, with identification of individual roles and responsibilities, a history of coping methods used in prior crises, and identification of the patient's and family's major concerns. Such questions as "Who is helpful to you when you are upset?" "How do you usually deal with problems?" and "What is your primary concern now?" supply information that is useful to the physician in anticipating the needs of the patient at home.[7] It may become apparent with this initial contact that child care, housekeeping, transportation, or financial needs must be addressed if the patient is to have the recommended treatment.

Referral to other members of the health-care team, such as the social worker, may facilitate a solution to problems such as transportation or may indicate that outside resources are necessary. Often, addressing these issues directly with the patient and family results in the development of a plan based on shared family responsibility. However, the patient and family may be so overwhelmed by the new medical status that they need the direction of an outside person to mobilize their existing resources.

It is useful during the first interview for the physician to ask the patient what his or her understanding is of the diagnosis.[8,9] This allows the patient to use the vocabulary that is most comfortable and enables the physician to determine the patient's perceptions of what is happening. The physician is also able to assess the degree of denial and determine the potential receptivity of the patient to new information. The different aspects of this psychosocial history, which are geared to improving communication between the physician and patient and family and developing a common language, are crucial in building the confidence that will enable the patient to deal with treatment at home.

With the initial diagnosis of cancer, the physician should facilitate the incorporation of the implications of the diagnosis for both the patient and family. The physician should be the educator, imparting an adequate knowledge base about the cancer and the treatment plan, emphasizing the potential benefits and risks balanced between the hope and the reality. Often at this time the families of cancer patients are receptive to issues of cancer prevention. Smoking reduction, breast self-examination, and review of the early warning signs are useful interventions for the family. Also, reassurance should be given that the patient's cancer is not contagious or, when appropriate, not inheritable.

## COMPLETION OF TREATMENT

Another significant point for the patient at home is the completion of treatment. The patient who has been at home for his or her course of treatment has maintained frequent contacts with the physician and the health-care system. Now the patient is expected to move completely back into the world of home, family, friends, and work. The physician must assess the dependency of the patient on the health-care system and determine how much anxiety the patient experiences at a time of withdrawal of medical support.[10] Concern about future symptoms and how to deal with them is of prime importance to patient and families. The physician must clearly define the time table of future medical contacts and reassure the patient that future symptoms will be addressed in a diagnostic way to determine what symptoms are potentially disease-related. The physician has the important role of providing technical information and support on an ongoing basis. In general, the physician should alert patients to early signs of recurrence, such as a fall in functional status, unintentional weight loss, pain, lump or bump, or loss of function, yet be reassuring that not every sign or symptom is a recurrence. The physician also needs a balanced perspective between the patient's lower threshold for seeking medical attention and the reality of the higher probability of developing medically important symptoms.

The physician must look for the reemergence of preexisting problems in the family or work place that have been put aside during the course of treatment. Family conflict, job dissatisfaction, and financial demands are examples.

### CASE STUDY

Mrs. S is a 45-year-old administrative assistant treated for 6 months for lymphoma. During chemotherapy she had been at home, worked part time, and had coped well. At the completion of treatment, Mrs. S became depressed. Discussion between Mrs. S and her physician about her shift in mood revealed that she had been dissatisfied with her job prior to becoming ill and that the treatment was in some ways a reprieve from having to make a decision about a job change. Mrs. S recognized that the diagnosis and treatment had altered her priorities, but she was overwhelmed at the prospect of making a change in job. She had survived her cancer, but was again faced with problems that she had thought would be unimportant in the context of having had this disease.

Referral for mental health intervention for this patient was appropriate at this time as Mrs. S now had the motivation to deal with preexisting psychological and social problems and the energy to move on to areas beyond the diagnosis of cancer.

This is a time at which problems in the mastery of normal developmental tasks occur. Life transitions such as career choices, marriage, and parenting are all affected by the fact of a cancer diagnosis, regardless of the status of cure. Job discrimination, denial of insurance, difficulty in social relationships, and barriers in educational endeavors are all realities that those cured of cancer face.[11,12] The physician should assess the significance of these common issues and help the patient anticipate potential obstacles. There are several possible interventions by the physician at this time. First, the physician can counter stereotyping of the cancer patient by supplying medical data to employers, insurers, and schools. Second, physicians should refer to those (such as vocational counselors and support groups) who can advocate for and assist the former cancer patient.

Reassessment of the physiologic and psychological effect of organ damage secondary to treatment is also necessary. Although these issues should be clearly discussed as treatment begins, they must be reviewed at treatment completion. The patient's and family's attention is shifted to the future away from the crisis of treatment. The long-term sequelae of the cancer and its treatment are now primary issues. As an example, the impact of treatment on sexual functioning must be readdressed and specialty referrals considered.[13,14]

Finally, the physician's intervention should focus on reinforcement of the patient's self-esteem and sense of mastery that treatment has been completed. Recognition of the patient's accomplishment includes acknowledgment of tolerance to the toxicity of treatment in order to achieve the therapeutic gain and the ability to cope with the treatment-induced life disruptions. Patients frequently express anxiety at the prospect of resuming normal life. Reassurance that this response is predictable and expected assists them in making the transition from their patient role to their premorbid role. These interventions by the physician at this time can help the patient to once again become an independent member of a family and community system.

## TERMINAL ILLNESS

Hopefully, the cancer patient remains free of disease and is not "the patient at home" but a person living in his or her normal environment. However, the natural course of the illness dictates that many cancer patients will have advancing disease and move into the stage of the illness called the *terminal phase*. At this point, the primary goal of treatment is symptomatic care rather than control or reduction of the underlying cancer. A consistent question is "Where can this patient best be cared for?" The answer, more and more frequently, is at home, because of hospital reimbursement policies, the influence of the hospice movement, and the availability of home care supports that can simulate a hospital environment.

The physician must define his or her own commitment and the patient's and family's commitment to home care. Are these adequate resources? What are the expected morbidities of the consequences of cancer and cancer treatment? The physician must assess the medical needs of the patient. Those factors to evaluate include pain control, nutritional concerns, need for respiratory care or wound care, and the patient's dependence on assistance for the activities of daily living. All these symptoms will be discussed in detail in the following section. Once the patient's medical needs are determined, the psychosocial characteristics and resources of the patient and family must be considered. The physician must assess the coping ability, particularly whether the patient and family can adapt to the patient dying at home. The physician often has to make this assessment in the context of an extremely ill patient who is dependent on the continuity of the health-care system, but whose inpatient terminal care plan is restricted by reimbursement guidelines.[15]

The physician must rely on the expertise of nursing, social work, and rehabilitation to determine the needs and resources for terminal care of the individual patient. Insurance coverage, resources in the local community such as hospice programs, physical set-up of the home, and the availability and motivation of family and friends as care partners are among the issues that must be evaluated. These other members of the health-care team assess individual needs and can work with the patient and family to develop a "package" of services that will enable the patient to remain at home. These include insurance-covered services for skilled nursing care, or home health-aide care, which perhaps can be afforded by the family or partially subsidized by community agencies. There is no limitation at this time to equipment available for the home, and the home, provided there is space, can offer most of the supports of the hospital.

These supports, particularly assistive devices, can encourage the terminally ill patient to participate in his or her own care. Maintaining the patient's energy and input into care can reinforce a sense of control and also sustain the patient's emotional connection with those who are close.[16, 17] For the patient living alone, volunteers can be recruited from a variety of programs to allow the patient some social link and also to decrease the number of hours a paid care giver is needed.

Education is a key service to both patient and family, focused on what the dying patient needs, how to talk with the dying patient, and how to anticipate what the actual death will be like. This information is available most importantly from the physician, who needs to communicate the anticipated symptoms prior to death and to deal with the predictable fears of emergencies. Management of these symptoms will be discussed in the next section. Widely available brochures, community-based workshops, and home visits by nurses or social workers can reinforce this information.

The family or friends who are caring for the patient at home need support and attention. Family members may experience physical and emotional exhaustion at the end of a long illness, be financially pressured, and be desperate for some normality in their lives.[18] The patient who is feeling dependent and helpless may become angry or express despair and a desire to die. This can predictably undermine the primary care partner, who may feel that he or she is not doing all that can be done. The physician who anticipates these expressions of guilt and self-doubt can ensure that the family members and care partners receive the support they require. The physician must emphasize the reality of the situation: "We are doing all we can." The guilt and anger can usually be reduced by bringing patients and family to the realization that in fact the best that can be done is to provide basic attempts at symptom control. The social worker or clergy can work with the care partners to recognize their efforts and determination. Volunteers, as mentioned earlier, can be used to give respite to the care partners, who often feel guilty about leaving the home. Paid help may be necessary, even if for short periods of time, to spell the care partner, particularly at night. The social worker can also help to organize a schedule for family members to share responsibilities. When there are young children or adolescents in the home, the physician should anticipate their needs, discuss with the well parent the importance of including children emotionally and intellectually, and refer to a mental health professional when indicated.[19]

The physician can help by predicting the time of death. This has a real value for the logistics of planning for the family. As an example, if relatives are to be called from out of town, the timing is important and can reduce the stress of the situation. The physician must also provide information in order to anticipate the sequence of events at the time of death. Important issues of how to contact the funeral directors, the completion of the death certificate, return of equipment, and probate should be discussed with the family at the appropriate time.

The issue of bereavement after the death of the patient is, unfortunately, very under-serviced. For the patient's primary physician the point of death usually marks the completion of the relationship. Reimbursement for professional services during the period of bereavement is not covered by the primary patient's insurance. In the setting of primary care by someone other than the family practitioner, the role of the physician is to be prepared to triage appropriate families to professional intervention. This issue is of much less concern for the family practitioner whose role as the primary physician for the family is maintained by offering bereavement counseling.

## SYMPTOM CONTROL

The home setting for the terminally ill patient can offer physical comfort, maintenance of the family unit, and familiarity and autonomy for the dying person. However, the home care situation works well only when the cancer patient's symptoms are able to be assessed and managed. For the patient at home the physician is responsible for symptom control, enlisting and directing support from other members of the health-care team, and providing guidance as to the realistic goals and outcome. The following section will discuss the symptoms of cancer by organ system with attention to what can realistically be accomplished in the home.

## PULMONARY

Pulmonary problems that arise in the cancer patient at home can be classified into four general categories: (1) progressive pulmonary involvement with cancer, (2) infection, (3) aspiration, and (4) pleural effusions.

Progressive pulmonary involvement can be due to either pulmonary parenchymal disease or endobronchial or lymphangitic involvement of the lungs. Presenting signs and symptoms of parenchymal involvement can be chest pain, particularly pleuritic chest pain, or increasing shortness of breath manifested by decrease in exertional tolerance and pneumonia. A plain chest x-ray film clearly offers the best single diagnostic tool; however, the clinical setting can help differentiate progressive pulmonary involvement from other etiologies that cause a similar symptom complex. As an example, progressive parenchymal involvement with cancer is generally a subacute process that evolves over weeks or months. If there is more rapid evolution of the symptomatology, then consideration should be given to other etiologies. Further diagnostic work-up for parenchymal involvement is only indicated if there are treatment options available for not only the pulmonary disease, but also the metastatic disease involvement.

Progressive endobronchial involvement with cancer can take the form of either postobstructive pneumonia or hemoptysis. In addition to primary bronchogenic carcinoma, a number of other cancers such as breast, melanoma, and renal cell seem to have a predilection to endobronchial spread. If there is clinical suspicion of postobstructive pneumonia, corroborating data can be obtained from physical examination and, when indicated, x-ray and bronchoscopy. The initial management in the home could consist of an empiric trial of antibiotics. Depending on the overall clinical setting, consideration should be given to palliative radiation therapy. If the patient has an estimated survival in excess of several months and if the postobstructive pneumonia is limiting, then strong consideration should be given to palliative radiation. If symptomatic shortness of breath is a clinical symptom, consideration should be given to home oxygen therapy.

Hemoptysis due to endobronchial involvement must be differentiated from hemoptysis from other sites. If the blood is mixed with sputum and appears to be darker in color, in all probability this represents an endobronchial source. The additional management should include cough suppression with a codeine-based compound. Oxycodone and acetaminophen compound is often a very effective choice. Alternatively, terpin hydrate with codeine might be considered. Superinfection is a significant problem. Recommendation could be made for a broad-spectrum antibiotic such as tetracycline or erythromycin. Another consideration is triage for palliative radiation therapy. In general, radiotherapy is very effective if the endobronchial source can be identified by bronchoscopy. The triage decision for radiotherapy must be based on the overall clinical setting. It is also important for the physician to educate the patient and family about the possibility of massive hemoptysis and the dire clinical implications.

Lymphangitic spread is often manifested by progressive shortness of breath and cough evolving over weeks to months. Exacerbating problems could be superimposed pneumonia or endobronchial progression. Symptomatic treatment should include oxygen therapy, and if there is a component of superinfection, a trial of antibiotics. If available, alternative systemic therapy should be considered. In addition, patients may be provided with significant symptomatic relief by home oxygen.

Primary pulmonary infection is a common clinical problem for the cancer patient at home. In the initial presentation the rate of development has triage implications. If the patient has relatively acute onset of signs and symptoms of pneumonia, then, depending on the clinical setting, consideration should be given to more aggressive intravenous antibiotics. If, on the other hand, there is a subacute evolution of the pulmonary process, then a more empiric choice of oral antibiotics should be considered. It is important to emphasize that bronchial pneumonia is often the final event for the patient with far-advanced cancer. In many settings it may be a welcomed natural death. The patient should receive symptomatic treatment with oxygen therapy, antibiotics if appropriate, sedation, and an attempt to maximize pulmonary toilet with the home team being trained in chest physical therapy and nasotracheal suctioning.

Aspiration may be caused by an impaired gag reflex, tracheoesophageal fistula, or excessive vomiting. Symptoms are usually progressive cough, shortness of breath, and occasionally chest pain. Management of aspiration includes careful attention to the position and level of alertness while taking substances by mouth. Consideration should be given to the availability of a suction machine to remove retained material from the aerodigestive tract. As an alternative, tube feeding should be considered. The treatment of a superimposed aspiration pneumonia may include the empiric use of steroids or antibiotics if superinfection is considered.

Pleural effusions are common manifestations of either progressive disease or infection. Depending on the clinical setting, intervention may well be appropriate. If a patient has progressive shortness of breath in the presence of a pleural effusion, strong consideration should be given to thoracentesis. In clinical practice, it is important to remember that large pleural effusions due to malignancy can often be readily tapped even in the home. If a survival in excess of three months is anticipated, strong consideration should be given to chest tube drainage and pleuradysis. Although there is no definitive literature, in general the preferred approach is either therapeutic thoracentesis for the patient with very advanced disease or alternatively an attempt at definitive pleural control with chest tube drainage and instillation of a sclerosing agent.

# CARDIAC

Cardiac symptoms that may be related to the cancer or cancer treatment include myopathy, pericardial effusions, and arrhythmias. The differential diagnosis of cardiomyopathy includes the cardiac toxicity of the anthracycline antibiotics, infectious cardiomyopathy, particularly viral, and radiation cardiomyopathy, which typically occurs 4 to 8 months after direct heart or mediastinal radiation. In addition to physical examination, the diagnosis of cardiomyopathy is supported by a gated-pool cardiac scan determination of ejection fraction. The necessity of diagnostic procedures must be weighed against the clinical realities. As an alternative for the patient at home, empiric treatment can be initiated in a standard manner including the use of diuretics, inotropic drugs, and salt and water restriction.

Malignant pericardial effusion is an important diagnostic consideration. These signs and symptoms are often very subtle and nonspecific and are difficult to distinguish from those of the systemic manifestations of progressive cancer. The main symptomatic manifestations of pericardial effusions are caused by a decrease in cardiac output resulting from the restrictive pericardial process. As an example, postural hypotension and dyspnea on exertion reflect this decreased ability to mount an increase in cardiac output. Pericardial effusions occur most commonly in those cancers that have major mediastinal involvement. The pathophysiology is by retrograde lymphatic flow of tumor cells into the pericardial tissue. The typical pathologic picture is one of a thickened pericardium causing tamponade. In contrast to more acute pericarditis, malignant pericardial disease is usually associated with small amounts of pericardial fluid. If pericardial tamponade is being considered, then an echocardiogram can determine the amount of pericardial fluid as well as the degree of restriction of wall motion. If there is a physiologically significant amount of fluid, consideration should be given to pericardial tap, which can result in dramatic symptomatic improvement. The same laboratory parameters used for pleural effusions can be applied to the diagnostic work-up of a pericardial effusion. The main treatment intervention for malignant pericardial effusions is drainage of fluid, but also there are anecdotal reports of the value of sclerosing agents in preventing recurrence. It is important to emphasize that with minimal removal of fluid, there can be major improvement in cardiac output. Pericardial tamponade must be considered as a diagnostic entity because of the palliative benefit of pericardial drainage.

The management of cardiac arrhythmias (in malignant pericardial disease) can be either directed toward the underlying heart disease or toward direct pericardial involvement by the tumor. Tachyarrhythmias are more common than bradyarrhythmias. Symptoms may include palpitations, syncope or near-syncope, and exertional intolerance. The diagnosis of arrhythmias may be made by standard physical examination assessments, or electrocardiogram, or may require Holter monitoring. The treatment may just be reassurance if the arrhythmias are incidental or are causing only minimal symptoms. Alternatively, drug intervention with antiarrhythmics may provide greater patient benefit.

# GASTROINTESTINAL

In discussing gastrointestinal complications, an anatomical approach can be used. One important cause of reversible esophageal dysfunction is infectious esophagitis secondary to candida or viral infiltration. Dysphagia may also be caused by external compression of the esophagus leading to mechanical obstruction. Radiation esophagitis is usually self-limited. Consideration must also be given to obstruction by a foreign body. Xerostomia and psychogenic-induced dysphagia may mimic these primary esophageal disorders.

The management of esophageal disorders includes the empiric use of antibiotics, adjustments in the texture of the oral intake, and, under specific circumstances, the use of endoscopy for diagnosis, removal of foreign bodies, and mechanical dilatation.

Gastric disorders to be considered include gastric outlet obstruction, due either to mechanical obstruction by tumor or by inflammation secondary to peptic ulcer disease. Chemotherapy and corticosteroids can exacerbate these gastric problems. Intervention includes treatment with antacids as well as H2 blockers.

An intestinal symptom that must be considered is bowel obstruction. Patients may initially complain of a change in bowel habits that cannot be explained by change in diet or medication, abdominal pain, and nausea or vomiting. Of particular concern is large volume vomiting, which suggests small bowel obstruction. Although surgery could be considered when there is a definable level of obstruction, surgery will in all probability not be of significant benefit in, as an example, ovarian cancer, given the diffuse nature of the peritoneal involvement. As alternatives to surgical intervention, palliative maneuvers that are of benefit include drug management with antiemetics, metoclopramide, antispasmodics, and maintenance of stool bulk. The relative palliation from the maintenance of oral intake versus nasogastric suction must be considered. Often it is the patient who can best judge the relative level of comfort of maintaining oral intake with persistent vomiting versus continuous or intermittent nasogastric suctioning.

Primary hepatic disorders that should be considered include the management of jaundice and hepatic capsular pain. In the jaundiced patient, the major distinction is between reversible jaundice secondary to extrahepatic versus intrahepatic involvement, which may require ultrasound assessment. Biliary drainage is of major palliative benefit for those patients with extrahepatic involvement. On the other hand, hepatic failure and coma may be a comfortable way to die. Symptom control includes the standard management of hepatic coma and the management of the pruritus with antihistamine lotions and cholestyramine. For the hepatic capsular pain due to the expanding hepatic tumor, consideration should be given to analgesics as well as palliative radiation.

The issues of ostomy care in this patient population are discussed in Chapter 14.

## GENITOURINARY

The relevant issues for treatment of genitourinary problems in the home can be divided into renal failure, urinary incontinence, and hematuria. As a differential diagnostic point, uremia should be considered in patients who have increased generalized weakness. In considering renal failure the reversibility is determined to various extents by defining the underlying etiology. In the home, prerenal azotemia is probably the most common cause of uremia. This is often associated with volume depletion. In the home setting, dehydration is most likely. Obviously, by rehydrating the patient, symptoms of renal failure may well be improved. Primary renal failure can be an accumulating effect of the nephrotoxicity of certain drugs such as antibiotics or cisplatin chemotherapy, or can occur in the more acute setting of acute tubular necrosis. There is no specific treatment for these causes of renal failure other than supportive care.

For postobstructive renal failure, major therapeutic and palliative benefit is achievable by urinary diversion; therefore, diagnostic intervention is often indicated. Postrenal obstruction generally occurs in the setting of primary pelvic tumors and those diseases that are prone to retroperitoneal spread. The mechanical obstruction and resulting postobstructive uropathy are best diagnosed by renal ultrasound. This is a noninvasive and highly reliable test. The palliative benefit is significant. If there is retroperitoneal obstruction then urinary diversion may offer dramatic symptomatic improvement. The method of urinary diversion depends on, among other things, the anatomical location of the obstruction. The urinary catheter may be sufficient to relieve bladder neck obstruction. Retroperitoneal ureteral catheters or nephrostomy may be indicated as a palliative maneuver for higher obstruction.

Urinary incontinence can be a major home care issue for patients with malignancy. Differential diagnosis of urinary incontinence should center around causes of polyuria and overflow incontinence. In considering the differential diagnosis of polyuria, one must consider metabolic causes such as hyperglycemia, hypercalcemia, and diabetes insipidus. Excess fluid intake and diuretic use must be considered in the differential diagnosis of polyuria. Alternative explanations for urinary incontinence must also include overflow. As an example, bladder obstruction secondary to bladder invasion by tumor, prostatic enlargement, debris from crystals, or tumor sloughing, all can cause urinary incontinence.

An alternative explanation for overflow incontinence is detrusor failure. Etiologies to be considered include primary causes of bladder irritation such as cystitis from urinary tract infections, radiation, tumor invasion, stones, or as a consequence of chemotherapy such as cyclophosphamide. Detrusor failure can also be caused by loss of afferent spinal nerve innervation as caused by tumor extension, neuropathy secondary to neurotoxicity to drugs or radiation, and decreased central nervous system input as seen with dementia. Iatrogenic causes of detrusor failure are anticholinergic drugs such as the tricyclic antidepressants or phenothiazines. A not uncommon cause of detrusor failure is fecal impaction.

The management of urinary incontinence includes maneuvers to increase the frequency of voiding. As an example, the logistics of voiding can be improved by the use of appliances and by maintaining a sufficient level of consciousness. An alternative would be to decrease fluid intake. If necessary, appliances should be considered. Diaper pads may offer a reasonable compromise. Catheter drainage should be considered but the risks and benefits must be carefully assessed. Catheter management in general is discussed in Chapter 13.

Specific interventions for detrusor failure include treating the underlying cause with local anesthetics such as Pyridium and, paradoxically, anticholinergic drugs such as Pro-Banthine, or tricyclic antidepressants.

Hematuria can be a very distressing manifestation of urinary tract involvement. Lower tract bleeding can often be corrected through the interventions discussed above for urinary incontinence. In reality, though, the major problem may be one of reassuring the patient and family as to the minimal amount of blood loss in spite of the color of the urine. Transfusion can be considered for those patients who over time have significant blood loss.

## NEUROLOGIC

The management of neurologic disorders in the home is an important part of rendering palliative care. Conceptually, one can think in terms of central nervous system disorders, cord compression, and neuropathies. In considering the central nervous system disorders, a clear distinction has to be made between brain metastasis and carcinomatous meningitis. The signs, symptoms, diagnostic maneuvers, and treatment for these two types of central nervous system involvement are different.

For brain metastasis the symptoms are varied. Focal neurologic signs are much less common than generally believed. In fact, often because of the multiple sites of metastatic involvement, clear-cut focal neurologic signs are less common. The most common presenting manifestations of brain metastasis include signs and symptoms of increased intracranial pressure. This can be very subtle and often difficult to distinguish from other symptom complexes. Characteristic headache, often occurring during the night and early waking hours, is a result of increased $pCO_2$ during sleep. This increase in $pCO_2$ leads to an increase in intracranial pressure. Nausea and vomiting ranging from mild nausea to projectile vomiting can often be the main manifestation of increased intracranial pressure. This very nonspecific symptom complex should always raise the suspicion of the possibility of increased intracranial pressure. Global dysfunction manifested by lethargy or change in personality or intellectual function may cause major morbidity. Careful consideration of brain metastases must be kept in mind.[11]

The clinical setting of brain metastases is usually one of hematogenous spread of tumor. The most common histologic types include lung cancer, breast cancer, melanoma, and renal cell cancer. Tumors that are less commonly spread hematogenously are colorectal cancer, pancreatic cancer, ovarian cancer, and prostate cancer, and thus less commonly cause parenchymal brain metastases.

The diagnosis and management of brain metastases are relatively straightforward. The computed tomography scan is the diagnostic procedure of choice. The treatment in the symptomatic patient consists of initiation of corticosteroids to reduce edema and intracranial pressure. Often the results of the reduction in edema can be seen in a matter of hours with dramatic improvement of symptoms. In some settings, it is even justified to consider an empiric trial of steroids if the clinical setting is not appropriate for more aggressive diagnostic work-up. Radiation therapy is the standard for palliation of brain metastases. In unusual circumstances consideration can be given to resection of the tumor mass.

Carcinomatous meningitis represents a distinct clinical problem. The main signs and symptoms of carcinomatous meningitis can be divided into three general components. At least two of these components should be present in order to entertain the diagnosis of meningitis. The patient may have manifestations of supratentorial change in function, specifically change in consciousness or intellectual functioning. Second, cranial nerve involvement can be multiple and asymmetric. Third, spinal root involvement can be manifested either by sensory, motor, or reflex changes. The diagnostic procedure of choice is a lumbar puncture with characteristic findings of increased opening pressure, high protein, low sugar, and on occasion positive cytology. The management of carcinomatous meningitis includes relieving the increased pressure, which can be done with a shunt. Alternatively, consideration can be given to the introduction of intrathecal chemotherapy. Corticosteroids may also be of some palliative benefit.

Spinal cord compression may evolve very rapidly and cause major morbidity of spinal cord dysfunction and pain. The pathophysiology of cord compression is very well worked out. It occurs in the setting of significant retroperitoneal disease or bone involvement, or both. The main cause of epidural masses is the retrograde flow of tumor into the epidural space with resulting growth of an epidural tumor. Signs and symptoms of cord compression can evolve very quickly because the pathophysiology is not so much tumor expansion but rather the vascular component. When the tumor reaches a critical mass, then the blood supply is compromised. Over a matter of hours it is not uncommon to have the patient evolve into full spinal cord compression. This is presumably due to the positive feedback loop of ischemia leading to more edema and more edema leading to ischemia and actual necrosis. In the management of patients with spinal cord compression, it is important to remember that the vascular necrosis is irreversible. Once a patient becomes paraplegic, the probability of improvement falls dramatically. For preservation of function it is essential to approach the diagnosis and management of spinal cord compression aggressively.

Another acute etiology can be subluxation or collapse of the axial skeleton. This occurs in the setting of bone metastases. Often the patient can pinpoint the moment of fracture by the onset of severe pain. The symptoms of spinal cord compression include long tract symptoms of motor dysfunction and sensory dysfunction with characteristic pain that is often radicular and position related. Parasympathetic dysfunction can also be seen in the bladder and bowel. For low-lying cord lesions, a characteristic cauda equina syndrome, which is manifest by perineal numbness and bladder dysfunction, can be observed. The diagnosis of spinal cord compression is made by physical examination with percussion tenderness over the involved area as well as long tract signs. A computed tomography scan and myelogram are required not only to make the diagnosis of spinal cord compression but also to determine the cephalad and caudad extent of the involvement. Treatment involves the early introduction of steroids to reduce the swelling, radiation therapy, and, in certain circumstances, surgical decompression.

Neuropathies can be the cause of significant morbidity in the cancer patient. Etiologies can either be part of a paraneoplastic syndrome or a result of drug-induced sensory neuropathy from vinca alkaloids or cisplatin chemotherapy. Unfortunately, there are few symptomatic interventions so that aggressive diagnostic approaches are not justified in the setting of home palliative care.

## BONE METASTASES

Isolated or diffuse bony metastases are a significant cause of morbidity for the cancer patient at home. Usually the main clinical issue is one of pain control, but consideration must also be given to consequences of pathologic fracture. The anatomical location of the bone metastases in the axial skeleton versus non-weight-bearing areas has an impact on the management. If there are bone metastases in weight-bearing areas, then prophylactic radiation or surgical fixation, or both, must be considered. Depending on the clinical setting, external immobilization or operative fixation can result in significant palliative benefit. This immobilization for pathologic fractures of the axial skeleton is of paramount importance to pain control. As discussed elsewhere, analgesics should be used liberally in order to provide symptomatic relief.

## DERMATOLOGIC PROBLEMS

Thrombophlebitis is an important clinical issue. The clinical presentation is usually one of erythema in the extremities, edema, and often pain. The diagnostic approach depends on the clinical setting. If the clinical suspicion is high, for example, if the patient has an adenocarcinoma, pelvic involvement, or inactivity, then if the clinical symptom complex is present, the clinical judgment of a deep vein phlebitis is adequate without requiring diagnostic intervention. The main palliative approach is symptom control with elevation and warm soaks. The issue of anticoagulation in the home setting is a very difficult one. Intravenous heparinization can only be done in the home under special circumstances. Alternatively, consideration should be given to oral anticoagulation with warfarin or parenteral subcutaneous low-dose heparin. The relative risks of the morbidity from the phlebitis and the risk of pulmonary embolization must be weighed against the clinical and logistical complications of anticoagulation.

Dermatologic problems that arise in the cancer patient involve the general principles of skin care. Special attention may have to be paid to skin care following radiation therapy, local skin reactions to chemotherapy, and the predisposition to cutaneous infection because of disease and treatment-induced immunosuppression. The specific issues of skin care are discussed in Chapter 16.

## PAIN

Unfortunately, pain must be accepted as a clinical reality for patients with advanced cancer. Statistics would support that approximately 60% of patients with advanced cancer have pain, but this rises to 85% in the hospice palliative care setting, and as many as 30% have unrelieved pain at death. It is also important to make the distinction between acute and chronic pain. In chronic pain, usually of more than 6 weeks' duration, there is little correlation between the source of the pain and the severity, and depression is a major component and dysfunction is significant. By contrast, in acute pain, usually of less than 6 weeks' duration, there is a clear correlation between the source and severity of pain, depression is much less a component, and there is minimal dysfunction. In contrast to chronic pain, if you treat the source in acute pain then there is symptomatic relief.

The clinical approach is to eliminate the cause of pain if possible. The most common etiology of pain is bone metastasis. As discussed in the preceding section, consideration must be given to the possibility of a fracture exacerbating the pain. The management includes the immobilization of the fracture if appropriate, and palliative radiation therapy. Another etiology to be considered is neuropathic pain. As discussed previously, spinal cord compression can cause significant pain that has certain characteristics. Alternatively, spinal root pain causes referred pain, which from a diagnostic standpoint must be localized so that if radiation is to be used, the appropriate site is treated.

In the differential diagnosis of headaches, consideration should be given to the possibility of central nervous system metastasis. If neuropathic pain is considered in the differential diagnosis and if diagnostic intervention is not clinically appropriate, consideration should be given to an empiric trial of corticosteroids. As an example, dexamethazone could be given orally at a dose between 8 mg and 32 mg per day for 2 days. If there is a clinically significant reduction of pain, then empiric continuation should be considered. However, if there is no significant improvement in pain, the steroids could be appropriately discontinued without any significant morbidity. If the patient has abdominal pain, consideration should be given to the possibility of a bowel obstruction. As discussed above, consideration could be given to diagnostic and possibly surgical interventions.

The treatment of pain, if the underlying cause cannot be treated, is pharmacologic management. In the context of home care, several important issues should be considered. There must be general acceptance of pain as a reality. The goal of care is palliation. Concerns about addiction and analgesic abuse are clinically insignificant compared to the morbidity of cancer-related pain.

The principles of the treatment of cancer pain are to believe the patient, think in a multimodality way, and aggressively use drugs in an analgesic ladder in interval rather than as-needed doses. Conceptually the analgesic ladder involves initially starting off with aspirin or acetaminophen for mild to moderate pain. For moderate to severe pain the analgesics of choice are generally an oxycodone preparation or morphine. For severe pain, oral morphine, particularly in the oral sustained-release preparation, has proven to be very effective. The importance of proper dose scheduling cannot be overemphasized. In general, cancer pain is constant. Patients should be encouraged to take their analgesics at regular intervals, anticipating rather than waiting for the return of pain as analgesic levels fall. The patient should be able to control the interval in such a way as to balance the analgesic effect with the toxicity of the analgesic.

For severe pain, the value of morphine as an analgesic must be emphasized. Although there are myths about morphine, including addiction, spiraling need, and admission of defeat, in reality morphine is a very effective analgesic with a very wide therapeutic index. A number of oral morphine preparations are in clinical use. Immediate-release morphine can be used at starting doses of 15 mg to 30 mg at approximately 4-hour intervals. Alternatively, sustained-release morphines are available for use at 8- to 12-hour treatment intervals. The advantages of 12-hour dosing of morphine include maintenance of a pharmacologic analgesic level, reduction in the number of pills, maintenance of the oral route, reduction in dependency and anxiety related to the reliance on others for dosing, and uninterrupted sleep.

Consideration can also be given to combining analgesics. As an example, if the patient becomes refractory to oxycodone compounds then morphine can be added to oxycodone compound. Coanalgesics to be considered include nonsteroidal analgesics such as ibuprofen. The tricyclic antidepressants are also useful, not only as analgesics but also as hypnotics. Initial doses of amitriptyline of 10 mg to 50 mg at bedtime have proven to be quite effective.

Consideration must be given to the treatment of narcotic side-effects. Of major clinical importance is constipation. This should be anticipated by the prophylactic use of stool softeners. In clinical reality, respiratory depression is a very unusual complication of narcotic analgesic use in the cancer patient. Dysphoria and drowsiness associated with narcotics can be dose-limiting problems. The clinical judgment must be made as to the relative risks and benefits of the analgesic effects versus the central depressive effects. Often the patient is in the best position to make this relative judgment.

## NAUSEA AND VOMITING

Nausea and vomiting as a symptom complex must be approached first to eliminate reversible causes and then to provide symptomatic relief. Reversible causes that must be considered in the home care setting particularly include peptic ulcer disease either as a primary process or iatrogenic secondary to drug use. As discussed earlier, bowel obstruction and central nervous system metastasis may produce a symptom complex of nausea and vomiting. Treatment-related causes include radiation sickness and chemotherapy-induced nausea and vomiting. In reality, these latter causes usually resolve within a matter of days after completion of treatment. Persistence of these symptoms should raise the concern of other etiologies.

The primary management of nausea and vomiting includes pharmacologic approaches. The standard drugs are the phenothiazines, particularly prochlorperazine. Alternatives include metoclopramide, which has both peripheral gastrointestinal and central antiemetic effects. Metoclopramide can be contraindicated when bowel obstruction is a diagnostic consideration, but in reality metoclopramide should be considered in those settings where there is considerable volume of vomiting. Although tetrahydrocannabinol has been used as an antiemetic in cancer patients, in fact its major benefit seems to be due to its central psychoactive rather than antiemetic properties.

## HEMATOLOGIC ISSUES

For the patient at home, the physician can use certain guidelines in assessment and intervention for hematologic problems. After myelosuppressive chemotherapy, the physician must be prepared to triage fever in the context of the probability of there being profound granulocytopenia. It is also appropriate for the physician to emphasize that there is no role for reverse isolation; rather, patients are infected by organisms previously colonized. Depending on the severity of the overall clinical setting, the degree of fever, and associated symptoms, the physician must judge whether or not a complete blood count and appropriate antibiotic intervention are indicated either with treatment in the home or by triage to the hospital.

Thrombocytopenia, induced either by treatment, consumptive intravascular or vascular coagulation, or marrow replacement, can be manifested by unusual bleeding or a hemorrhagic petechial rash. The indications for platelet transfusion for thrombocytopenia would be dependent on the clinical situation. Similarly, for anemia, the physician must be aware of the signs and symptoms of profound anemia and again the indications for transfusion would be dependent on the clinical setting.

## MOUTH CARE

Careful attention to the mouth can greatly improve quality of life of the cancer patient at home. Careful attention must be paid to maintaining oral hygiene with the use of cleansing mouthwashes, such as one part sodium bicarbonate mixed with hydrogen peroxide, and brushing and flossing. The judgment must be made whether or not to continue to use poorly fitting oral appliances.

Important reversible causes of mouth symptomatology include overgrowth oral candidiasis, which can be easily treated by antifungal medications such as ketoconazole. Symptomatic management of xerostomia includes simple maneuvers such as frequent moisturizing with ice, liquids, moisturizing agents such as mineral oils, and topical remedies such as dyclonine and lidocaine applied to the sore areas.

## CONCLUSION

Home care offers advantages for cancer patients and their families at all stages of the disease. Unfortunately, few families are able to cope with the variety of problems home care creates without the support of their attending physician and other members of the health-care team. A multidisciplinary approach to home care that focuses on anticipating physical and psychosocial problems, and intervening before a crisis arises, is a prerequisite of effective home care. Although each patient's situation will differ somewhat from another's, the assessments and interventions described in this chapter will hopefully facilitate the adjustment of the cancer patient and his or her family at home.

## REFERENCES

1. Weisman A: Coping with Cancer. New York, McGraw-Hill, 1979
2. Lewis C, Linet MS, Abeloff MD: Compliance with cancer therapy by patients and physicians. Am J Med 74:673–678, 1983
3. Groves J: Taking care of the hateful patient. N Engl J Med 295:883–887, 1978
4. McCue JD: The effects of stress on physicians and their medical practice. N Engl J Med 306:458–463, 1982
5. Schnaper N, Hahn AP, Devries R: Specialty rounds: Psychosocial roles in the cancer drama. Am J Med Sci 276:249–261, 1978
6. Koocher G: Adjustments and coping strategies among caretakers of cancer patients. Soc Work Health Care Winter:145–150, 1979
7. Weisman A: Coping with Cancer. New York, McGraw-Hill, 1979
8. Novak D, Plumer R, Smith R et al: Changes in physicians' attitudes towards telling the cancer patient. JAMA 241:879–900, 1979
9. Goldberg RJ: Disclosure of information to adult cancer patients: Issues and updates. J Clin Oncology 2:948–953, 1984
10. Mullan F: Re-entry: The educational needs of the cancer survivor. Health Educ Q 10:88–94, 1984
11. Feldman FL: Work and Cancer Health Histories: A Study of the Experience of Recovered Patients. San Francisco, California Division of the American Cancer Society, 1976
12. Burton L, Zones JS: The Incidence of Insurance Barriers and Employment Discrimination Among Californians with a Cancer Health History in 1983: A Projection. Oakland, CA, California Division of the American Cancer Society, 1982
13. Schain WS: Sexual problems of patients with cancer. In DeVita VT, Hellman S, Rosenberg SA (eds): Cancer: Principles and Practice of Oncology, pp 278–291. Philadelphia, JB Lippincott, 1982
14. Schover LB, von Eschenbach AC: Sexual and marital counseling with men treated for testicular cancer. J Sex Marital Ther 10:29–40, 1984
15. Bayer R, Callahan D, Fletcher J et al: The care of the terminally ill: Morality and economics. N Engl J Med 309:1490–1494, 1983
16. Wanzer SH, Adelstein SJ, Cranford RE et al: The physician's responsibility toward hopelessly ill patients. N Engl J Med 310:955–959, 1984
17. Rosenbaum EH, Rosenbaum MA: Principles of home care for the patient with advanced cancer. JAMA 244:1484–1487, 1980
18. Billings JA: Outpatient Management of Advanced Cancer: Symptom Control, Support, and Hospice in the Home. Philadelphia, JB Lippincott, 1985
19. Adams Greenly M, Moynihan R: Helping the children of fatally ill parents. Am J Ortho-psychiatry 53:219–229, 1983

# 21

# The Pediatric Patient

ROBERT M. GREENSTEIN
SUZANNE STEFANOWSKI HUDD

Following an uneventful planned pregnancy, Christopher was born at full term weighing 7 lb 6 oz to healthy parents. There are two other children, a girl age 2½, and a boy, age 5, both in good health. Christopher was noted immediately to have respiratory distress secondary to a cleft palate associated with a small jaw (micrognathia), the Pierre Robin anomaly. He also had minor facial anomalies (dysmorphic features) including hypertelorism, upturned nose, and low-set ears, as well as bilateral simian creases of the palms and dysplastic toenails. There were no abnormalities of heart or kidneys identified, but the neurologic examination revealed generalized hypotonia, including difficulty sucking. In view of these findings, a genetic syndrome was suspected. A chromosome analysis was obtained, which revealed a normal karyotype, 46,XY; no specific syndrome diagnosis was established.

The major management problems for Christopher were his airway and nutrition. By 5 weeks of age in the neonatal intensive care unit, he continued to have frequent apneic spells despite scrupulous attention to maintaining a chest-down position, even during feeding. Feeding was also a problem because of his poor suck, and he finally required nasogastric tube feeding followed by a gastrostomy tube. After a particularly severe apneic spell, he received a tracheostomy. His parents had visited almost daily and participated in all major management decisions.

At 8 weeks of age, Chris developed a generalized seizure disorder with an epileptogenic (abnormal) EEG. The seizures responded well to phenobarbital, but his neurologic status continued to reveal hypotonia, delayed development, and probable cortical blindness. His nutritional status was stabilized by continuous gastrostomy tube feeding by pump. His respiratory status is complicated by frequent suctioning of the tracheostomy and position changes. He received daily occupational and physical therapy and weekly visits by the ophthalmologist, neurologist, and otolaryngologist. At 4 months of age, Chris's parents requested his discharge to home care with the expectation that the hospital staff and appropriate community services would be available to develop a comprehensive, coordinated management program to meet Chris's and the family's needs.

It is not unique today to find a child born with multiple handicapping problems. It is now more common that many of these "high-tech" children will survive to leave the neonatal

This work is funded in part by the National Institute on Disabilities and Rehabilitation Research, U.S. Department of Education, Grant #G0084C0043.

intensive care unit (NICU) and pediatric surgical suites. High-technology advances in the NICU have lowered the infant mortality rates and improved survival rates, particularly for low-birthweight infants and those with congenital abnormalities. So, it is not surprising that Christopher survived. The survival of infants such as Christopher is not unusual. The number of children "graduating" from NICUs has dramatically increased during the past decade. Concurrent with this improved survival of handicapped and low-birthweight infants, the demand has grown for home-based services that will enable families to care for their technology-dependent children in their homes and communities. As families continue to express a willingness to care for these children at home, the primary-care physician must develop an understanding of the service system that has developed in response to their needs.

The purpose of this chapter is to acquaint the primary-care provider—pediatrician or family medicine physician—with the essential elements of home-based care for children and their families. Specifically, the focus will be on the physician's role in caring for multihandicapped or disabled children on a long-term basis, rather than the treatment of short-term, acute illnesses. A model for providing home care for the "multiple needs" of a pediatric patient will be described and this model will be applied to a number of practical treatment situations. We believe that the primary-care physician should be a leader in the development, implementation, and maintenance of home-based care programs for handicapped children.

## WHAT MAKES CHILDREN DIFFERENT

While it is true that many of the principles and disease models addressed in preceding chapters apply equally well to children, there are additional, unique features about the pediatric age group that must be considered in developing a home care program. First and foremost is the consideration of the family unit itself. Planning for the needs of a handicapped child at home will certainly impact on the interdependence and dynamics of the family unit. There are three basic concepts to consider when addressing the needs of disabled or handicapped children.

### HABILITATION

When an adult becomes disabled or handicapped, programs are employed that are directed at returning the individual to his or her previous level of function. This is the concept of *rehabilitation*. However, infants and children born with birth defects or who suffer serious acquired conditions (*e.g.,* meningitis, birth anoxia, accidents, or trauma) have not yet reached their full level of function. These disabled or handicapped children have a potential that remains relatively unfulfilled. The concept of *habilitation* implies that supportive programs are directed at helping the child and family achieve the best possible outcome, realizing that full or normal function may never be realized. This principle applies to both motor and cognitive function of the child. Likewise, the importance of stabilizing the family for long-term support of the handicapped child must also be considered.

### GROWTH AND DEVELOPMENT

From birth, children rapidly change over a time continuum that operates across the dimensions of growth and development. Growth is measured in three major areas: head circumference, reflecting brain growth and intellectual competence; linear growth, which is largely a function of the genetic endowment of the parents; and weight, which reflects nutritional and environmental stability. The dynamic changes over time and the interrelationships of these measurements may be documented on longitudinal growth curves.

Development implies a complex set of skills, attainments, competencies, and behaviors that change over time along a predictable schedule of events. This time course reflects activities in the areas of social adaptation, gross and fine motor ability, and communication skills, including language and cognitive functioning. The interaction of the developing child with family members and environmental experiences shapes the child's personality.

Thus, congenital abnormalities or trauma during infancy that results in handicaps has the potential to cause widespread deficits in both the growth and development of the child. These deficits may impart a lifelong reduction in the ability of the child to reach a normal level of function, even with an aggressively applied habilitation program.

## CRITICAL TRANSITIONS

The lives of children and their families are intimately entwined over time by their shared experiences, which define the nature of family relationships. In essence, the family itself experiences a developmental sequence, a series of *critical transitions:* (1) the birth of a child and transition from hospital to home; (2) early childhood development; (3) beginning school; (4) adolescence and separation from family; and (5) marriage and the birth of grandchildren. For the handicapped child, these transitions may be delayed or complicated by more "extreme" experiences (*e.g.,* transition from NICU rather than the normal nursery), or these transitions may never occur at all. The occurrence of a child's disability or handicap is thus superimposed on the family's expected developmental sequence. As the child and family progress through these milestones, changes may occur that magnify and stress the nature of family relationships. We will use this concept to highlight specific examples later in this chapter. Through the remainder of the chapter, the unique qualities of children must remain in the forefront: habilitation, growth and development, and critical transitions. Each of these concepts poses additional challenges in the management and care of children in a home-based model.

## MAKING THE DECISION TO PROVIDE CARE IN THE HOME

The term *home care* has been defined as an attempt to normalize the life of a child who has a significant handicap or disability (often one that requires major technological intervention) in the family unit and community setting, in order to minimize the disruptive impact of the child's condition and to foster the child's maximal growth and development.[1] The concept of normalization is the key issue in providing home care to children. The provision of home care services connotes a holistic philosophy, that of providing comprehensive medical treatment to the child while minimizing disruptions to normal family life.

A variety of factors have been described as critical to the development of an effective home care program including (1) patient factors (potential benefits and risks, and care needs); (2) community factors (medical, social, and community supports); (3) family factors (the presence of involved family members and an appropriate home setting, including, wherever possible, two family members who understand the nature of the child's medical treatment); (4) the designation of a case coordinator; (5) the establishment of a defined back-up system for medical emergency; (6) ensuring family access to a telephone; (7) the development of a plan for monitoring and making adjustments in the care plan; (8) assigning the child and family to a primary-care physician; and (9) obtaining educational services for school-aged children.[2]

The primary-care practitioner committed to providing home-based care for a pediatric patient must be willing to become involved in issues beyond the basic medical needs of the child. Patient, community, and family resources must be similarly assessed, and the treatment protocol must address the limitations and potentials in each of these areas. For example, if medical technology and respite services are available but the family is not emotionally able to entrust the child's care to another individual, it is not likely that respite services will be used appropriately. Ultimately, the inability of parents to access appropriate services will affect the habilitation of the child. Their willingness and commitment to provide continued home-based services might also be diminished. Thus, the well-being of the family is an integral component in the "success" of the child's home treatment program.

## MODELS FOR PROVIDING HOME CARE

Most home care models cited in the literature are designed in a manner to suggest that the pediatrician does *not* directly provide services in the home. Rather, allied health professionals are primarily responsible for the direct delivery of medical treatments. The pediatrician sees the family regularly at the tertiary-care facility and maintains frequent contact with the primary-care providers. Such models have been very effective in terms of reducing costs while maintaining high standards of care. None of these models, however, is appropriate for the private-practice, primary-care physician who may not have easy access to a tertiary-care facility or agency-sponsored home care program to facilitate the provision of home-based medical treatments. The *physician–manager* model is presented here as a method by which the private practitioner (who does not have immediate access to an institutionally based or other program) may effectively address the home care needs of his pediatric patients and their families.

### THE INSTITUTIONALLY BASED MODEL

Stein's program[3] is most commonly cited as a model for providing home care to an inner-city pediatric population. In this program, the physician is based at a single tertiary-care institution that sponsors the home care program. Center-based nurses and allied health professionals conduct both hospital-based (prior to discharge) and in-home training with family members who assume primary responsibility for the medical care of the child at home. The physician sees the family in the hospital on a regular basis. Nurses and allied health professionals maintain contact with the patient and family in the home, and regularly update the pediatrician. The institutionally based home care model provides an excellent integration of primary-care and tertiary-care systems.

### THE "REACH" MODEL

A second model through which home care has been effectively provided to pediatric patients is exemplified in the REACH program (Rural Efforts to Assist Children at Home).[4] Through REACH, nurses serve as "choice managers" providing direction, coordination, interpretation, and other support to families caring for their medically involved child in the home. The program is intended to encourage appropriate utilization of tertiary-care facilities and consequently reduce costs. REACH has demonstrated that the primary-care physician is less apt to hospitalize the patient when he knows that the family is receiving appropriate professional support in the home. REACH has reduced institutionally based outpatient encounters by 40% and inpatient days by 9%.[5]

### THE PHYSICIAN–MANAGER MODEL:
### A ROLE FOR THE PRIMARY-CARE PHYSICIAN

The primary-care physician treating a medically involved or handicapped child at home must be willing to assume a more active role in nonmedical issues pertaining to the child's treatment. The physician should be prepared to coordinate the multiple services that comprise the child's overall plan of treatment. Whether the physician employs support staff (*e.g.,* a nurse practitioner) to conduct home visits or whether he assumes full responsibility for carrying out home-based therapies, he must be willing to commit a percentage of his time to management of the case, ensuring that all the necessary services are being delivered.

Figure 21-1 portrays the relationships between each of the crucial contributors to a successful home care program. The primary-care physician, whether institutionally based or in private practice, works in collaboration with members of the health-care team to mobilize community resources around the needs of the child and the entire family. Community resources may include individuals or organizations that are enlisted to address a single aspect or multiple aspects of the child's treatment, for example, parent support groups, respite services, or a for-profit home care agency that provides a variety of therapeutic services. While the institutionally based physician may have immediate access to ancillary medical services, the private-practice physician will need to assume the dual roles of team member and team leader, service provider and service coordinator. The physician in private practice must determine the availability of community resources and organize these to meet the specific needs of his patients.

The most *crucial* function the practitioner can fulfill is that of "personalizing the system" for the patient and family. The literature abounds with accounts of physician insensitivity and lack of concern for the needs of handicapped children and their families. Parents of a handicapped child are forced to negotiate with nursing agencies, insurance carriers, equipment supppliers, and the educational establishment. The practitioner must demonstrate sensitivity to the multitude of demands that the parent and, consequently, the family unit with a handicapped child continually face. The physician will be looked to for guidance and advice in many areas beyond the immediate medical needs of the child.

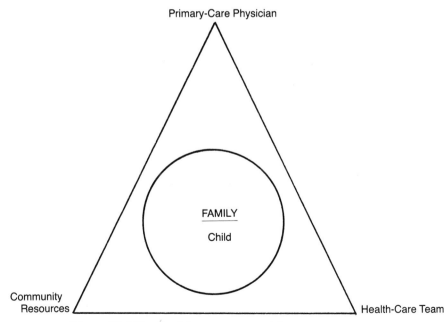

**Figure 21-1** The physician–manager model.

## Coordination of Services

Kanthor and co-workers have recommended that a single individual should assume responsibility for both the *specific* health services and *overall direction* of the child's treatment.[6] These authors designate nine "areas of responsibility," which are important in the management of children with chronic disabilities, including evaluation and treatment of the disease; advice; future planning; genetic counseling; coordination; support; education; acute illness care; and well-child care. The importance of the physician's role in providing coordination for the multiple services needed by the handicapped child has been reiterated the most frequently.[7–10] The primary-care practitioner has consistently been encouraged to assume the role of case coordinator. Some programs have provided the physician with financial incentives to fulfill this function.[11] Generally, the physician is regarded as having the greatest ability, knowledge, and access to the medical system, and so is most able to negotiate for the multiple needs of the child and family. Certainly, the coordination of multiple services that are typically required for the comprehensive treatment of the multi-handicapped child demands a unique set of skills that the general-practice physician must master.

## Management of Services

The physician must make an equal commitment to treatment and management.[8] While not necessarily serving as case coordinator for every child he sees, the physician must be sensitive to the multiple needs of the patient and family. Breslau[10] compared satisfaction with medical care of families of disabled children with other randomly selected families. She found that continuity of physician had a greater positive impact on parental satisfaction in families with a handicapped child. Thus, the physician must be committed to providing consistent and comprehensive treatment in order to minimize the family's frustrations.

Pless[12] and associates conducted a regional survey of private-practice pediatricians and general practitioners to determine which services were provided directly and which services were obtained from specialists or others. The data in this study demonstrated that while referrals to specialists were made on a somewhat regular basis, primary-care practitioners tended *not* to utilize other support services (*e.g.,* social worker, psychologist, vocational rehabilitation). In general, responsibilities seemed to be divided such that well-child care and the treatment of episodic illnesses were left to the primary-care physician, and treatment of the disease itself was left to the specialist.

In response to questions regarding services received, the parents in Pless' study reported that neither the specialist nor the primary-care physician had provided guidance or advice about the daily care of the child, making plans for the future, or genetic counseling. About one third of the parents studied indicated that they received insufficient assistance with coordination, support, and problems related to schooling. Thus, the physician needs to look beyond the basic medical needs of the child, to develop a multidisciplinary approach to meeting the interrelated needs of the family caring for their handicapped child at home.

## IDENTIFYING NEEDS AND RESOURCES

Once the decision has been made to provide home treatment, the needs of the handicapped child and the family must be determined. The major needs or "burdens" for the family can be divided into four major categories: socioemotional, financial, medical, and educational. The family with a handicapped child faces potential short-term or long-term crises in each of these areas throughout the course of the child's development. Likewise, a "crisis" or critical transition in any one of these areas may limit the family's ability to carry

**TABLE 21-1. FAMILY CONCERNS**

| | Medical | Educational | Socio-emotional | Financial |
|---|---|---|---|---|
| ***State Agencies**** | | | | |
| 1. Health services to handicapped children | X | | X | X |
| 2. Department of mental retardation | | X | X | |
| 3. Department of education | | X | | |
| 4. Department of income maintenance | | | | X |
| 5. Department of human resources | X | | X | X |
| 6. Department of child and youth services | | | X | |
| ***Private Agencies*†** | | | | |
| 1. Visiting nurse associations | X | | X | |
| 2. Easter Seals Association | X | | X | |
| 3. Association for Retarded Citizens (ARC) | | X | X | X |
| 4. United Cerebral Palsy | X | X | X | |
| 5. Technology-based services | X | | | |
| ***Other Groups*** | | | | |
| 1. Tertiary-care facilities | X | X | X | X |
| 2. Specialists | X | | | |
| 3. Parent-to-parent support groups | | X | X | |
| 4. Information services | | X | | |

*Each agency has various programs that may or may not effectively meet the needs of a home-care program. These programs vary state-to-state depending upon federal support and state legislation.

†These agencies are representative of *national* organizations that may provide critical resources in support of a home program.

out a prescribed medical treatment. This section will briefly describe each "burden" and the services that may be accessed to alleviate concerns in a particular area (see Table 21-1).

## Information Resources

Access to up-to-date and pertinent information about specific disabilities, programs, and services is a basic need of both families and primary-care physicians. A good deal of information on prevention programs, nutrition, and health issues is now available for display and distribution in the office. However, specific information on handicaps is not readily available. Parents frequently comment that they would prefer to have and read such materials rather than listen to complicated explanations. It is important to remember that parents may not be able to understand materials taken from technically oriented, medical textbooks. They require specially developed materials with reduced technical content in order to assimilate the information.

## Local Sources

There are limited sources for parents to seek information about specific handicapping conditions. Public libraries are not well equipped to maintain this type of current information, but they could access national databases by computer linkage, such as the National Rehabilitation Information Center (NARIC) at the Catholic University of America.* Hospital libraries may have similar linkages as well as current scientific publications, but these are not well suited for public access. There may be a local medical school library with a dedicated interest in public access information.

Other local sources include categorical disease groups, the state or community association for retarded citizens (ARC), and state developmental disabilities council, usually found associated with the state department of mental retardation. The state department of educa-

* 4407 8 Street, NE, Washington, DC 20017

tion may also sponsor a special education resource center or library that both professionals and consumers may access. The local chapter of the National Foundation–March of Dimes has developed an entire series of publications on birth defects that is useful to display in the office. Many medical genetics services collect a wide range of consumer- and parent-oriented publications for distribution.

The state may also maintain a central information service (*e.g.,* INFOLINE) and provide direction in accessing programs and professional services.

### National Sources

A brief listing of various national organizations and information sources may be found in the Appendix. This is only a partial listing and emphasizes the wide-ranging diversity of the sources along with its unfortunate lack of centralized coordination.

## SOCIOEMOTIONAL ISSUES

The birth of a handicapped or medically involved child poses a crisis to any family. Psychologists have described a series of predictable stages through which the parents of a handicapped child typically progress in order to resolve this crisis.[13] Others argue that differences among family reactions are greater than commonalities.[14] As Blacher[15] notes, "the impact of a severely impaired child on the family appears to be profound, pervasive and persistent, and these effects can endure into the child's adult life." Throughout the process of familial adjustment, stress can impair many aspects of the family's functioning, including the marital relationship, siblings' relationships, finances, relationships with friends and relatives, and the ability to plan for the future.[15]

### The Marital Relationship

Having a chronically ill family member has been linked to reduced marital integration and increased conflict and tension between parents. The presence of a hemophiliac son has been shown to contribute to the withdrawal of the husband from family relationships and to marital break-ups. Hemophilia has also been shown to contribute to increased financial strain, limited family mobility, heightened feelings of resentment and guilt between parents, and a more strained relationship between healthy siblings and the hemophiliac child.[16]

### Effects on Siblings

Seligman[17] summarized research on the reactions of brothers and sisters to living with a handicapped sibling. Some siblings exhibited an increased tolerance of others and certainty about their own futures, while others were harmed by the experience, demonstrating resentment and guilt. Caldwell and Guze[18] noted that the type of living arrangement selected for the retarded child was not crucial for the adjustment of siblings. Rather, the views of brothers and sisters mirrored the family decision. Where the parents are capable of accepting the child, the family unit is more able to adapt. By providing emotional support for family members, the physician will enhance the ability of the family to focus their emotional energies on tasks other than those related to the treatment of the child.

### Mother's Adjustment

Research has demonstrated that the maternal concerns for the handicapped child are typically both emotional and pragmatic. A mother may feel guilt, shame, or anger after giving birth to a handicapped infant.[19] Additionally, she may feel frustrated and overburdened, in that she may perceive her care taker role as perpetual.[20]

## Father's Adjustment

Fathers have been described as more focused on the long-term potential of their handicapped child and the financial problems that will ensue as a result of the child's disabilities.[21] Marital problems may frequently be exacerbated by the father's tendency to become less involved with the family. Fathers also tend to be more concerned about the adoption of socially approved behavior by their children, specifically, their social status and occupational success.[22] Because of these higher expectations, they typically report greater disappointment with their retarded children.[23]

## Familial Adjustment

Familial adjustment to the presence of a handicapped child may be exacerbated by any number of environmental factors. For example, Pless and Roghmann[8] have demonstrated that chronically ill children, compared with healthy children, are more frequently perceived by their teachers as truant, troublesome in school, and socially isolated. At both primary-school and secondary-school levels, these children are also more apt to be described by their teachers as having poor attitudes toward their work. Such issues are related to increased levels of stress for the parents of handicapped children and, consequently, have an impact on the entire family.

## Stresses of Daily Life

In addition to the emotional issues that must be resolved by the family with a handicapped child, family members are subjected to an increased number of pragmatic concerns as well. In an interview with 400 families of handicapped children, Blachard and Barsch[24] found that families typically expressed that they felt more burdened by financial and time constraints than by psychological issues. The primary-care physician should not stress the need for psychological consultation without first considering ways in which the pragmatic demands might be reduced.

## Helping the Family to Maintain the Child at Home

Irrespective of the family's degree of involvement in directly administering medical treatments, the child's adaptation and integration in the home environment is highly dependent on familial support and acceptance. As Stein and Jessops[25] note

> The care of an ongoing condition is heavily dependent on the family. The pediatrician is not in control of the situation to the same degree as in the acute inpatient setting. . . . If the condition cannot be eliminated and if there are a variety of possible interventions of potential but uncertain value, individual preferences may play a role in the decision about whether a given intervention should be undertaken. This may be influenced by the short- and long-term tradeoffs, by the sense of how much the problem is bothering the patient, and how acceptable or unacceptable the intervention is in terms of family values. Moreover, in order for the family to function optimally for the child, the well-being of the family unit itself has to be taken into consideration.

Thus, when providing care directly or coordinating care in the home, the concerns and capabilities of the individual family must be taken into account. As Turnbull[26] notes, by failing to recognize the feelings and needs of a particular family, the professional may "force" the family to comply with a treatment or program that is intrusive to the family structure. The recommended treatment must be based on a knowledge of the services that are available and prescribed with a sensitivity to the family's willingness and capability to obtain and utilize these services.

The priorities for effective home care are perhaps best summarized by Karen Buck-holtz,[27] the parent of a child with bronchopulmonary dysplasia, who has received home care since the age of 2 years:

I believe everyone considering home care for their child should have the following: 1) a supportive primary care physician; 2) dependable and responsible nurses; 3) coordinator assistance; 4) therapy services (CPT, OT, ST, etc.) as needed; 5) an educator to assist in getting schools involved; 6) a social worker to assist with community and financial resources; and 7) a psychologist to provide help with emotional stress.

It is noteworthy that the need for a supportive primary-care physician is listed as most important. The physician who becomes involved in the delivery of home care should be prepared to meet these expectations.

A variety of resources are available to help the family cope and adjust to the demands and stresses associated with bringing the handicapped child home. State agencies, such as the department of mental retardation, human resources, child and youth services, and health services to handicapped children provide support for parents and families with handicapped and medically involved children. The availability of specific services for specific types of problems varies from state to state. The primary-care practitioner is encouraged to investigate the resources that are available through state agencies and to convey this information to the family.

Private agencies are generally equipped to provide the family with additional socioemotional support. Disease-specific organizations (*e.g.,* United Cerebral Palsy) frequently sponsor parent support groups and provide up-to-date information on therapies and other such services. There are also more "generic" groups such as the Association for Retarded Citizens (ARC) and Easter Seals that sponsor supportive activities for families of children with a variety of disabling conditions. These organizations may also encourage and facilitate the involvement of family members in advocacy activities for the child. The organizations may also provide services such as sheltered workshops or respite care.

In many cases, tertiary-care medical institutions may provide additional family support services, such as a support group for families of children with Down syndrome, genetic counseling services, or an early intervention program. Thus, the primary-care practitioner is encouraged to become familiar with the availability of such programs through hospitals, clinics, and visiting nurse associations in his area. The physician might begin to generate a list of available agencies by checking the "social services" section of the Yellow Pages in his area.

## FINANCIAL ISSUES

In caring for the handicapped or medically involved pediatric patient at home, consideration must be given to the cost of treatment as well as the extent to which services are reimbursable. In contrast to other therapies discussed in this book, public and private coverage for *pediatric* home care services is extremely limited. Most private insurers fund home care therapies for an acute illness, in transition from hospital to home. In the process of prescribing a home treatment program for the child, the practitioner must develop *with the family* and other qualified persons a plan for financing the child's medical treatment.

While the cost-effectiveness of delivering home health services to a medically involved child has been documented,[28] a variety of "disincentives" encourage the utilization of tertiary-care facilities. Castellani[29] notes that in assessing the child's eligibility for Medicaid and Supplemental Security Income, parents' income is deemed "available" to a child residing with the parents but is *not* available to the child who is institutionalized. Delays in reimbursement or lack of coverage for specific problems will cause frustration and additional stresses for the family and will ultimately impact on the family's willingness and ability to continue to maintain the child in the home.

Perrin and Ireys[5] provide an excellent breakdown of sources of payment for medical services utilized by families with a handicapped child. This section will highlight each of these with respect to their applicability to home care. For information on state and federally sponsored financial assistance programs for home health care, the physician should contact his state's departments of income maintenance, health services to handicapped children, and human resources. As the cost-effectiveness of home care becomes increasingly recognized, financial incentives in both the public and private sectors are likely to become more available.

## Medicaid (Title XIX)

Medicaid is the largest public program for providing health care services. Eligibility for families to receive services for their handicapped child is tied to the family's eligibility for Aid for Families with Dependent Children (AFDC) funds. Thus, for any family where the need for Medicaid funds to subsidize their child's treatment is expected, the practitioner should ensure that the paperwork for enrollment in the AFDC program is processed.

Twenty-eight states have enacted the "medically needy option," which is particularly crucial for families of handicapped children. In these states, a family with dependent children or a family with an unemployed or incapacitated parent can receive Medicaid coverage for their handicapped child as long as the family income falls below the poverty level once medical expenses have been subtracted.[5] However, a large percentage of children in low-income families do not meet the eligibility requirements for Medicaid coverage, and any number of needed services may not be available. In the case of the handicapped child, coverage may be confounded by the dual need for medical and educational services.

With respect to providing home care services, six states currently participate in the 2176 Medicaid waiver program. The waiver permits states to finance long-term care services for pediatric patients who are eligible for Medicaid reimbursement and who would otherwise require nursing home care at the intermediate care level or greater.[28] The services included under the waiver plan are case management, respite, personal care, homemaker care, transportation, home repair, home health aide care, and rehabilitation. It is noteworthy that the waiver has been applied to populations not traditionally served under Medicaid programs (*e.g.*, mentally ill, mentally retarded, and disabled children). The availability of Medicaid reimbursement for pediatric home care services will doubtlessly increase as the cost of providing institutionally based therapy continues to soar. Thus, the practitioner should remain abreast of department of income maintenance programs in his state.

**Supplemental Security Income (SSI).** SSI is a national program. The purpose of the program is to provide minimum income for disabled and needy blind children. The child must meet specific criteria as to what constitutes a disability. The array of services provided under this program may include home health services. Referrals to this program must be made through the Social Security Administration. The agency typically requires proof of the family's income and resources, as well as medical documentation of the child's disability. Once deemed eligible, the child will receive medical coverage through Medicaid. SSI will either assume responsibility for providing services, contract for the services with appropriate agencies, or refer the child to existing resources. The primary-care practitioner should ensure that comprehensive and coordinated services are being provided.

### Crippled Children's Services (CCS) and Special State Programs

As the predecessor to Medicaid, CCS was mandated by the federal government to locate, diagnose, and provide medical services to handicapped children. Since the enactment of the Maternal/Child Block Grant in 1981, CCS has provided services through the initiative of state governments. Thus, within individual states, CCS may play a more or less significant role in providing and coordinating services for handicapped children. In some states, CCS may assist the community-based physician with the coordination of care for the handicapped child.[30] The future of the role of CCS without a federal mandate to provide services is questionable. Still, the community-based practitioner is advised to investigate the availability of CCS services in his state, and their applicability to his pediatric patient population. Additional special programs may also be available through CCS on a state-by-state basis (*e.g.,* services for children with a specific genetic disorder).

### Private Insurance

Seventy-five percent of all children in the United States are covered by private insurance. Sixty-eight percent are covered through group insurance as dependents of working parents. Private insurance plans typically provide reimbursement for hospital and physician costs, as well as expenditures for some laboratory and drug services. Most insurance plans do not reimburse for home renovations, work compensation, and counseling. Private insurance does not usually include coverage for children who have limitations in activity and whose income is below the poverty level.[28]

Home care reimbursement plans have generally been applied to patients with chronic and catastrophic illnesses. In more recent years, there has been a shift toward the development of programs for the disabled population. Innovative programs have begun to consider reimbursement for a variety of services, such as case management, physical and speech therapy, nutrition counseling, medical equipment, barrier removal, and visiting nurse services.[31] Although Blue Cross/Blue Shield remains somewhat restrictive in providing reimbursement for home care (prior hospitalization is usually necessary, and services must be directed toward providing acute or short-term care), the proven cost-effectiveness of home treatment has inspired the development of pilot programs.[28] Wherever possible, the primary-care practitioner should work with parents in the selection of the most appropriate insurance coverage. Likewise, therapies should be prescribed with a recognition of the type and amount of coverage for each particular family. In summary, while reimbursable services are presently somewhat limited, there is a continued trend toward expanding coverage for home care.

### Disease-Oriented Voluntary Organizations

Perrin and Ireys[5] note that disease-oriented voluntary organizations (*e.g.,* United Cerebral Palsy) frequently provide financial support to families in need. These organizations tend to pay for services that are *not* reimbursable through the regular system of care (*e.g.,* prostheses). In addition, they provide funds for research, patient education, medical services, community services, public education, and professional education and training. The primary-care practitioner should investigate which organizations operate in the area and encourage parents to utilize the services offered by these organizations.

### Out-of-Pocket Expenditures

In the delivery of home care services, the expenses that are *not* reimbursed by alternate sources are frequently high and unpredictable.[5] The prescription of certain therapies may impose immense financial burdens on the family. It is important to note that home care is frequently *less* cost-effective for the family (*i.e.,* it may actually cost the family *more* to keep the child at home rather than in the hospital or another institutional setting since fewer services will be reimbursed). A comprehensive financial package for the family should include all public programs for which the family is eligible. A home program should *not* be undertaken unless the cost of services is determined to be within the family's financial means.

## EDUCATIONAL ISSUES

As coordinator of the child's overall plan of treatment, the physician must be concerned with the educational services the child receives. The pediatric patient receiving home care may or may not require special education services, depending on the nature of his disability. Children with functional impairments may need adaptive equipment, removal of architectural barriers, or special transportation services, while children with intellectual impairments will require a more comprehensive special education program. Developmentally disabled children commonly exhibit multiple handicaps, which require specialized services that consider both their physical and intellectual capabilities. In general, the educational plan for the child with special needs must provide enrichment and challenge, must work toward normalizing development and preventing secondary disabilities, and must periodically assess the pupil's educational remediation.[32]

The problems associated with the education of handicapped and chronically ill children are varied: school attendance may be interrupted; the visibility of symptoms can lead to withdrawal and isolation; school buildings may not be adapted to meet the child's special needs; or school teachers and programs may pose obstacles that prevent the child from receiving appropriate educational services.[33] As medical team leader, the physician must be concerned that the child's educational program is flexible enough to meet the child's special needs.

Unlike the child's medical diagnosis, the assessment of a developmental disability may be vague and ambiguous. Alternative interventions may be debated, and the treatment strategy that is selected may not be agreed upon unanimously.[34] The primary-care practitioner must be prepared to assist the family in obtaining appropriate educational services. Likewise, he must be available to special education personnel to provide medical consultation for the development of the child's educational program. Wherever feasible, the child should be encouraged to attend school. Opportunities for interaction with his peers throughout the school day enable the child to develop social skills and behaviors appropriate for his age.

### Education for All Handicapped Children Act

In 1975, PL 94-142, the Education for All Handicapped Children Act, was passed. Under this law, handicapped and chronically ill children are eligible for special education services on the basis of an existing learning disability, developmental delay, perceptual handicap or some other learning problem. Handicapped children who do not fall into one of these categories may still be eligible for services under the auspices of the "other health impaired" category.

Hobbs, Perrin and Ireys[33] delineate the services that are typically provided to handicapped and chronically ill children (see Table 21-2). The role for the primary-care practitioner relative to the child's education is clear. The physician must ensure that the school system receives an accurate assessment of the child's medical condition and the extent to which the child's medical needs may impact on his intellectual or physical capacity to participate in regular education programs. Ultimately, as is mandated by PL 94-142, the child must receive services in the "least restrictive environment."

PL 94-142 also requires that "related services" be provided to the special needs child. Related services include school health services, speech therapy, psychological services, physical and occupational therapy, counseling services, medical services for diagnostic or

**TABLE 21-2. EDUCATIONAL PLACEMENTS FOR HANDICAPPED
AND CHRONICALLY ILL CHILDREN**

| Grouping | Regular Education | Special Education |
|---|---|---|
| Chronically ill child with intellectual impairments | Not placed here | Always placed here |
| Chronically ill child with impairments only in physical mobility | Occasionally placed here | Usually placed here |
| Chronically ill child without intellectual or physical impairments | Frequently placed here | Sometimes placed here |

(Hobbs N, Perrin J, Ireys P: Chronically Ill Children and Their Families, p 112. San Francisco, Jossey-Bass Publishers, 1985)

evaluation purposes, and parent counseling and training. Special education and related services are delivered in accordance with the child's individualized education program (IEP), which is developed jointly by parents, teachers, and other appropriate individuals (*e.g.,* guidance counselors and school nurses).

The IEP presents an ideal means through which the physician can become involved in the development of the child's educational program. While the physician may be called on to conduct medical evaluation or diagnosis, the IEP meeting provides a formal mechanism for the physician to assume an active role in the child's education. Although a private-practice physician may not be able to attend every IEP meeting for every special needs patient he sees, he can ensure his availability by providing a telephone number where he can be reached during the meeting, should additional medical information be needed. Where feasible, the physician might be able to participate in the meeting via a telephone conference call.

Once the IEP has been developed, the primary care physician should request a copy to be included in the child's chart. The practitioner should remain informed as to changes in the IEP and the child's educational progress, as a part of his regular follow-up with the child and family. Updated information should be obtained from the parents or school officials. The physician should serve as a source of information and support for the parents. Parents may need to be reminded that their involvement in the IEP process is welcomed, and where parents demonstrate an interest in participating, they should be encouraged to do so.

The development of an IEP presumes that the child who is receiving home-based medical services will be capable of being transported to and from school each day. However, the provision of special education services is relevant to the homebound child as well. Unfortunately, the service system is less well organized for the child who receives out-of-school instruction. State policies regarding the provision of homebound instruction are inconsistent. According to Hobbs, Perrin, and Ireys,[33] some states report no minimum absence requirement before home instruction can be administered, while others require that absence be "anticipated over 30 days." Eligibility for home instruction may also depend on physician recommendation. The physician is advised to check with the state department of education to determine the specifics of PL 94-142 as it is applied to homebound instruction for the handicapped or medically involved child in his state.

### Early Intervention

For the child below school age, the pediatrician should become familiar with the availability of early intervention services in his area, and this information should be conveyed to parents. Early intervention involves the identification of a child's developmental problems at the earliest possible age, and the prescription and delivery of appropriate therapies to minimize the deleterious effects of the problem. Early intervention programs also attempt to prevent the occurrence of secondary problems.

There are various types of early interventions that can be prescribed for children with different disorders. These include (1) newborn screening, diagnosis, and treatment for metabolic disorders; (2) identification of major sensory impairments; (3) early intervention for children with adverse environmental conditions; (4) interventions for premature, low-birthweight or at-risk infants; and (5) interventions for infants with established developmental delays and disabilities.[35]

States differ as to the age at which the provision of services is mandated. Most states are mandated to provide services for children above the age of 5 years. A number of states provide services for children aged 3 to 5; and a few states provide services for children below the age of 3. Many states are currently considering lowering the mandate for services to birth. These mandates typically involve the collaborative efforts of health and education professionals, and thus early intervention services may be more able to address the young child's needs in a more comprehensive manner.

Irrespective of whether state-funded programs are available, early intervention services are typically provided through (1) *center-based programs* (services that require parents to bring the child to an organized class); (2) *combinations of center-based and home-based programs* (parents are trained at the center, and return periodically for ongoing professional evaluation of the child); and (3) *home-based programs* (parents receive instruction on working with their child in the home).[35] Information on the availability of early intervention services can be obtained through medical staff in the hospital nursery or by contacting the state department of education or mental retardation.

## MEDICAL

Home care programs are most effective when there is a complete array of services to meet the complex needs of the handicapped child and the family. Medical services are but one component of this system (see Table 21-1) and may be obtained directly or indirectly. The *physician–manager model* emphasizes the need for the primary-care physician to fill the roles of both case coordinator and case manager.

As *coordinator,* the physician ensures that necessary resources are in place, such as visiting nurses, home-based early intervention, visits to specialists, and continuing insurance reimbursement. This is accomplished by compiling written reports from all participating professionals. Regular office or home visits with the child and family will verify the progress of the child and reinforce the central role of the physician.

The *manager role* calls for a more active participation with the community-based multidiscipline team. This includes convening periodic meetings of the team in order to address and resolve ongoing problems; being available for conference calls with public school officials or other agencies; and maintaining up-to-date office records of the patient's management. There are additional duties to pursue on behalf of the patient and family.

### Problem-Oriented Record

Handicapped children, especially those with multiple problems, present the physician with the need to organize a complex database. The use of the problem-oriented record is one approach that permits focused management for a patient with a wide variety of problems.[36,37] According to the problem-oriented model, an active, complete listing of *all* of the patients' medical, social, and educational and financial problems ("problem list") is maintained in the front of the patient record, each one keyed by an identifying phrase (*e.g.,* problem #3 *Gastrostomy feeding,* Problem #6 *Early Intervention Program,* etc.). All clinical notes should be problem-specific in order to permit optimal organization of information, reduce the length of notes, and encourage ease of retrieval when reviewing the chart.

### Professional Relationships

Consultation from multiple specialists will be needed, but this requirement is frequently episodic and not always well coordinated. The community physician should firmly establish a central managerial role by consistently requesting *timely, written* records of these visits which should contain clear recommendations for therapy, further evaluation, and follow-up visits. Telephone calls to specialists to gain verification of recommendations is a useful method to improve communication. In this respect, your consistency will become the hallmark of the relationship.

### Tertiary-Care Centers

Depending on the nature of a patient's problem, specialized care teams may be sought on a local, regional, or even national basis. Many of these services are housed in medical schools, children's hospitals, or medical centers that, by the nature of their subspecialty focus, could preempt the natural relationship of the family and community practitioner. There is a need to balance the availability of expertise at a center with the local, day-to-day programmatic needs of the child and family. The practitioner should establish a working, collegial relationship with such teams by expressing appropriate expectations for timely communication and shared responsibilities. The specialty team should be expected to support the practitioner in his role as service coordinator.

### Administrative Agencies

Personnel from public and state organizations (*e.g.,* public schools, public health, income maintenance [welfare]) have criticized physicians for failing to provide information that is adequate and up to date. Frequently, these agencies are responsible for establishing a family's eligibility for public services, as well as offering additional supportive services for families undertaking a home care program. While their administrative procedures are at times tedious, they cannot be avoided. By developing effective working relationships with agency personnel, especially through telephone contact, the child and family will become the beneficiaries of needed services and entitlements on a timely basis.

## ILLUSTRATIVE CASE EXAMPLES

In the preceding sections, we attempted to provide background information about practice models, the unique features of the pediatric age group, especially the handicapped child, and the "burdens" faced by handicapped children and their families, as well as the organization of the service delivery system to address these issues.

In keeping with the *critical transitions* model, several illustrative examples of handicapping conditions will be discussed with regard to diagnosis, family support services disposition planning, and home care management.

## TRANSITION FROM NICU TO HOME: THE CHILD WITH TRISOMY 18

One in 200 liveborn infants will have a chromosomal abnormality involving either the *number* of chromosomes (*e.g.,* trisomy, an extra chromosome), or the *structure* of chromosomes (*e.g.,* unbalanced translocations).[38] The most commonly occurring *sex* chromosome abnormalities are Klinefelter's syndrome (XXY) and Turner's syndrome (XO). *Autosomal* abnormalities usually involve chromosomes 13 (trisomy 13), 18 (trisomy 18), and 21 (Down syndrome).

The infant with trisomy 18 is usually low birthweight at full term, has distinctive (dysmorphic) facial features, typically clenched fingers with the thumb and fifth fingers overlapping the other three, rocker-bottom feet, and congenital heart disease. They are neuro-developmentally abnormal, feed poorly and slowly, frequently have seizures, and exhibit primary or genetic growth retardation resembling failure to thrive. The average life span of these children is 6 months. Apnea may be a prominent component and breathing must be electronically monitored.

**Diagnosis.** The diagnosis is suggested by the clinical examination and confirmed by chromosome analysis on peripheral blood. Consultation with the neonatologist or clinical geneticist is appropriate, especially if the infant's condition is precarious. The family should be involved *before* diagnostic testing is begun. The initial meeting with the family should involve *both* parents, whenever possible. The suspicion of a genetic disorder should be suggested immediately, preferably by as familiar a health professional to the family as possible (*e.g.,* the obstetrician or primary-care provider). Thereafter, a complete delineation of the infant's problems should be undertaken and specialists consulted, as needed.

**Supportive Activities.** In addition to the medical determination of the child's problems, steady attention to the family's coping needs is essential since it should be anticipated that, in general, there will be grief, sadness, depression, and withdrawal. Since these are normal reactions to stress and the "loss" of the expected child, other resources from both the hospital and the family's community should be identified. These include the nursery staff, social service, siblings and grandparents (who themselves will need supportive counseling), clergy, and possibly the availability of a parent-to-parent support program from the community. There is a natural desire on the part of professional staff to shield the family from "too many cooks." The family also tends to withdraw into their own coping strategies, which may take the form of anger, hostility, or debilitating grief. However, it is essential that the family be counseled about the resources that are available, if only to permit them to be more future-oriented.

**Disposition Planning.** Although the role of the primary-care physician in the modern high-technology NICU has been diminished, he should remain very involved with the family and receive regular updates on the child's status. The physician should expect daily reports from the NICU staff and take an active role in assisting the family to interpret data, management decisions, and discharge planning. It is appropriate to call the attending neonatologist in order to establish this professional-to-professional role. In most cases, the child with trisomy 18 will be stabilized for discharge, in spite of the expected neurologic, cardiac, and nutritional complications. The primary-care physician should play a major role in the decision to discharge the child home by ensuring that medical services, home nursing, and other needed resources are made available to the family. The NICU may have delineated the problems very well, but they may not be aware of resources, or may not be prepared to coordinate and obtain the services that are needed by a particular family in their community.

The hospital discharge coordinator, usually from the nursing service, should meet with the parents and the physician. If case management will be handled by someone other than the physician, this should be determined beforehand. A complete *problem list* of the infant's needs should be developed and specific individuals, agencies, and resources identified to address each one. Many states have well-developed early intervention programs for handicapped infants. These professionals may be invited to meet with the family before discharge in order to establish linkage and transition for the family.

In addition to the medical needs and community resources inventory, the family should receive financial counseling from a knowledgeable and experienced staff person. This may be the hospital's patient advocate representative, the social worker, or the physician. There are usually many issues to review, including the availability of insurance reimbursement and eligibility for home care programming. It may be possible to negotiate directly with the third-party payer for coverage of the "prescribed" program for home care, including nursing, physical therapy, transportation, and medications. In our experience, it is not advisable to discharge the infant until the critical array of resources for home care are confirmed to be in place. In this instance, the primary-care physician must serve as advocate for the family by ensuring that the child's and family's needs will be met. Before the child is discharged, the physician is advised to make a home visit to determine if the home environment is adequate (*e.g.,* heat, space, electrical outlets, etc.).

**Home and Community Management.** The child with trisomy 18 will likely have significant problems in a number of areas.

*Medical.* The child should be seen at regular intervals in the office, usually as need dictates. However, there may be extensive technical equipment, such as an apnea monitor, infusion pump, or suction machine. Here, office personnel, such as a nurse practitioner, or the visiting nurse service may be more appropriate for home visits. If the child has either congenital heart disease or seizures, continued consultation from appropriate specialists will be needed. The primary-care physician should maintain the central care function. Without this, the family will experience diffused responsibility and be forced to make frequent visits to perhaps more than one tertiary care site.

If the medical center offers a case management team, it may be reasonable for the primary-care practitioner to play a peripheral role until the child's medical problems are stabilized in the home setting. Once the service network is in place, and the child is at home, the *case coordinator* function is best maintained by the community physician. This includes arranging for the purchase or rental of necessary equipment with local agencies, reviewing the complete problem list at regular intervals, and meeting with the parents to discuss their understanding of the complex changes that will occur on a day-by-day basis.

The infant will feed slowly, perhaps requiring nasogastric feeding or even a gastrostomy. The parents will need instruction and ongoing support to carry out this function. The visiting nurse may provide continued instruction and assistance to parents with respect to feedings. The nutritionist at the local hospital may act as a resource.

*Early Intervention.* If contact with early intervention services was initiated in the hospital, then the program should be in place within a few weeks. If not, it is important to determine whether the program meets parental needs as well as being concerned with the infant's development.

*Family Support.* Trisomy 18 is a terminal illness. Parents, siblings, family members, and neighbors need to understand the nature of the genetic diagnosis and natural history, including complications. The family will be under constant stress to cope with their own adjustment, as well as their feelings of inadequacy and helplessness to deal with the child's impending death. Likewise, the child's medical problems will constantly be changing. New problems may arise, and chronic ailments will go through acute phases. For example, the child may experience aspiration pneumonia, apnea associated with seizures, or an intercurrent infection superimposed on failure to thrive.

In spite of these complexities, most parents will opt to attempt home care *if* the necessary array of supportive resources is in place. The availability of parent-to-parent counseling is all the more essential. This may represent a local program, a religious group, or, as frequently seen, the identification by the physician of another family that has experienced the same or a similar event. This selection should be done carefully since the other family may not yet have resolved their own problems. The risk to the new family of now coping with someone else's problems is self-evident. Established parent advocacy programs generally have access to "prepared" parents who act as helpers or advocates without intensifying the family's adjustment problems.

The physician should establish advocacy for the child and family. This is done in many ways: making an occasional home visit; being readily available by telephone; orienting office staff to the multiple needs of the family; and, most importantly, compassionately understanding and accepting parental behaviors through anticipatory guidance. In addition, the physician should make himself accessible to other professionals who are participating in the team care of the child and be ready to compromise on management issues, such as physical and occupational therapy prescriptions and local educational recommendations.

*The Dying Child at Home.* The death of an infant or child is always a shock to the family. It generates a series of reactions that reverberate throughout the family and neighborhood. When the child is identified to have a terminal illness because of a birth defect, cancer, or any chronic illness associated with medical complications, the process of grief, denial, anger, and resolution/acceptance may fluctuate at different periods of time, depending on the child's immediate health status.

There should be open discussions with the parents about the impending death, the expected terminal events, and the issue of pain and suffering. Certainly not all parents will feel comfortable with this approach. They will experience feelings of guilt and inadequacy and wonder if the child had been in the hospital, would he have lived longer or suffered less. They will also feel a sense of panic about needing to intervene but not knowing how to perform cardiopulmonary resuscitation, for example. There may also be a need to relieve discomfort by suctioning or positioning, or for medication to be given to relieve pain.

The physician will be of greatest assistance if he is present at the time of the child's death, or at least shortly thereafter. In many communities, bereavement groups have been developed to comfort families after the death of the child. These programs provide group counseling and are frequently attached to a local NICU or hospital. There may also be a local hospice group to provide guidance and assistance. There is also the availability in most communities of pastoral or clerical counseling. This avenue of support should probably be pursued before the child's death.

For those parents who appear to have chronic sorrow or prolonged, even debilitating, grief, professional counseling should be sought with either a psychiatrist or psychologist.

## EARLY CHILDHOOD DEVELOPMENT

### Bronchopulmonary Dysplasia

The incidence for prematurity (weight < 2500 g at birth) varies widely for different populations, especially those designated as "at-risk" (*i.e.,* teenage pregnancy, poor prenatal care, maternal illness, etc.). Improved pregnancy surveillance and high-technology advances in the NICU have improved the survival of low (< 1500 g) and very low (< 1000 g) birthweight infants. However, while the proportion of survivors has increased, the complications associated with low-birthweight infants extract a significant toll, including intraventricular hemorrhage, respiratory distress syndrome (RDS), retrolental fibroplasia, and metabolic instability. Potential long-term complications include cerebral palsy and developmental delay.

**Diagnosis.** Bronchopulmonary dysplasia (BPD) is a chronic respiratory disease of infants, manifested by tachypnea, dyspnea, hypoxemia, and hypercapnia with characteristic chest x-ray features. The disorder commonly follows the treatment of RDS with mechanical ventilation, but may occur occasionally following pneumonia, meconium aspiration syndrome, tracheoesophageal fistula, and congenital heart disease.[39] Some infants may require tracheostomy and become ventilator dependent. An average of 7% of premature admissions to the NICU have BPD. Expressed relative to RDS, BPD occurred on an average in 20% of infants. There is, of course, a wide range of severity and chronicity, but an increasing number of these infants will be discharged home.

Clinically, there is airway obstruction without hyperinflation, as well as reactive airway disease. Pulmonary hypertension and cor pulmonale occur from hypoxic pulmonary vasoconstriction. Chronic oxygen therapy associated with bronchodilators, digitalis, and diuretics may be necessary, as well as increased fluids and caloric intake. Chronic lung disease is frequently accompanied by failure to thrive and recurrent hospitalization.

**Supportive Services.** Similar to infants with birth defects, families with BPD infants require the same intensive professional and parent-to-parent support. Many hospital NICUs maintain ongoing support groups while the infants are hospitalized, and even thereafter, as needed. Ventilator-dependent or tracheostomy-dependent infants may remain in the hospital for even longer periods of time. The SKIP program (Sick Kids Need Involved People, 16 Newport Drive, Severna Park, MD 21146) is a parent-run organization that provides support to families with ventilator-dependent children at home. They are prepared to provide technical assistance to local groups wishing to establish chapters.

**Discharge Planning.** Depending on the severity, intensity, and stability of BPD, a variety of services may be needed, including home respiratory services, total parenteral nutrition, oxygen, visiting nurse, home pharmacist, respiratory or physical therapist, and electronic monitoring of cardiopulmonary status. Parents will need to be taught cardiopulmonary resuscitation and the local emergency medical service needs to be alerted to the child's presence in the home and the possible need for emergency transportation to appropriate facilities.

**Home Management.** Oxygen-dependent BPD infants may be cared for at home with great financial savings.[40, 41] Low-flow oxygen therapy increases $PaO_2$ and can diminish pulmonary artery hypertension. Taussig[42] reports a savings of $618,000 for 20 BPD infants cared for at home versus in the hospital. The infants received oxygen for a mean duration of 132 days (range, 30–335 days). In addition to the amount of savings, home therapy provides psychological advantages to family life and stabilizes the home environment.

The primary-care physician will be responsible for the meticulous coordination of the child's care needs at home. As case manager, and later case coordinator, the physician must maintain open, available communication with parents and specialists in order to "fine-tune" the complex daily care of the child. This care program will develop its own rhythm and pace and should be monitored using a *problem-oriented* approach. It is likely that an NICU–pulmonologist team will also monitor the child. The primary-care physician, however, will provide one of the most important elements for the family—that of viewing the multiple needs of the child (immunizations, early intervention, first-line monitoring of symptoms) in the context of the whole family and home environment.

At times, the home will take on certain hospital-like qualities. Schedules will need to be maintained for medications, therapies, professional visits to the home, family visits out of the home to specialists' offices, and blood tests. The management of medical services for the child will require frequent telephone calls and much coordination by the parent in spite of professional input from the case manager. Under these circumstances, parents tend to lose freedom of involvement in personal activities, spontaneity, and privacy due to this ongoing stressful situation. Wherever possible, respite care should be sought, but admittedly, this is difficult to arrange and finance.

**Early Intervention Programs.** The primary-care physician should investigate with the family the availability of state programs through the departments of mental retardation, public health, or education, and private programs through agencies such as Easter Seals, United Cerebral Palsy, or the Association for Retarded Citizens (ARC). State agency programs are usually free if the child meets defined eligibility criteria set by the agency and based on both federal and state guidelines. The private agencies usually charge a fee that is covered by some insurance companies under a "rehabilitation" definition.

Enrollment in IEP provides opportunity for regular professional evaluation and assessment of the child's development needs in physical and cognitive areas. It is also an introduction to structured educational programming for the family and acts as a transition into public school programs after the age of 3. For the child with BPD at home, the best program would provide home-based visits by a qualified developmentalist or teacher on a weekly basis. Center-based programs that require parents to transport infants to receive 30 to 60 minutes of physical therapy a week are of questionable value unless there is a need for a specific prescription to address impairment as opposed to cognitive deficits (developmental delay).

**Children in Foster Care.** Many families volunteer as foster parents or group home managers, or to use their home as a community training home. For a variety of reasons, handicapped infants may be temporarily placed in such settings awaiting resolution of administrative or legal complications. Some of these children may also be awaiting adoption proceedings. A community physician may be called on to provide home care to the foster child in concert with the agency that has legal guardianship. The principles of home care programming are no different, but the process of prior acknowledgment for treatment would be an added consideration. A representative from the agency of record should be a member of the case management team.

**Respite Care.** Most families who accept the responsibility for their child's home care program do so willingly, anticipating that the constellation of resources so effective in the hospital will now be available in their community (*e.g.,* three shifts of nurses and other support personnel). Once home, the real impact of 24-hour care and the associated responsibility may overwhelm the family. However, with appropriate nursing staff and other medical professionals to help on one or two shifts a day, the family will still function effectively if the resources are consistent. There are many unforeseen difficulties that the family may face because of changing insurance coverage, the lack of available nurses each day, sibling care requirements, difficulty in arranging for transportation, and the need to maintain employment.

These stressors might be buffered by periodic opportunities for respite care, which will enable the family to go out to the movies, shopping, or away for the weekend. Local and regional agencies or organizations *may* offer such programs, but usually at cost and without reliable insurance reimbursement. Some families are eligible for this option on the basis of their home care program or Medicaid waiver, but most would have to pay for the service, especially when it involves special care.

Before utilizing a particular respite program, the physician should investigate its appropriateness for the family with respect to cost and the potential for insurance reimbursement. In the absence of organized, professional respite services, the physician must remain attentive to family members' needs to "take a break" from the daily routine of caring for the medically involved child. The use of trained members of the extended family or other trained sitters might be one possibility.

## TRANSITION TO PUBLIC SCHOOL: THE CHILD WITH SPINA BIFIDA

In continuing with the critical transitions model, this section will discuss the home care treatment of the school-aged child with spina bifida. In addition to cerebral palsy and muscular dystrophy, spina bifida (neural tube defects) is one of the more frequently occurring handicapping conditions in childhood. The treatment of these conditions requires a long-term care program that considers the child's immediate needs along with those that will evolve as the child continues to develop. The physician will need to work closely with the public school system to coordinate the child's care such that the child will receive the "most appropriate" placement in the "least restrictive" setting (PL 94-142).

**Diagnosis.** Spina bifida occurs in approximately 1 per 1000 live births. Of these cases, 85% involve either anencephaly or myelomeningocele, with the former being uniformly lethal. Children with myelomeningocele may exhibit a variety of disabilities and handicaps, especially when there is involvement high on the spinal cord, significant bone deformity, and associated hydrocephalus. In 1975 there were estimated to be 58,000 children under 21 years of age in the United States with spina bifida.[43]

Today, survival of spina bifida infants has improved significantly with early aggressive treatment. However, a large proportion of these surviving children will have physical and intellectual handicaps, including reduced cognitive function and ambulation, restricted mobility, orthopedic complications, genitourinary dysfunction, hydrocephalus with shunting, and limited access to social and educational environments.[44, 45]

Prenatal diagnosis using maternal serum alpha-fetoprotein (MSAFP) screening of *all* pregnant women will reduce the incidence of cases gradually, but this approach finds only 75% to 80% of affected pregnancies. For families with a previously affected child, the recurrence risk is 1% to 3%, but may be further reduced by the use of supplemental preconceptual and prenatal multivitamins; folic acid may be the critical element.[46]

The range of physical complications includes the following:

| Complication | Management |
| --- | --- |
| • Hydrocephalus (75%–80%) | Ventriculoperitoneal shunt; monitor for obstructors and ventriculitis; need may spontaneously remit |
| • Paralysis (90%) | Prevention of complications (hip dislocation, knee contractures, and foot deformity) by position, physical/occupational therapy, bracing, and surgery |
| • Spinal deformity (15%–25%) | Closure of defect; removal of deformed vertebrae; bracing; and surgery |
| • Neurogenic bladder (90%) | Teach family and child Credé maneuver; straight metal catheterization; monitor for infection |
| • Bowel control (50%–70%) | Avoid overdistention; stool softeners, nutritional counseling, and suppositories, as needed |
| • Mental status | Wide range of cognitive ability; needs regular school placement (PL 94–142); maintain socialization with peers |
| • Sexual function | Family and peer group counseling; regular urologic or gynecologic examination |
| • Mobility | Major goal is ambulation, but some may be wheelchair bound; evaluate upper extremity function |

It is important to carefully evaluate and delineate the potential complications outlined above. However, the *main* goal of the habilitation program is to integrate the child into the family and community to the greatest degree possible. This includes attention to social and emotional reactions that may be caused by frequent hospitalizations, the potential segregation of the child from peer and sibling activities, and the quality of family coping with critical transitions.

There are many regional spina bifida clinics that have developed multidisciplinary teams to address these interrelated complications. They may be located in medical schools or rehabilitation centers of children's hospitals. These programs represent a tertiary center-based model in comprehensive care and are very effective in coordinating multiple specialists to address ongoing problems. However, there is still the real need for the practitioner to maintain the primary-care role in the child's community. The practitioner should establish this role with the team coordinator in order to receive timely reports and coordinate local community activities relating to school, recreation, and transportation.

**Adaptive Equipment.** Many children will require specially engineered equipment designed to meet both their current and changing needs. Some centers coordinate their orthotic and prosthetics services with rehabilitation engineering, but not consistently. It may be necessary to coordinate seating and wheelchair needs, braces, and adaptive devices (*e.g.,* computers) with the daily living activities and structural conditions of the child's home. The home should be made barrier-free to maximize the child's independence in activities of daily living. A home visit by the physician with an adaptive equipment consultant will facilitate the family's planning to meet these needs. Most insurance companies and Medicaid programs will cover the expenses incurred in the process of implementing structural changes.

**Family and School Environment.** Managing the needs of a child with spina bifida is challenging, but very satisfying as both the child and family progress toward independence and self-reliance. The goals of the program must be clearly delineated, organized by a problem list, and coordinated with the multidisciplinary team. Most importantly, the physician's role as advocate for the child in the community is essential. Dealing with community attitudes that tend to isolate children at school or insurance policies that attempt to withhold needed services may be effectively countered by the physician-advocate who is a part of that same community.

## SUMMARY

Throughout this chapter, we have highlighted a variety of issues that are essential to the development of comprehensive home care programs for medically involved and handicapped pediatric patients. In summary, it is important for the primary-care physician to consider each of the following:

• *Identification of existing programs, services, and resources within your service area*

The physician preparing to commit himself to providing home-based care for medically involved pediatric patients should become familiar with resources that are available in his region to address the family's major needs. Up-to-date information on the programs offered by state, local, and private agencies should be maintained at his office. The physician might identify a staff person in his office to be responsible for performing this function.

• *Addressing the multiple needs of the family*

The family and child's socioemotional, financial, educational, and medical needs must be addressed simultaneously, *prior* to the child's discharge from the hospital. The physician is advised to develop a working relationship with hospital discharge departments in his area to ensure a comprehensive, problem-oriented discharge plan for each child and family.

• *Home visits*

Ideally, the physician should make a predischarge home visit and should continue to see the family in the home as needed. We recognize that the time commitment required for a home visit is significant; in the case of comprehensive home care, "more is better." The information gathered in a single home visit will be invaluable and will enable the physician to plan more appropriate medical interventions for the child. It will also allow the physician to develop a sensitivity to the needs and capabilities of family members to participate in the home care program.

- *Physician as coordinator*

We recommend the use of the *physician-manager model* because it permits maximum involvement of the physician with the multiple aspects of the child's medical and associated treatments. The physician will need to maintain frequent contact with other professionals and paraprofessionals involved in the child's treatment. The child's chart should contain a comprehensive, up-to-date documentation for all related services the child is receiving, irrespective of whether the physician has prescribed them himself. It is recommended that the problem-oriented record be used for this purpose. Appropriate medical interventions must recognize all related issues for the family and child.

- *Periodic meetings with family members*

Periodic meetings can serve as a means for discussing the course of the child's home treatment, as well as any changes that may be required. Such meetings are particularly important during periods of *critical transitions* where new issues may be arising for the family. In the case of the pediatric patient, it is important to remember that a home care program will only be as successful as the family's willingness and capability to maintain the child at home.

## APPENDIX
### ADDITIONAL READING

The Association for the Care of Children's Health has published resources that address the needs of families caring for their handicapped child at home, including

The Chronically Ill Child and Family in the Community (1984)

Home Care for Children: An Annotated Bibliography (1984)

For information on these and other publications, contact: ACCH, 3615 Wisconsin Avenue, NW, Washington, DC, 20016; telephone (202) 244-1801.

Cohen S, Warren RD: Respite Care: Principles, Programs and Policies. Austin, TX, Pro-ed, 1985

Fewell R, Vadasy P: Families of Handicapped Children: Needs and Supports Across the Life Span. Austin, TX, Pro-ed, 1986

Gallagher J, Vietze P: Families of Handicapped Persons: Research, Programs, and Policy Issues. Baltimore, Paul H Brookes, 1986

Jones ML: Home Care for the Chronically Ill or Disabled Child: A Manual and Sourcebook for Parents and Professionals. New York, Harper & Row, 1985

Seligman M: The Family with a Handicapped Child: Understanding and Treatment. Orlando, FL, Grune & Stratton, 1983

### NATIONAL INFORMATION SOURCES

National Rehabilitation Information Center (NARIC)
Catholic University of America
4407 8th Street, NE
Washington, DC 20017

National Information Clearinghouse
  for Handicapped Children and Youth
PO Box 1492
Washington, DC 20013

Association for Child Advocates
3615 Superior Avenue
Building 31, Suite 2B
Cleveland, OH 44114

Spina Bifida Association of America
343 S Dearborn Street
Chicago, IL 60604
Telephone (312) 663-1562 or 1-(800) 621-3141

Sibling Information Network Newsletter
Department of Educational Psychology
Box U-64
University of Connecticut
Storrs, CT 06268

The Exceptional Parent
296 Boylston Street
3rd Floor
Boston, MA 02116

Library of Congress
Division for Blind and Physically Handicapped
1291 Taylor Street, NW
Washington, DC 20542

National Easter Seal Society
2023 West Ogden Avenue
Chicago, IL 60612

Office for Handicapped Individuals
United States Department of Health and Human
 Services
200 Independence Avenue, SW
Washington, DC 20201

## NATIONAL TOLL-FREE TELEPHONE NUMBERS

| | |
|---|---|
| American Council for the Blind | 800-424-8666 |
| Better Hearing Institute Hearing Helpline | 800-424-8576 |
| Center for Special Education Technology (in Northern Virginia) | 800-345-TECH 703-750-0500 |
| Children's Defense Fund | 800-424-9602 |
| Epilepsy Information Line | 800-426-0660 |
| Job Opportunities for the Blind | 800-638-7518 |
| National Cystic Fibrosis Foundation | 800-344-4823 |
| National Down's Syndrome Society | 800-221-4602 |
| National Easter Seal Society | 800-221-6827 |
| National Health Information Clearinghouse | 800-336-4797 |
| National Information Center for Educational Media | 800-421-8711 |
| National Rehabilitation Information Center | 800-34-NARIC |
| National Spinal Cord Injury Hotline | 800-526-3456 |
| Spina Bifida Hotline | 800-621-3141 |

## REFERENCES

1. Stein REK: Home care: A challenging opportunity. Children's Health Care 14(2):90–95, 1985
2. Ad Hoc Task Forces on Home Care of Chronically Ill Infants and Children: Guidelines for home care of infants, children, and adolescents with chronic disease. Pediatrics 74(3):434–436, 1984
3. Stein REK: Pediatric home care: An ambulatory "special care" unit. J Pediatr 92:495–499, 1983
4. Pierce P, Freedman S: The REACH Program: An innovative health delivery model for medically dependent children. Children's Health Care 12(7):86–89, 1983
5. Perrin JM, Ireys HT: The organization of services for chronically ill children and their families. Pediatr Clin North Am 31(1):235–257, 1984
6. Kanthor H, Pless B, Satterwhite B, Myers G: Areas of responsibility in the health care of multiply handicapped children. Pediatrics 54(6):729–785, 1974
7. MacKirth H: Editorial: The buck stops. Dev Med Child Neurol 11:691–692, 1969
8. Pless IB, Roghman KJ: Chronic illness and its consequences: Observation based on three epidemiologic surveys. J Pediatr 28:387–392, 1971
9. Battle CU: The role of the pediatrician as ombudsman in the health care of the young handicapped child. Pediatrics 56(6):916–922, 1972
10. Breslau N: Continuity reexamined: Differential impact on satisfaction with medical care for disabled and normal children. Med Care 20(4):347–359, 1982
11. Carlova J: Make the most of the home care boom. Medical Economics February:129–141, 1986
12. Pless IB: Individual and family needs in the health care of children with developmental disorders. Birth Defects 12(4):91–102, 1976

13. Solnit AJ, Stark MH: Mourning the birth of a defective child. Psychological Study of the Child 16:523–537, 1961

14. Allen DA, Hudd SS: Are we professionalizing parents? Weighing the benefits and pitfalls. Ment Retard, *in press*

15. Blacher J: A dynamic perspective on the impact of a severely handicapped child on the family. In Blacher J (ed): Severely Handicapped Young Children and Their Families, pp 3–50. Orlando, Academic Press, 1984

16. Salk L, Hilgartner M, Granich B: The psychosocial impact of hemophilia on the patient and his family. Soc Sci Med 6:491–505, 1972

17. Seligman M (ed): The Family with a Handicapped Child: Understanding and Treatment. New York, Grune & Stratton, 1983

18. Caldwell BM, Guze SB: A study of the adjustment of parents and siblings of institutionalized and noninstitutionalized retarded children. Am J Ment Defic 64:845–861, 1960

19. Baum MH: Some dynamic factors affecting family adjustment to the handicapped child. Except Child 28:387–392, 1962

20. Laborde PR, Seligman M: Individual counseling with parents of handicapped children: Rationale and strategies. In Seligman M (ed): The Family With a Handicapped Child: Understanding and Treatment, pp 261–284. New York, Grune & Stratton, 1983

21. Lamb ME: Fathers of exceptional children. In Seligman M (ed): The Family With a Handicapped Child: Understanding and Treatment, pp 125–146. New York, Grune & Stratton, 1983

22. Lamb ME: Paternal influences in child development: An overview. In Lamb ME (ed): The Role of the Father in Child Development, rev ed. New York, Wiley, 1981

23. Grossman F: Brothers and Sisters of Retarded Children: An Exploratory Study. Syracuse, Syracuse University Press, 1982

24. Blackhard MK, Barsch ET: Parents' and professionals' perceptions of the handicapped child's impact on the family. Journal of the Association for the Severely Handicapped 7(2):62–69, 1982

25. Stein REK, Jessops DJ: Issues in the care of children with chronic physical conditions. Pediatr Clin North Am 31(1):189–198, 1984

26. Turnbull AP, Turnbull HR: Parent involvement: A critique. Ment Retard 20:115–122, 1982

27. Buckholtz K: Fragile children: Brandon. Caring 4(5):8–10, 1985

28. Cabin B: Private health care coverage for children. Caring 4:53–56, 1985

29. Castellani PJ: Policy perspectives on the economics of mental retardation: The new environment of developmental services. Ment Retard 24:5–7, 1986

30. Dixon MS: United States health programs for children. Pediatr Clin North Am 27:633–640, 1981

31. Agosta J: Personal communication, 1985

32. O'Connor FP: Education for the handicapped child. In Downey JA, Low NL (eds): The Child With Disabling Illness: Principles of Rehabilitation, pp 579–604. Philadelphia, WB Saunders, 1974

33. Hobbs N, Perrin JM, Ireys HT: Ill Children and Their Families. San Francisco, Jossey-Bass Publishers, 1985

34. Shonkoff JP: A perspective on pediatric training. In Mulick J, Pueschel SM (eds): Parent-Professional Partnerships in Developmental Disabilities Services, pp 75–88. Cambridge, MA, Academic Guild Publishers, 1983

35. Bennett FC: Early Intervention: Rationales and Practical Guidelines to Prevent or Ameliorate Developmental Disabilities. Children Are Different: Behavioral Development Monograph Series: Number 10. Columbus, OH, Ross Laboratories, 1984

**36.** Weed LL: Appendix. Medical Records, Medical Education and Patient Care. Cleveland, OH, Case Western University Press, 1971

**37.** Bjorn J, Cross H: Problem-Oriented Practice. Chicago, Modern Hospital Press, 1970

**38.** Thompson J, Thompson M: Genetics in Medicine, pp 142–180. Philadelphia, WB Saunders, 1980

**39.** Farrell P, Palta M: BPD and Related Chronic Respiratory Disorders. 90th Ross Conference on Pediatric Research, pp 1–6, 1986

**40.** Pinney M, Cotton E: Home Management of BPD. Pediatrics 58:856, 1976

**41.** Campbell A, Zarfin Y, Groenveld M, Bryan M: Low flow oxygen therapy in infants. Arch Dis Child 58:795, 1983

**42.** Taussig L: Long-term Management of BPD. 90th Ross Conference on Pediatric Research, pp 126–133, 1986

**43.** Paul MA, Piazza F: Costs of treating birth defects in state CCS. Public Health Rep 94:420–424, 1979

**44.** Myers GJ: Myelomeningocele: The medical aspects. Pediatr Clin North Am 31(1):165–175, 1984

**45.** Bowser B, Solis I: Pediatric rehabilitation. In Halstead LS, Grabois M (eds): Medical Rehabilitation, pp 265–277. New York, Raven Press, 1985

**46.** Smithells R, Sheppard S, Schorah C et al: Apparent prevention of neural tube defects by periconceptual vitamin supplementation. Arch Dis Child 59:911–918, 1981

# PART 4

# Issues in Home Care

# 22

# Psychosocial Issues

## MACK LIPKIN, JR.
## SARAH WILLIAMS

This chapter presents an overview of the psychosocial issues that primary-care personnel face in providing home care. It begins with a brief overview of psychosocial aspects of care in general. It then identifies and describes those generic aspects of home care that present distinct issues of assessment and management. It closes with a discussion of psychosocial aspects of special home care situations such as the care of the dying patient, the infectious patient, acquired immune deficiency syndrome (AIDS) patients, and the like. The chapter is designed to be clinically useful. As such, it avoids theoretical discussion and controversy, and instead attempts to focus the reader to deal usefully with the practical complexities of this increasingly important modality of general medical care.

## PSYCHOSOCIAL ASPECTS OF PRIMARY CARE

Primary care is defined as ongoing, continuous, first-contact, general care in which the physician acts as advocate for the patient, coordinates all care, and engages in acute and chronic illness care, preventive care, and health maintenance.[1] Paramount in primary care is the doctor–patient relationship since this is the "medium" in which all care occurs.[2] Home care, whether for a severe or debilitating chronic illness such as severe rheumatoid arthritis or a demyelinating disease or for a terminal illness such as breast cancer or AIDS, is a form of primary care but with a difference. For in home care the primary-care provider and team must focus not only on the patient's needs but also, in order to make it work, on the needs of the home environment as well. Thus, the psychosocial aspects of primary home care include care for the psychological aspects of the patient with respect to the illness, attention to the homeostasis of the patient in the home environment, and attention to the needs of those at home required for the care of the patient.

## PSYCHOLOGICAL AND SOCIAL ADAPTATIONS TO ILLNESS

Every illness includes psychological and social dimensions. The skilled practitioner recognizes that these include both predictable reactions to the objective situation and personal and idiosyncratic reactions based on the prior experience of the patient and his or her personality style. Each of these passes, over time, through a series of stages and adaptations. Since the significance of an illness may be more painful or distressing to the patient than the actual physical aspects, it is a central part of care to ascertain the patient's psychological reactions to the illness and to intervene skillfully to promote the most comforting and growth-producing adaptation possible.

In this section, we will address the general, predictable reactions to illness. In a later section, we focus on specific personality styles and how they help determine *individual* reactions to illness.

**319**

### Grief, Fear, Loss

Every illness beyond the trivial is accompanied by some degree of loss. The patient at the very least loses a personal image of invulnerability; at worst, he or she becomes aware of severely threatened mortality. In between is a spectrum of losses, such as loss of attractiveness, of an important role (*e.g.,* breadwinner, parent, pillar of community, etc.), or even of a body part. With such, there is deviation from one's idealized sense of self and with this also comes loss. This concept of loss is an important aspect of reaction to illness, which is often not sufficiently recognized.

Every loss results in grief.[3,4] Unlike depression, discussed below, grief is a normal and not a pathologic response. It is a natural response to loss, which includes stages of initial shock or numbness, denial, anger, questioning, bargaining, and acceptance. Affects observed and experienced during grief are numerous and labile. The "stages," typically, are not linear but rather mixed together. It is natural to expect sadness, tearfulness, anger, withdrawal, and shame. To a lesser extent, these same reactions occur with recurrent episodes of the same illness and to progressive events in a deteriorating illness.

The reason for stressing the normality of grief is that, in healthy persons, grief is handled healthily and does not require specific intervention. In fact, the appropriate role of the primary-care provider is to facilitate the patient's and others' approach to healing grief rather than to exacerbate, prolong, or inflame it through excessive or invasive examination or through denial.

In order to facilitate natural healing of grief, certain information is useful, namely, what is the patient's normal response to and mode of management of grief. The best index of this is prior response. If one has known the patient a long time, this will be known from prior experiences shared mutually (one more advantage of the primary-care relationship). If it has not been previously shared, inquiry concerning prior losses will reveal how the patient reacted, for example, to loss of a parent or grandparent, to prior severe illness, and so on.

Some but not all patients also respond to illness with fear. This too is natural, especially when the prognosis is serious, includes pain or loss of function or life, or is unknown. Again, normally patients respond to fear appropriately in ways that contain and manage it. In doing so, they may draw on varied resources. Some find knowledge useful (the unknown being frightening for these persons). Others find faith useful, feeling the doctor, fate, or God will take care of future problems. Many simply use denial in a healthy way.

Here, the physician's role is to ascertain how the patient is reacting, and to learn what is the patient's way of coping with such reactions. Then it is possible to "prescribe" or "administer" what is needed, be it clarification, reassurance, confidence, or support for denial by avoidance of the feared issues. The key point here is that the basic approach to grief and to fear is to enhance the patient's own healthy responses. It is not helpful to introduce one's own needs into the situation, for example, by denying sadness or shame in an effort to get on with medical matters or to unnecessarily confront the *patient's* denial due to one's own need to confront difficult issues.

### Anxiety and Depression

While loss, grief, and fear are normal reactions to illness that usually are self-limited and require modest intervention, anxiety and depression are psychopathologic reactions that demand more definitive diagnosis and treatment.

Depression is a potentially serious complication of illness, occurring in 35% of hospitalized patients and in an uncertain but high percentage of nonhospitalized patients with chronic diseases. Depression is best understood as a disease with biologic, psychological and social aspects. The biologic aspects include any disturbance of sleep (*i.e.,* not just early morning awakening but difficulty falling asleep or frequent wakening), loss of libido, and appetite disturbance with possible weight loss. Psychological aspects include, most importantly, anhedonia (loss of ability to experience pleasure), guilt and remorse, and dysphoria or sadness. Social aspects include withdrawal, elimination of contact with subsequent isolation, and consequent loss of social functioning. Depressed patients frequently somaticize, so that evaluation of symptomatology in such patients is complicated.[5]

Suicide also occurs in depressed patients and is always to be borne in mind. Suicide is most likely to occur in patients in the middle decades who are recovering from depression, who have a suicide plan and the means to execute it, who are isolated, who use alcohol or drugs excessively, who have poor impulse control, or who are very angry.[6]

As depression and normal grief have many features in common, they can at times be difficult to distinguish, particularly because sick people may have many of the classic "vegetative" signs of depression that are caused by the illness itself. The problem is compounded by the common response to a depressed and ill person that "anyone in that situation would be depressed." While anyone in an illness situation may be *sad and grieving,* he or she will *not* be *depressed* unless there are other intervening factors. Usually this happens when the loss created by an illness has an idiosyncratic, symbolic, and painful significance for the patient or the patient is vulnerable to depression due to heredity or a depression history. In any case, as noted above, it is very important to make this distinction and several concepts help. First, while the sick person may be sad about the illness situation, he or she does not express the generalized feelings of self-blame and unworthiness common in depression. Second, one usually comes away from contact with a sad and grieving person feeling touched and empathetic. However, despite the unrelenting woe expressed by depressed people, one sometimes comes away feeling annoyed and as if there were a "willful" quality to their suffering. This subjective response, when recognized, can be a useful guide. Finally, further explanation of how the patient is perceiving and interpreting the illness may reveal that some aspect of the illness is interacting with previous unresolved painful experiences to produce depression.

Care for depression in physically ill patients has three elements: pharmacotherapy, psychological care, and environmental manipulation. First-line pharmacotherapy is indicated if the patient has prominent biologic aspects of the depression, if the depression is not apparently reactive, and if other interventions are not working. The usual first-choice drugs are the tricyclic antidepressants. The tricyclic with the fewest side-effects should be chosen unless one wishes to utilize one of the side-effects for therapeutic benefit. Thus, one would use desipramine initially for most patients. In those who require an effective hypnotic, however, amitriptyline might be chosen. Doses are begun low, especially in older patients, and titrated upward. Response does not occur immediately but takes from 2 to 4 weeks. If one tricyclic fails, a second may be tried before seeking a different class of drugs. In cases in which an immediate response is indicated, a phenothiazine (such as thioridazine) may be used in the period in which one is awaiting effect of the tricyclic. Electroshock therapy is very useful when reserved for patients in whom drugs are contraindicated, in whom drugs fail, or in life-threatening situations. Of course, it is essential to review for and eliminate drugs that cause depression.[7]

The psychological treatment of the depressed physically ill patient, although a complex matter, essentially consists of systematic support and acknowledgment of the depressed feelings while reframing them in a nondepressed mode. That is, depressed patients tend to view problems as insurmountable, as their fault, and to see themselves as inadequate to live an effective and pleasurable existence. These perceptions must be systematically and gently corrected. The key is frequent, supportive discussion. While explorative or psychodynamically oriented psychotherapy may be useful in the long term to deal with underlying problems, it is not helpful in the short term for depressed patients.

The central social intervention in depressed patients is to prevent or alter their patterns of isolation. Finding ways for the patient to see others and to be involved with them helps enormously and is central to stable recovery. Clearly, the home care patient has a special need in this regard. Attention to prevention of social isolation is a key feature of effective prevention in home care. Steps to accomplish this include careful elicitation of who will be visiting, checking to see that they are in fact doing so, and assessment of the patient's reactions to his or her new social position after the patient has been in home care for several weeks and again after several months. The patient's views of these issues will vary as a result of the stage of reaction to illness. Hence, this must be ascertained and factored into interpretation of the patient's reactions to the illness and must be done repetitively.

Anxiety, like depression, is a pathologic response to illness that needs to be distinguished from normal fear. It results typically from a conflict, created by the illness situation, with which the patient is unable to cope. It may be fear of such proportions that the patient feels he or she will panic or decompensate if expression is given to the fear. It may result from feelings that the patient will be abandoned, will be unable to prevent shameful occurrences, and so on. Usually, discussion of the fears and concerns of the patient will reveal the origins of the anxiety and provide the basis for its relief. In general, in primary care, most anxiety is related to phobic fears and this may also be the case for illness-related anxiety. If so, simple discussion may not suffice and the patient may require some form of desensitization, a therapy some primary-care physicians are trained to provide but that often requires the services of a mental health specialist.

In general, use of anxiolytics for illness-induced anxiety is a misuse. It is far safer, definitive, and curative to explore and intervene psychologically. However, if anxiety is acute, incapacitating, creates detrimental insomnia, or the like, then short-term anxiolytic therapy may be appropriate. Panic attacks sometimes occur and may be manifest as somatization. For these patients, tricyclic therapy may be appropriate.[8]

### Stages of Reaction to Illness

The stages of reaction to illness have been briefly described above and are well known to most practitioners: shock or numbness, denial, anger, bargaining, "why me," and acceptance and accommodation. What is less clear to many is that these are not linear stages. That is, each patient does not go through each stage sequentially. Rather, the patient is in different reaction modes with respect to different aspects of his life, psychology, and social system. A person may be angry at loss of work, denying loss of sexual ability or attractiveness, numb concerning potential loss of life, and angry at pain. Nor does a patient necessarily progress from one reaction mode to the next. Hence, assessment of a patient's reactions must be recurrent and must be made specifically in regard to the specific area of importance for a particular discussion or decision process.

### Social Support and the Support System

The support system of a person includes all those persons and institutions with which the patient has significant positive and negative interaction. Typically this includes family, friends, neighbors, work and co-workers, the relevant government systems, and financial and other institutions. Interestingly, each of these shifts significantly when a person becomes ill. Work, for example, becomes a setting that may be threatening to the patient since there is a need from those at work that the patient either return to work or not drain their resources unduly.

Friends typically shift during illness. Normally, each person has a balance among friends between those who primarily give and those who primarily take from the patient. When the patient becomes less able to give due to illness, or is less able to be depended on and instead must depend on others, those who used to take from the patient fall away and those who mainly like to be depended on or to give become more prominent. Thus, assessment of the social system must also be made initially and recurrently as it shifts. Patients may feel strongly about the changing balance among their friends and may feel hurt or bereft that some have abandoned them. It is very useful to anticipate and discuss this as a normal process. The patient, however, may also have difficulty accepting the altered dependency relationships occasioned by the illness. In this case, work on these issues will be necessary over time, including allowing the patient to grieve the changes, in order to move through the stages of grief and come to accept them.

Likewise, the patient frequently must establish relationships with the family that are altered or new. For those with whom family ties are close, warm, and healthily interdependent, the adjustment should be allowed to develop naturally. However, often such is not the case. Prior knowledge of the family relations is the best guide to the need for family interventions. Prior history (as elicited from patient and family in the present) is next best. An approach to elicitation of this history should be established and practiced. It begins with open-ended and structural inquiry ("tell me about your family...." "Who is in the family...." "Tell me about...."). Direct questions about caring behaviors are useful, such as "What happens in your family when someone takes sick." Questions about problems and sensitivity to indirect cues about problems are paramount in importance, since one does not want to make untoward assumptions about caring relationships that will embarrass the patient or family or make the patient feel that you are unable to accept the realities of family conflict. Further discussion about the interaction with the family is given below.

There are no useful generalizations about the make-up of the functional support system of the home care patient. Rather, one has to find out from experience who will be useful. This applies not only to the family but to friends, neighbors, and all classes of health personnel. Some are useful, others not. While role definitions may be important, commitment and availability are more so and seem to us to be independent of discipline or title. The primary-care team must therefore attempt to ascertain those who will be helpful and involve them, and quickly move past those who are not.

Finally, each case, illness, and individual requires unique constellations of involvement with public and private agencies in the community, as discussed in Chapter 5. However, in addition to agencies related to paying for and procuring basic medical and nursing needs, self-help and support groups in the specific disease category are important to be informed about and to access for or with the patient. Also, groups that provide ongoing social contacts may be very useful to some patients.

## MENTAL DISORDER

The occurrence of mental disorder in home care patients has not been well studied. Therefore, we must rely on general and hospital experience, tempered by knowledge of the illness types involved in home care. In general, due to the isolation, stress of the illness, enhanced dependency, and the complexity of treatments with their own toxic psychosocial effects, home care patients are at risk for mental disorder.

### PSYCHIATRIC PROBLEMS IN GENERAL

The recent studies emanating from the National Institute of Mental Health (NIMH), the Epidemiologic Catchment Area (ECA) studies, give us our clearest picture of the general occurrence of mental disorders.[9,10] Overall, the lifetime prevalence of mental disorder in the general United States population is about 32%; that is, one is likely to find that one of the thirteen most common mental disorders has occurred at some time in 32% of adults. The lifetime prevalences of the individual disorders are shown in Table 22-1. Note that anxiety disorders, substance abuse, and depression are the most prevalent. Among anxiety disor-

**TABLE 22-1. LIFETIME PREVALENCES (PROPORTION OF SURVIVORS AFFECTED) OF MENTAL DISORDER**

| Disorder | Percent Affected |
|---|---|
| Any disorder | 32.8% |
| Substance abuse | 16.7% |
| Alcohol | 13.6% |
| Drug | 5.6% |
| Affective disorders | 7.7% |
| Major depressive | 5.2% |
| Manic | 0.9% |
| Anxiety (two thirds phobia; 10% panic) | 15.9% |
| Antisocial personality | 2.6% |
| Schizophrenia | 1.6% |
| Cognitive impairment | 1.2% |

Epidemiologic Catchment Area Study (NIMH); n = 9543 (Baltimore, St Louis, New Haven)

ders, phobias are most common; alcoholism is the most significant substance abuse; and unipolar depression accounts for most of the depression seen in the population.

Table 22-2 shows that the 6-month prevalences do not alter the picture significantly. The table gives the frequencies in the last 6 months of the listed disorders in the general population. The results are probably a more accurate picture of what to expect in the home or the office. Here, the most important observations are that anxiety-related problems are most prevalent, the affective disorders include primarily depression, and depression is most prevalent in women, whereas alcoholism and antisocial personality disorders are more prevalent among men.

There are several reasons that detection of mental disorder is of importance in home care. Foremost, of course, is that specific treatment may be of help to the patient's sense of well-being and for the relief of suffering. Secondly, it may be essential for adequate pursuit of care in other domains. The phobic or anxious patient may be unable to attend to self-care. The depressed patient with pseudodementia or psychomotor retardation will be unable to participate consistently in difficult routines or self-monitoring and may contribute to self-destruction through omission of aspects of care. These are problems treatment will erase! Of course, the home care patient is at risk for problems associated with isolation and

**TABLE 22-2. SIX-MONTH PREVALENCES OF MENTAL DISORDER (OVERALL, 19%)**

| Disorder | Percent Affected |
|---|---|
| Anxiety | 8% |
| Phobia | 5.5% |
| Panic | 1.5% |
| Alcoholism | 5.5% |
| Major depression | 6.5% (female/male = 2) |
| Schizophrenia | 1% |
| Antisocial | 1% |
| Sex | Women (phobias, depression, dysthymia) |
| | Men (alcohol, phobia, drug abuse, antisocial, dysthymia) |
| Age | Depression greatest age 18–44, least over age 65 |
| | Substance abuse decreased after age 44 |
| | Drugs greatest age 18–24 |

Epidemiologic Catchment Area Study (NIMH); n = 9543

decreased stimulation such as transient psychosis due to disorientation (the home equivalent of "sun downing"). In such situations, confidence about the baseline mental condition of the patient can circumvent much unnecessary uncertainty about preexisting psychosis, for example. Finally, most patients with mental disorders are at risk for somatization, which may complicate evaluation. Here again, awareness of increased probability of somatization will be helpful. (Somatization is discussed in detail below.)

## GENERALISTS AND SPECIALISTS IN MENTAL HEALTH CARE

One of the major areas of uncertainty in the care of patients at home concerns the relative responsibilities of practitioners of diverse disciplinary backgrounds. It is now the case that about 25% of patients with defined mental disorders obtain care from mental health specialists. Yet, because of their personal preferences and their models of care, most mental health specialists will not get involved in home care. Also, about 60% of patients with mental disorder are cared for only by primary-care personnel. In short, it is very likely that much of the care of psychological difficulties of home care patients will fall on the shoulders of primary-care personnel. Thus, it is important that the roles of the members of the team be defined with respect to the care of any identified problems and that explicit discussion occur between physicians, nurses, social workers, and others involved in the case. Items to agree about include how monitoring of psychosocial adjustment will be accomplished; what definitions of problems will be used (*i.e.,* it is important everyone call the same problems by the same names so as not to confuse or upset the patient and the family); how support will be given—since it is futile to have one group of providers fostering independence at the same time another group is fostering dependency; and how problems will be solved. Clear communication of these decisions among the team members, clear liaison with the family or other supporters, and clear lines for further communication also greatly facilitate the successful development of the care over time.

## PSYCHOSOCIAL COMPLICATIONS OF CARE

### MENTAL STATUS

As noted above, alterations of mental status, particularly the acute and potentially reversible alteration known as delirium, are common in sick patients. Since there is much confusion about the definitions of the various types of organic mental syndromes, we will start with some brief definitions.

### *Organic Mental Syndrome*

The hallmark of organic mental (or brain) syndrome is a deterioration in mental status, involving intellectual function, personality, and affect to varying degrees, that is caused by known or postulated physical changes in the brain or its environment. The organic brain syndromes are generally divided into those states that are chronic and irreversible (the dementias) and those that are acute and, at least potentially, reversible (delirium). However, there is some overlap between these states in that certain conditions that are at first treatable may cause a delirium or a dementia-like picture that ultimately becomes chronic and fixed if not treated (*i.e.,* $B_{12}$ deficiency, chronic alcoholism).

### *Dementia*

Dementia is a deterioration of mental status caused by irreversible, pathologic changes in brain tissue. The mental impairment, which may be mild to severe, affects a wide range of functions, including intellect (impairment of memory, orientation, logical thinking, and judgment), personality, and affect (most commonly inappropriateness or lability of affect).

Unlike delirium, dementia does *not* involve a change in the level of consciousness, nor do the patients hallucinate. They are, however, liable to have delusions, especially paranoid ones, which are very distressing to the family.[11]

### Causes of dementia include

Alzheimer's disease

Multi-infarct dementia

Communicating hydrocephalus

Alcoholic (Korsakoff's)

Post-traumatic

Huntington's disease

Parkinsonism

Uncommon causes: infections (syphilis, Creutzfeldt-Jakob, etc.), inflammatory vascular diseases, degenerative diseases (Pick's, multiple sclerosis, ALS, etc.)

The first two causes listed account for about 60% of dementias, followed in frequency by hydrocephalus and Korsakoff's dementia. As noted above, a number of other deficiency states and metabolic abnormalities can lead to chronic dementia if left uncorrected.

**Diagnosis.** While a severe and even moderate dementia is obvious to everyone, early or mild cases may be quite subtle. Early diagnosis is important for several reasons. First of all, if the dementia is due to an ongoing insult, such as alcohol or multiple cerebral (*e.g.,* hypertensive) infarctions, its progression may be arrested by stopping the insult (*e.g.,* abstinence, control of blood pressure). Secondly, if superimposed reversible insults are identified, these can be treated, with consequent improvements in the patient's status (see Delirium, below). Thirdly, the family can be prepared for probable further deterioration. Finally, one can begin to manage the patient and the environment and to improve and maintain function as much as possible. Diagnosis is made mainly by mental status evaluation, both formal and informal. Formal tests of mental status include memory, orientation, and tasks requiring concentration and calculating ability. Equally useful are informal, but careful, observations of the patient's communication. Such things as vagueness with lack of detail and description, circumstantiality, perseveration, and word finding problems are all good clues. (Early on, one may also see the converse: an obsessive attention to details with list-keeping, and so on, in the patient with early dementia who is desperately trying to cope with loss of memory.) Finally, those who know the patient well may observe subtle changes in personality or a lack of concern for social appropriateness and grooming.

A frequent problem in diagnosis is "pseudodementia," an apparent dementia that is really caused by severe depression (particularly because depression itself is common in dementia). Differentiating these two is difficult; it may be helped by a specialized psychiatrist and frequently also requires a trial of antidepressants.

Problems caused by dementia follow from the deficits: depression, apathy and withdrawal, disorientation (often with agitation and especially at night), tendencies to wander (which may require constant supervision), and incontinence. In addition, witnessing the deterioration of a loved one is usually quite distressing to the family, and care of such patients exhausts the most caring homes. (See Management of Dementia for recommendations for care of patients.)

### Delirium

Delirium is an acute, potentially reversible alteration of mental status that *does* involve a change of consciousness (from simple sleepiness to obtundation, stupor, and even coma). Other prominent features of delirium include hallucination, marked variability in degree of

## MANAGEMENT OF DEMENTIA

1. Search for and correct contributing factors.
2. Maintain a familiar and constant environment, with the same care givers as much as possible.
3. Frequent orientation by care givers ('My name is . . . , it's 12 o'clock, time for lunch . . . , today is . . . ,'' etc.). A radio or television is also helpful, as is an easily seen calendar.

4. Keep a night light on at night.
5. If patients are very agitated, small doses of a phenothiazine (such as Stelazine) or Haldol are effective and preferable to other sedatives, which may worsen confusion.

(Reproduced by permission of Mack Lipkin, Jr.)

---

impairment and level of consciousness, and deficits of all intellectual functions (because of the global changes in brain function).

Like dementia, delirium can be flagrant or subtle and may require considerable attention to diagnose, especially in the patient who responds by becoming withdrawn. In such cases, diagnosis is made by repeated examinations of mental status, especially of level of consciousness, orientation, and memory. The patient should also be specifically asked about hallucinations.[12] Confirmatory neurologic findings are asterixis and multifocal myoclonus. The list of conditions that can cause delirium is long (see Causes of Delirium). Fortunately, most can be quickly ruled out by the history, physical examination, and basic laboratory tests.

Since drugs and medications are among the commonest causes of delirium, the evaluation of a homebound patient with delirium must always include a review of the bedside table and medicine cabinets (as well as assessment of alcohol and other drug use). Benzodiazepines are frequent offenders, particularly those with long half-lives (*e.g.,* Valium and Librium), which accumulate in the body and therefore lead to delirium only after several days of use. For this reason, if benzodiazepines are used, the shorter-acting ones (*e.g.,* lorazepam, oxazepam) are preferable.

A final important point is that the traditional teaching of "one cause to one disease" does not always hold in delirium. Sometimes delirium may result from the additive effects of a number of smaller deficits, none of which would be sufficient in itself to impair mental status. Thus, an elderly patient (already operating at the limit of mental capacity) who has a

---

## CAUSES OF DELIRIUM

Intracranial
  Epilepsy and postictal states
  Trauma
  Infection
  Hemorrhage
  Neoplasms

Extracranial
  Drugs (and drug withdrawal)
  Poisons

Endocrine dysfunction (hypofunction or hyperfunction)
  Pituitary
  Pancreas
  Adrenal
  Parathyroid
  Thyroid

Disease of nonendocrine organs
  Liver (hepatic encephalopathy)
  Kidney (uremic encephalopathy)
  Lung (hypoxia, hypercarbia)
  Cardiovascular (heart failure, persistent arrhythmias, hypotension)

Deficiency diseases
  Thiamine
  Vitamin $B_{12}$

Systemic illness or stress (fever, sepsis, anemia, dehydration, starvation)

Electrolyte imbalance

Postoperative states

mild anemia and a slightly decreased $PO_2$ who gets a viral gastroenteritis and becomes slightly hyponatremic, may become temporarily delirious.

Treatment for delirium involves, first and foremost, identifying and treating the cause or causes as quickly as possible. Other measures for managing the delirious patient while the cause is being sought and corrected are those given under Management of Dementia.

### Depression

Depression has been dealt with earlier. We mention it again here simply to emphasize that it is a not uncommon complication of chronic illness that needs to be differentiated from the normal grief reactions to the losses involved in being ill.

### Pain

Pain is ubiquitous in patients with both acute and chronic illness and its skillful management can make a great difference to the patient. Therefore, we deal here with the basic principles underlying effective pain treatment. The technical details of management are well described in standard literature.

Pain is a subjective phenomenon that cannot be measured objectively. The same stimulus will cause different amounts of pain in different people and even in the same person at different times. The subjective pain experienced is very dependent on the significance of the pain. For example, if the patient fears that a new pain signifies a progression of disease or has other frightening implications, the pain will feel much more severe.

Pain is also influenced by other emotional variables as much as by the pain stimulus itself. These other variables include depression, anger, fear, and anxiety. This has been well illustrated by the large number of studies demonstrating that preoperative preparation for surgery (reassurance, description of what is going to happen, etc.) consistently reduces postoperative analgesic requirements by 30% to 50%.[13] A major and avoidable source of fear and anxiety in patients with pain is the fear that their next dose of pain medication will not be there when they need it!

There are several implications for treatment derivable from these principles. First, the patient's subjective experience of pain needs to be taken seriously as significant for that patient. One way to get a more generalizable picture is to ask the patient how the present pain compares to common pain experiences such as breaking a bone or giving birth. Whenever possible, the source of pain should be explained to the patient in a way that is constructive and demystifying. For instance, a patient with cancer may interpret the pain as a sign that "the cancer is eating away at my stomach," accompanied by an appropriately horrifying vision of what this means. The care giver can explain that the pain is caused by the tumor putting pressure on the nerve endings or stretching the covering of the stomach, thus providing understandable and manageable images that do not signify disaster.

Secondly, while the onset or escalation of pain may be due to a pathophysiologic change, it is just as likely to be due to psychosocial factors. Fear or anxiety about the illness or its treatment, approaching death, grief about a deterioration in function, loneliness or other interpersonal difficulties, and unresolved conflicts and depression can all lead to a worsening of pain. Thus, any unexplained increase in pain or analgesia requirement should lead to an exploration of these factors. An empathetic discussion of the patient's feelings or an improvement in the social environment (as well as pharmacologic treatment of depression or anxiety as indicated) can save many milligrams of narcotic.

An often overlooked option in the treatment of pain, especially chronic pain, is the use of nonpharmacologic measures such as relaxation training. Use of self-hypnosis, meditation, or the relaxation response can provide self-mastery and good pain control.

A third important aspect of pain treatment is the effective use of the placebo effect. Irrefutable major studies have shown that a consistent 30% to 40% of patients get significant relief from placebos, *regardless* of pain etiology. This does *not* mean that such patients do not have real pain, but rather that for many people the positive expectation of relief is in itself capable of producing relief.

The treatment implication of this is that the caring, confident, and positive expectations on the part of the care giver create a powerful "placebo effect" that can and should be used whenever pain, or any symptom, is treated.[14]

Finally, the proper amount, timing, and scheduling of analgesics are crucial for getting maximum benefit. Many people fear that providing an adequate amount of pain medication on a regular basis will lead to the creation of addicts. In fact, the converse is true. The most powerful reinforcer of drug-seeking behavior is this cycle:

pain—anxiety—drug-obtaining behavior—relief

However, if patients are provided with adequate medication on a regular schedule (instead of "prn"), the escalating pain and anxiety are avoided, as is the need for whatever behaviors the patient has evolved to try to convince those in charge of the medicine that he or she is truly in pain. Regular use of analgesics may in fact reduce analgesic requirements.

It is usually better to start on the higher side with analgesia when treating significant pain; once the patient is relaxed and confident that the relief is available and the medicine works, the amount can be decreased as appropriate. This works much better than the opposite approach of starting with an insufficient amount and building up.

## PERSONALITY STYLE

While many of the problems imposed by serious or chronic illness are universal, there is a great deal of variation in the ways people respond to and cope with these. Therefore, variation in the management style is needed to help each particular person cope. Much of this variation is a function of the personality style of the patient. Personality style refers to a constellation of behaviors, feelings, ways of thinking about and perceiving the world, and of interacting with others that characterize the person described. We have found that an acquaintance with the major personality styles helps the clinician understand why a given person is relating to an illness in the way he or she is and what kind of interventions will be most helpful. While most people have a mixture of styles, one usually predominates in a given area (such as responding to an illness).[15]

## HYSTERICAL STYLE

One of the more common personality styles, the hysterical, is characterized by a strong focus on feelings by the patient. Such persons have little interest in facts or tedious details. Instead, they focus on overall impressions usually conveyed in extreme terms (the "best doctor," the "worst pain"). While usually charming, always engaging, and relating well, the hysterical person is very afraid of genuine intimacy and may flee when a relationship gets too close. Because of their overwhelming desire to please, they can be very misleading historians, as they will say whatever they think you want to hear (such as a perfect description of ischemic chest pain if they sense that is what you are getting at!). Therefore, one important aspect of dealing with hysterical patients is to ask open-ended questions and avoid leading them in interviews. Another aspect is that, unlike obsessives, hysterical people are made very anxious by being given a lot of factual information about their illness, upcoming tests, and so on. They do much better with general reassurance in the climate of a warm, caring relationship with the care giver. While they do flourish with an interested care giver, care must be taken not to go beyond the amount of closeness they can tolerate, even though they may seem to be wanting this closeness (by asking the doctor about personal matters, complimenting his or her clothes, etc.).

One additional characteristic of hysterical patients that makes their recognition even more important is that they frequently somatize.

## OBSESSIVE–COMPULSIVE STYLE

Another of the more common styles, the obsessive–compulsive patient is familiar to all practitioners. This is the patient who arrives in the doctor's office with a carefully prepared list of problems and proceeds through the list of symptoms in tedious and maddening detail. In contrast to the hysteric, the obsessive person is *highly* focused on facts and details, sometimes to the exclusion of feelings, impressions, or of "seeing the whole picture." Obsessive–compulsive patients are generally neat, organized, and very careful about time, and in fact rely on a sense of order in all aspects of life. When functioning well, they make model patients because of their scrupulous compliance. (They also make excellent engineers, accountants, clerks, and doctors.) However, when their sense of mastery is threatened by the helplessness and loss of control involved in illness, they may decompensate and react with severe anxiety, inability to make important care-related decisions, or self-destructive attempts to control their environment.

In treating obsessive–compulsive patients there are several important aspects to keep in mind. The first is that obsessive patients cope with stressful events primarily by intellectualization. They are helped by being given logical, detailed information about their illness and its treatment. Also, particularly when decompensating, obsessives are tremendously helped by changes that give them a sense of control and mastery. For example, a post-myocardial infarction patient who refuses to stay at bedrest, in order to feel "control," might be asked to design for himself an exact schedule of rest and sitting-up periods.

Both patient and care giver will benefit if the patient's obsessiveness is enlisted in constructive ways. The patient who is perseverating over his or her symptoms when the practitioner has stopped in for a brief visit can be asked to make a complete list for the next visit.

## PARANOID STYLE

The paranoid style is a more pathologic style related to the obsessive–compulsive style. The outward manifestations of this style are familiar to everyone. Paranoid people are guarded, suspicious, and frequently appear hostile or arrogant (though they may also at times act obsequious). Paranoids are vigilant, observant, and very often perceptive. However, they usually do not get a complete picture of what is going on because they focus exclusively on those things that confirm their fears. Paranoid people are extremely rigid, with tremendous fears of loss of control and autonomy. In addition, they project their own "negative" qualities onto others.

The best approach to managing paranoid patients is to avoid getting into struggles about control with them by giving them as much autonomy and control as possible. Because of their suspiciousness (and acuity), one must be as straightforward as possible with them about their illness and one's thinking about it. It is important to create a safe environment for them, but one must be very respectful of their need for emotional distance. Paranoids feel very threatened with loss of self-control in situations of too much intimacy or dependence. Despite their apparent arrogance, they are actually very unsure of their true worth. Therefore, it is helpful to subtly praise their qualities of perception, acute observation, and vigilance. It can also be extremely helpful to enlist these qualities in their treatment (*e.g.,* ask them to observe carefully for symptoms or side-effects).

## DEPENDENT PATIENTS

Dependent patients are the favorites for some practitioners. Other feel like running the other way when they see them coming! These patients expect the care giver to fill all needs and to be endlessly fascinated with their every belch and bowel movement. On the other hand, they are very devoted patients and usually are very compliant.

The key in caring for dependent patients is to set firm, realistic, but nonpunitive limits on what you are willing to give and then stick to your limits. Within these limits, one is then free to be concerned and caring without feeling taken advantage of.

## NARCISSISTIC PATIENTS

Narcissistic patients act and feel as if only they matter. They demand the best service from the most important physician and describe their place in life grandiosely. They seem arrogant and superior, whereas actually they are riddled with doubts about their own adequacy and safety. They usually respond promptly to recognition of their importance, explanation of how well they are being safeguarded, and to explanations of how their own actions can make them even more superior patients.

## IMPULSIVE PATIENTS

The impulsive personality is characteristic of patients with many psychiatric (and derogatory) labels including sociopaths, alcoholics, addicts, and others. Such persons act impulsively, on whim, often against their own intentions or self-interest. An example is the alcoholic who sincerely intends not to take another drink but is unable to refuse the first one offered. Often their impulses are flamboyant, immediately self-gratifying, or destructive to themselves or others. Practically, there are several implications of this style for practitioners; most important, once this style is recognized, one can expect impulsive behavior. This will minimize disappointment and frustration on the practitioner's part when the impulsive behavior (inevitably) occurs. Expectations of the patient's ability to comply must therefore be realistic and one should save one's struggles with the patients for only the most important issues.

Because these patients are superb at manipulating practitioners, one should decide clearly on one's limits and stick to them (knowing they will be repeatedly tested). Within these limits, one can then be on the patient's side as fully as possible. From this position, it is possible and sometimes useful to explicitly discuss the impulsive behavior with the patient; occasionally it will help this type of patient change.

## BORDERLINE PATIENTS

Borderline patients are probably the most difficult because they have severe psychological disturbances. Their most basic problem is a very poor sense of self; they have a strong need to merge with others but are then terrified by the loss of self that intimacy engenders. They are also liable to intense and irrational rage that can erupt 30 seconds after they have finished telling you that you are the only doctor they've ever trusted. This quality of "splitting" can make treating them an emotional roller coaster. These patients also tend to "split" various care givers into "good" and "bad" nurses, doctors, or social workers, and to set them against each other. Borderline patients are frequent somatizers and are also the predominant personality type seen in factitious or self-induced illness. Other self-destructive acts (drug abuse, suicide, etc.) are also common among these patients.

Management of borderline patients is difficult, especially if the personality type is not identified. Recognition of the diagnosis is crucial since it will help the practitioner protect both parties from the harmful relationships these patients otherwise engender. Instead, with an attitude that is consistently positive, supportive, and firm, the practitioner can provide a stable "anchor" for the patient. Because of their tendency to somatize, treatment for somatization disorder may also be indicated for borderline patients. In addition, careful documentation of signs and symptoms is needed to detect factitious illness. If more than one professional is involved in caring for a borderline patient, all members of the team need to have frequent, open discussions with each other to prevent "splitting" of the team by the patient and to formulate a consistent approach.

## PSYCHOSOMATIC PROBLEMS IN GENERAL

Recently, there have been major advances in our understanding of the interactions of brain and body in disease. These have come from three main sources. First, epidemiologic surveys have shown increased rates of illness after bereavement and after major life change (positive or negative). These have been prospectively validated. Second, specific studies of neuroendocrine and immunologic mechanisms have shown that psychosocial "stresses" are related to physiologic change. For example, in bereaved spouses, significant impairments of immune function have been demonstrated. Similarly, Ader has been able to produce durable immunosuppression using a conditioned stimulus.[16] A third line of evidence comes from psychologists, who have documented a variety of "stress" responses, a number of physiologic changes (*i.e.,* muscle tension, changes in blood pressure and flow, and endocrine changes) that occur in response to psychosocial stresses.

Therefore, we now recognize that psychosocial factors are important in all illnesses (*e.g.,* the amount of pain in postoperative patients is related to the amount of fear and anxiety) and may be causative in some (*e.g.,* tension headaches).

An additional important dimension of the mind–body interface is the group of syndromes in which psychosocial factors are expressed as bodily symptoms (without the patient being conscious of the role of psychological factors in his or her illness). These *psychogenic syndromes,* which will be described in more detail later, include

Somatization disorders and the less extreme forms of somatization

Somatic symptoms as signs of depression

Hypochondriasis

Psychophysiologic reactions

Conversion disorders

Although the actual *mechanisms* of most of these disorders are still not understood, there have been major advances in clinical observation and description of these syndromes.

## PSYCHOLOGIC PROBLEMS PRESENTING AS MEDICAL ILLNESS: PSYCHOGENIC SYNDROMES

In this group of disorders, psychological, interpersonal, or environmental problems, rather than being expressed as such, are manifested as physical symptoms. They can be manifested as the disordered physiologic function seen in psychophysiologic disorders (*e.g.,* functional bowel disease), as unusual or bizarre sensations or pains in somatization disorder, or as the heightened sensitivity to *normal* bodily functions that is seen in hypochondriasis. All of these syndromes, which will be described individually below, have common features. The first and most important of these is that psychosocial factors are causative in the meaning, timing, and nature of the symptoms. Despite this, the patients are generally unaware of the role of psychosocial factors and strongly identify themselves as having *medical* rather than *psychological* problems. They are usually very resistant to psychiatric referral, but, ironically, among patients with severe psychogenic illness there is a high rate of associated psychiatric illness.

These patients, especially those with severe problems, are high utilizers of medical care. If their true diagnoses are not recognized, they are usually treated inappropriately with extensive diagnostic testing (including invasive procedures), which is clearly detrimental to both the patients and the health-care system.

Although we tend to focus on the patients with severe psychogenic illness because of their high visibility, these syndromes actually cover a range of severity; mild or transient psychogenic symptoms (fatigue, headaches, diarrhea, atypical chest pain, etc.) are common in primary care and familiar to all practitioners.

Although these symptoms or illnesses may create advantages for the patient in his or her environment, such as avoidance of work or other responsibilities, this so-called "secondary gain" is rarely a *causative* factor. However, once established, it may perpetuate the symptoms even when other "primary gains," such as resolving psychological conflict, become less needed.

## *Somatization*

Somatization is best thought of as a process in which psychosocial matters are experienced and expressed as physical symptoms for which there is no exclusively physiologic or other organic etiology. The symptoms (which can be multiple and bizarre) may have a symbolic meaning, most often modeled on a past illness experience of the patient or someone significant, or expressive of a wish or conflict. They may also function as punishment for unacceptable feelings (as postulated for pain-prone patients), as a way of "keeping within" someone who has been lost and not sufficiently grieved (as in the patient who presents with "hysterical paralysis" after her husband died of a stroke), or as a communication of need for

## GUIDELINES TO TREATMENT OF SOMATIZATION

1. The relationship is paramount (although the patient generally is not conscious that this is what he or she is seeking).

2. Frequent, regular visits or contacts not contingent on symptoms (generally every 2 to 4 weeks). In home care patients, some "visits" will be done by phone; these too should be regular and scheduled.

3. Medical work-up, as indicated, should be gradual with care to avoid unnecessary tests.

4. Conservatively evaluate new or changing complaints, but do not dismiss them (somatizers do get sick and at a higher rate than controls).

5. Behavioral prescriptions to
   a. Reduce self-destructive patterns (*i.e.*, social isolation, inactivity)
   b. Substitute healthy behavior (*i.e.*, exercise, hot baths)

6. Gradual exploration of past psychologic history and present homeostasis
   a. Search for a model for symptoms (*i.e.*, an experience in the patient or a significant other on which the present symptoms are modeled (for example, chest pain in a patient who as a child had witnessed his mother having angina).
   b. Exploration of present psychosocial stresses, particularly their relation to timing of onset or changes in symptoms (Note that it is the significance of the event for the patient that counts, not its "objective" significance.)
   c. Work through clear problems such as unresolved grief or sexual conflicts.

7. Provide corrective (*i.e.*, *healthy*) relationship over months to years to promote healthy development, that is, a respectful interest in the patient that does not encourage dependence but allows the patient to feel cared for.

8. Treat underlying psychiatric disorders (depression, schizophrenia).

(Reproduced by permission of Mack Lipkin, Jr.)

a caring relationship in a person whose fears of closeness and dependency do not otherwise allow this, as well as many other intrapsychic and interpersonal issues.

In somatization, as in all disorders in this group, the patient is generally unaware of the psychosocial etiology of the symptom and in severe cases will go to great lengths, including such invasive procedures as cardiac catheterization or exploratory laparotomy, to find a "physical reason" for his symptoms. Somatization covers a broad spectrum of severity, from a process common in everyday life to most people (such as the gastrointestinal symptoms commonly experienced by husbands of pregnant women) to the severe multisystem disorder known as Briquet's syndrome. In Briquet's syndrome, a patient must have 24 or more symptoms, from at least 9 to 10 symptom groups, with onset before age 35. A slightly modified version is listed in the *DSM III* as somatization disorder.[17]

For guidelines to the treatment of somatization, see below.

## *Hypochondriasis*

Like somatization, hypochondriasis is common and covers a spectrum of severity. It is defined as the exaggerated response of a patient to a normal bodily function with undue preoccupation concerning the threatening meaning of such "symptoms." The patient transforms normal physical sensations into symptoms or very minor symptoms into major ones. The preoccupation with such "symptoms" is usually accompanied by anxiety, care seeking, and medication. Sometimes a particular symptom has a symbolic value but most often it is a nonspecific symptom choice in response to anxiety or depression that the patient is unable to experience directly. Hypochondriasis may be transient (as in the young woman who suddenly discovers "swollen glands" in her neck one year after her mother died of cancer) or it may become the patient's normal way of coping with painful affects.

As in somatization, a major goal of management is to protect the patient from unnecessary and invasive work-ups (and to protect the health-care system from misuse). (See Suggestions for the Management of Hypochondriasis.)

## PSYCHOPHYSIOLOGIC DISORDERS

Psychophysiologic disorders are those in which the physical symptoms, although the result of emotional factors, are postulated to also have a true physiologic basis (although the actual physiologic mechanisms are not always known). In general, psychophysiologic symptoms are very closely related to the physical manifestation of anxiety:

---

### SUGGESTIONS FOR THE MANAGEMENT OF HYPOCHONDRIASIS

1. Respectful medical evaluation of major complaints. Like somatizers, hypochondriacs *do* get sick.

2. Avoidance of unnecessary testing provoked by patient's complaint

3. Clear explanation of what is found without undue emphasis or deemphasis

4. Accurate and descriptive names to symptoms that give the patient security and do not mislead other doctors (e.g., idiopathic left anterior chest pain)

5. A statement of optimistic but reasonable prognosis ("Symptoms will persist, may gradually get better, and will wax and wane.")

6. Emphasis that nothing worrisome to you as a clinician has been found

7. Explain that certain things may help with prescription of healthy and safe activity

8. Prescription of activity that improves self-esteem and mastery

9. Specific treatment of anxiety or depression if present but avoid excessive or prolonged use of anxiolytics

10. Psychiatry referral if significant mental disorder present *and* patient can accept it

11. Continued relationship with medical practitioner regardless of psychiatric referral

(Reproduced by permission of Mack Lipkin, Jr.)

*Acute anxiety:* sweating, palpitations, "atypical" chest pain, dry mouth, tremulousness, feelings of choking or tightness in the throat, abdominal pain (mild). In general, these are thought to be secondary to the catecholamines released in the course of the "fight or flight" response.

*Chronic anxiety:* mainly manifestations of chronic muscle tension and disordered autonomic tone, tension headaches, low back and other musculoskeletal pains, nausea and other stomach-related complaints, and functional bowel problems

Psychophysiologic reactions, particularly the "chronic" forms, occur in everyone, usually temporarily in response to various psychosocial "stresses." In such cases they are generally amenable to simple measures such as exploration of the precipitating stress, exercises (*i.e.,* for low back or neck pain), and, in some cases, relaxation training. However, in some patients both the acute and chronic forms can become severe and persistent problems, such as recurrent anxiety attacks or repetitive care-seeking for chest pains, severe functional bowel disease, or musculoskeletal complaints. In many such cases, there is an overlap between the psychophysiologic symptoms and somatization, so that these symptoms, while having an apparent physiologic basis, also take on a symbolic meaning. These cases require a combination of the treatment methods described for somatization and those described for psychophysiologic disorders.

## PSYCHOSOCIAL ASPECTS OF HOME CARE

Home care poses unique issues for patient and providers alike. Overall, for many it is a much preferable solution to care elsewhere. It allows the patient to be spared the discomforts and dangers of hospital or institutional care; to be in familiar and appreciated surroundings; and to be spared the pain of travel for those in pain. Yet, problems also occur. These relate to lack of mobility, the increased pressure of the illness on those in the home environment, and the reactions they have to this, especially at times of crisis. Patients also usually have doubts about the adequacy of care in the home, especially, again, at times of crisis. Thus, it is our experience that most home care patients will feel a need to test this at some time to be sure hospital care is available if needed and that the systems of home care really are working. We have found that allowing modification or exception to home care facilitates acceptance of it. For example, many patients who want comfort care for cancer still need a day or two in the hospital at some time when they begin to have constant severe pain. If given this, they readily accept subsequent management at home. If denied this, it is much harder to manage their care at home.

The specific issues of psychosocial aspects of home care are discussed in the following sections.

### THE PSYCHOLOGICAL SYSTEM

The patient's view of the illness, its nature, prognosis, and special aspects (*e.g.,* infectiousness for AIDS, stigma for cancer, repulsiveness for debilitating or disfiguring diseases) must be known to the primary-care team. Obviously, if a decision has been made to withhold information, there must be consistency. If the prognosis has been couched in specific ways for sound reasons, such as with uncertainty for the cancer patient, each health worker relating to the patient should be aware of the terms in use, their agreed-upon meanings, and the reasons behind these choices.

In addition, the patient's views of the illness may be critical to adaptation to the stages of reaction to the illness. Some patients harbor serious misconceptions that may alter their ability to develop acceptance, may inhibit participation in self-care, or prevent establishment of reasonable monitoring or reporting of new problems. Rarely, the patient may feel that the home care is a withdrawal of treatment or a punishment. This is a distortion, and it is important that it be revealed as such and corrected.

The patient's adaptation to the illness is affected by home care in several respects. Positively, the acceptance of loss of function is facilitated by absence of loss, also, of the home. That is, patients who are hospitalized or institutionalized may suffer not only from the reasons requiring their removal from their home, but also from the loss of their home. This loss includes decreased contact with loved ones, disruption of stabilizing and orienting routines, as well as pleasurable routines, and loss of control. These losses are minimized with home care.

On the other hand, the patient's view of the home setting now changes. The patient may have to make changes, such as where he or she sleeps, what he or she can do or accomplish, who does what, and so on. In some aspects, the persistent stay in the home is a reminder of losses of function.

The patient will also experience the reactions of the setting; that is, having a home care patient creates issues for the others present. They are never free of the presence of the patient. They may have to make accommodations such as moving rooms, taking up the living room, altering the bedroom from a haven to a hospital-type setting, and such other changes. Home care also introduces a series of strangers into one's homes—nurses, aides, self-help group visitors. To some extent, privacy is always compromised.

These issues, or others like them, may concern the patient. The critical factor for the primary-care provider is to give the patient opportunity to express and explore his reactions and to accommodate realistic concerns, correct distortions, solve problems that can be solved, and work toward acceptance of the rest.

## THE SOCIAL SYSTEM

In the best of all worlds, the family and significant others will be without conflicts, fears, or mixed feelings about the patient, the treatment goals, and the decision to care for him or her at home. They will have no conflicts between them and will all be selflessly united in their desire to provide loving and competent care for the homebound patient.

This situation is, of course, rare; in most situations, each member of the household will have complex reactions to the presence of the patient and a number of problems may need to be addressed in the social system.

To some extent, altruism, love, and generous feelings will permit the family members (or others) to experience satisfaction in the heroic efforts they are making for the patient. However, some resentment, conscious or not, is likely. This must be anticipated and eased through recognition and acknowledgment that it is normal and human. Guilt should be minimized.

Family members (or significant others) often have discomfort with or disagreement about the philosophies or goals of treatment. For instance, while a patient with terminal cancer and his or her physician may have decided to pursue comfort care instead of aggressive medical care, family members may be troubled by this decision for varied reasons (such as fear of losing the sick person or guilt). Similarly, some care partners may not be comfortable with providing home care. As noted above, when patients are being cared for at home a much larger responsibility is placed on the family and significant others, who may have discomfort with this for a number of reasons in addition to those changes of routine already mentioned. They may be fearful of the patient's illness (particularly if it may be contagious) or they may fear witnessing the patient's deterioration or death. On the other hand, they may have ambivalent feelings toward the patient or may be resentful of the amount of responsibility or feel unsure of their ability to carry it out.

Another common problem is conflict about roles, responsibilities, and authority within the social system, with various people wanting more or less of certain tasks, decision-making power, or importance to the patient. Usually this represents preexisting dynamics within the system that are exacerbated or altered by the issue of caring for the sick person.

Exhaustion of the household is also a common occurrence in home care. Suddenly family members have a new job. They are night nurse, home health aide, and social worker in addition to the usual roles of, for example, spouse and fulltime day worker. These tasks are in addition to the task they have of adapting to and accepting their losses due to the illness of the patient. Thus, they often become drained physically and emotionally and increasingly become unable to respond creatively or lovingly to the situations presented over time.

This is why *respite* is critical for the household. The regular scheduling of rest, recreation, and freedom from the night-in night-out burdens of home care is important for everyone, including the patient. Therefore, it is the responsibility of the primary-care provider to ensure that these are being done and that the nonprofessional persons contributing to the home care effort are kept healthy and reasonably fresh, and do not come to feel exploited or burned out.

Deterioration of the patient's condition becomes a focus around which home care succeeds or fails. The patient and family will typically have fears centered on such things as seizing, bleeding, loss of continence, or development of delirium. Losses of function such as inability to accomplish chores previously within the patient's province also challenge homeostasis. The key to management of such events lies in several steps.

First, anticipation of problems is of value. For example, AIDS patients with encephalopathy will eventually lose ability to communicate. By discussing this and its management, in advance, with the significant other of the patient the coming event loses its fearful aspect (but this does not mean it loses the necessity for grieving).

Second, clear "rules of reaction" to changes are critical. The persons at home should know who to call and how to get them in the event of any significant or worrisome change. Most crucial is a failsafe system for getting in touch with the primary care giver or a substitute. It should be clear that no problem is too small or insignificant to lead to using this system of calling. For example, how should the nurse's aide react to a new fever? How should the family report moderate blood in the feces of a patient with colonic herpes? Detailed instructions relieve anxiety, obviate the necessity for panic and trips to the emergency room, and eliminate insertion of unnecessary care or cost.

Third, gentle preparation for distressing events is useful. Anticipatory grief does help patient and family get ready. The fine line is between worrying them prematurely and helping them adapt. Usually, a useful approach is to ask what is worrying them since they will often have thought of the worst already. Then, showing how to be useful in the situation, how to cope with it practically, and how to be sure to maximize the comfort and care of the patient will frame the events as constructively as possible and maximize the adaptation and satisfaction that if things must go badly one has coped well.

## HOME CARE PROFESSIONALS

Home care professionals include visiting nurses, home aides, social workers, and physicians, who, ideally, are working as a team. However, all the problems described for the family can and do occur within the home care team as well as between the professionals and members of the family. Thus, there may be disagreements about philosophies and goals of care and—particularly in this case—technical aspects of care. In addition, similar struggles about roles can arise; competition is common.

A specific and frequent problem is disagreement about the level of care to be provided. For instance, a nurse or social worker who has spent a lot of time in the patient's home may feel that comfort care is indicated and be resentful of the doctor who is pursuing more aggressive care from a more detached viewpoint. Conversely, it may be the doctor who is attempting comfort care while the nurse or aide, who is upset by this approach, continues to take vital signs 4 times a day and reports them anxiously to the doctor even though a decision has been made that nothing will be done should the condition deteriorate.

Other disagreements concern such matters as the extent of a patient's disability or care needs or need for analgesics or other medications.

Finally, the presence of a medical professional within the home is a change that requires adjustment on the part of the family. Furthermore, the family may have complaints or questions as to how well the helpers are doing their jobs.

A unique feature of home care is that it involves a number of persons in the details of the care process who are not normally initially involved and who feel entitled to their own views and opinions. In the office or hospital, the primary-care team sets the rules and procedures. In the home, others may be the owners, may be dominant, or may have personal or private concerns that do not normally fall within the realm of "straightforward" medical or nursing concerns.

This raises several crucial considerations for the practitioner who, first of all, assumes a more advisory role in relation to the family. At that same time, he or she is providing care outside the "safe" medical environment and must therefore rely on "untrained" family members to deliver much of the actual care and to make many day-to-day on-site decisions. Clearly, this all adds up to a complex and challenging situation.

While the patient is still the dominant concern for the team, in a sense the entire social situation becomes "the patient," and the roles and needs of others may make or break the success of planned approaches. Thus, they need to be known, understood, and managed effectively in the interest of the patient. Solomonic judgments are needed. Compromises may be called for that allow overall benefit not able to be accomplished otherwise.

Effective management of the social system requires careful assessment of each important member's roles, strengths, and problems. One also wants to assess interactions *between* caretaking people. All of this assessment is best done by careful observation. An additional and very important assessment that must be made is to determine which family member is in charge and how responsibilities are to be divided, and especially who is the person who will make important decisions (*e.g.,* in an emergency). Who this person is usually is obvious but should be made explicit and should be agreed upon. In some settings, the real decision-maker is covert, using influence and indirection (*e.g.,* the grandmother in a Hispanic household). If so, this should be understood.

Exploration and addressing of fears, problems, and resentments of the various care-takers are also extremely helpful. It is best to do this individually at first, followed by a group conference to make whatever compromises are needed and to agree on goals and plans as much as possible.

Especially when dealing with the family it is always best to frame arrangements positively; for example, taking care of the patient at home is a positive good, not a second best alternative to hospital care; having the home health aide come less often is a sign that the patient is improving (or is being left unbothered), not that care is being withdrawn. One wants to show by one's manner that this is a good and right thing to do and that high-quality care is being delivered. Show confidence, caring, and attention to detail. Similarly, provide support and praise to the family for their care, emphasizing that what they are doing requires love and strength.

One of the trickiest aspects of home care is to give as much responsibility to the care partners as possible (avoid taking over) *yet to know when they need you to take over* (this is a fine line).

As noted above, preparation for and discussion of possible anticipated problems can be crucial. At the same time, care givers (*e.g.,* home health aide, visiting nurses, and family members) must have the best tools for use in these situations, so they have real care to provide (*i.e.,* symptomatic medications when needed, range-of-motion exercises to prevent contractures, home respiratory care for deteriorations in chronic obstructive pulmonary disease, and so on).

All of the above-described approaches are also appropriate and useful for the person coordinating the home care team. In addition, each member of the team has the responsibility to try to work effectively with the others, to allow the various perspectives to complement each other, rather than compete with each other, and to avoid being set in opposition to each other by the patient or family, which is sometimes a risk.

A final problem is the situation in which there *is no* social system (or a very inadequate one). This situation, while often tragic, is unfortunately not rare. In this case, the deficit must be made up as much as possible by professional services and community organizations. While the available services differ greatly from one place to another, the range of options may include visiting nurses, home health aide or homemakers, social workers, transportation systems, Meals on Wheels, community companion and buddy systems, and others.

In this situation not only medical and physical care must be provided by professionals or volunteers. For optimal care, the patient's social and environmental needs must also be addressed; otherwise the person may receive excellent medical care, but die of loneliness. This is obviously a very difficult problem requiring much ingenuity and dedication from all members of the team and enlistments of such things as "buddies," companions, and activity programs.

## SPECIFIC SITUATIONS

### AIDS and Other Infectious Diseases

With the increasing number of AIDS patients, more and more of whom are electing to remain at home, the question of risk of contagion for the family and other care givers is being raised increasingly. Fortunately, we now have data on this. Friedland and associates studied the families of 39 AIDS patients who received their care at home, including extensive contact with bodily fluids. Careful examination including HIV testing did not show any case of AIDS transmission in the 101 family members studied.[18] Thus, we can now reassure care givers that their risk of contracting AIDS in this situation is extremely low and that only minimal precautions need be devised, such as wearing gloves when handling body fluids and feces. Nevertheless, people's fears should not be trivialized, but should be explored and answered in detail with whatever information we have.

### Terminal Care

Many of the principles of home care for the terminally ill patient have been included in the preceding sections of this chapter. There are, however, several areas specific to this situation that we will deal with briefly here.

**Comfort Care.** If the terminally ill patient is being cared for at home, this generally means that a decision has been made to provide comfort care versus aggressive care. Usually such a decision is made when the patient is considered to have an incurable illness or when cure is doubtful and treatment involves extensive pain or discomfort. Comfort care involves a change from disease-oriented treatment to symptom-oriented treatment, with attention to psychological, interpersonal, and physical needs of the dying patient. It includes all medications and treatments that offer a hope of maintaining or increasing comfort without unnecessary prolongation of life or increased disability.

**Psychological Care of the Dying Patient.** Initially, this involves assessment of where the patient is in his or her adjustment to dying. Subsequently, continued work on coping with death may be needed, with the patient alone and sometimes with significant others as well. The dying person may also need judicious pharmacologic treatment of anxiety, depression, and insomnia, although this should never substitute for help with the psychological work of dying.

Much of this work may have been done while the patient was in the hospital and prior to initiation of home care. Nevertheless, one needs to touch base about it periodically, particularly about any new issues of dying brought up by being at home.

Legal matters should be attended to early on while the patient is still competent (if possible), but not, of course, so early that it is inappropriate and frightening. These include

Appointment of a person who will be legal guardian if the patient does become unable to make decisions (because of deterioration in mental status) and who will also act as executor

Creation of a will

Arrangement with a funeral home to pick up the patient's body after death and for signing of the death certificate. While this may seem trivial or morbid, there is little more distressing to the family than to have to sit for 12 hours with the dead body of the loved one while waiting for a busy medical examiner to arrive to sign a death certificate.

## THE HOME VISIT

The major medium of home care delivery is the home visit. Depending on the length of time a patient is cared for at home, practitioners may make one, several, or many visits and will also be in touch by telephone. It is desirable, at least during one visit, to have as many members of the patient's social system present, so that the problems and issues noted above under Social System can be most effectively addressed.

The following is a suggested approach to an initial home visit. The approach can be modified, as appropriate, for follow-up visits. (See also Outline of Home Visit.)

1. Assessment of patient
   a. Obtain interval history from patient (if able), nursing personnel, or other care givers.
   b. Examine patient; generally one proceeds as for an office or hospital visit, checking general status of the patient, looking for signs of a change in status, and new problems possibly needing evaluation. However, if the patient is terminally ill and getting comfort care, the examination will have a very different emphasis. In this case, the focus will be on careful assessment of symptomatic or potential problems. Thus, if the problem does not hurt or cause some other discomfort, you do not need to do anything about it or even assess it. You *do* want to know specifically about the following, as there are remedies for these:
      Eye care
      Mouth care
      Incontinence
      Nausea
      Itching
      Pain
      Cough
      Delirium
      Psychosis–hallucinosis
      Insomnia or other sleep disturbance
      Thorough knowledge and skill in these matters are important.
2. Assessment of setting
   a. Comfort of room (air, noise, etc.). Is it actively pleasant and *not morbid*?
   b. Distance to bathroom and other areas if patient is ambulatory
   c. Specific items as needed such as bedside commode; nasogastric tube; catheters; hospital bed; oxygen, and other supplies
3. Observation/assessment of care partners
   Needs, abilities, who is capable of what. What is the state of coping of each person? What needs to be done? Who will do it?

## OUTLINE OF HOME VISIT

1. Greetings, introductions
2. Obtain recent history.
3. Examine patient.
4. Assess environment (physical, psychosocial).
5. Speak individually with care partners as needed (to elicit and attend to individual problems and needs).
6. Group conference: discuss patient's physical needs, symptoms, and their solutions; clarify responsible persons, decision-making plans, and procedures for contacting doctor.
7. Post telephone numbers.
8. If patient has not been included in group conference and is alert, summarize plans and treatments with patient. Also give patient opportunity to discuss thoughts and feelings about what is happening.
9. Make arrangements for next contact and anything to be attended to subsequently (*i.e.*, obtaining equipment or medicine, arrangements for diagnostic testing, etc.).
10. Document visits and plans.
11. Write prescriptions as needed.

(Reproduced by permission of Mack Lipkin, Jr., Sarah Williams, and Adina Kalet)

---

**4.** Legal matters (for terminally ill patients)
See above.

**5.** AIDS patients and other communicable diseases
Discuss risks, precautions, hygiene.

**6.** Discuss supply lines (how to get medications, appliances, etc.).

**7.** Discuss and arrange diagnostic testing if needed (*e.g.,* patient with known cancer may need x-rays or computed tomography scan to assess a new bone pain). Make transportation arrangements as needed. Patients may also be receiving certain therapies (radiation therapy, physical therapy) that cannot be provided at home and arrangements may need to be made for these services.

In essence, the process described here is a succinct integration of the principles described earlier. First, you use the occasion of the home visit to complete or update your physical and psychological assessment of the patient. This is done with an eye to fine-tuning your own observations as your increasing knowledge of the home site informs your understanding of the patient's needs and situation.

Second, you use the home visit to recognize and begin to manage potential and real barriers to home care present physically, psychologically, or socially in the home. This is done through a thorough "physical," psychological, and social assessment of every aspect of the setting. Most of this can be done subtly, indirectly, and without creating self-consciousness or embarrassment on the part of the persons in the home. Some of it genuinely may seem "nosy" but still may be important. For example, it is often very useful to have a look at the medicine cabinet. Similarly, it is important to inquire about materials disposal and cleaning and bathroom arrangements in the home visit to an AIDS patient. This also can become the time for a useful discussion of the fears of the attendants or others about infectiousness in these patients.

Finally, the home visit is of great value in setting the tone of home care. If done with professional elegance, in which caring, competence and painstaking thoroughness are visible to all concerned, it creates a feeling of confidence in those at home. They then will be freer to invest themselves in making it work. The persons taking part in any home visit, through their manner, can convey that this is, in fact, optimal care. Similarly, the visible involvement of the whole team, their effective conferencing, their mutual problem-solving, and their coherent consideration of the full range of problems, shows all present that this is an effective, inspiring process.

The frequency and timing of home visits are surprising to most physicians used to hospital-based care. It is essential to make an early definitive visit to accomplish the three central goals described above. Thereafter, however, most of the care can be by telephone or through the various professional intermediaries who need to be there frequently (such as the visiting nurse or the nursing aides). The key is to go often enough in the beginning to be certain the problems are worked out, to be sensitive to when calls about minor or inappropriate issues really reflect a need for a personal visit, and to go occasionally when it is not absolutely necessary to reinforce the notion that this is *not* minimalized care.

## SUMMARY

Psychosocial aspects of home care are fundamentally important to its success. It is critical to understand and assess the psychological and social adaptation of the patient to the illness process. This always includes grief due to loss of function and independence and may also involve pathologic reactions of anxiety and depression. The ability of the patient to accept and manage home care rests on effective or at least compensated psychological and social functioning and so assessment of overt nonreactive or reactive mental disorder is important. Somatopsychic complications such as delirium and dementia must be assessed and managed.

In home care, the patient is not the only person critical to the success of care. Home care alters relationships in the home, places extra demands on the family and friends, and changes the physical and psychosocial homeostasis of the home environment. Understanding of how these changes are occurring and effective management of them are needed if home care is to persist and pass successfully through the predictable crises of exhaustion and physical deterioration or emergency. Thus, the care team needs to have accomplished cogent assessment of the adaptation and attitudes of the significant others involved and to monitor their acceptance and tolerance of the process.

Doing home care is not in the repertoire of every physician, especially those used to the extensive and physically concentrated resources of the hospital. Nor is it to every practitioner's taste. It is extremely useful, even for those interested and committed to the ideas in support of home care, that they accompany someone who is accomplished at doing it on an initial home visit. We find that having seen it done with finesse once, our primary-care residents can then do it themselves and are willing and eager to get started. It is also extremely useful, once it is started, to have a back-up person to discuss it with subsequently. We have found that those managing home care programs, such as supervising visiting nurses, often have a wealth of useful experience to bring to bear on particular problems. Also, those running the agencies usually know how to do such things as find surgical supplies on the weekends, get complex drugs or narcotics to the bedside in a timely fashion, and so on.

There are several ways in which home care appeals to primary-care practitioners especially. It is often the most appropriate modality of care. It is a setting one can genuinely control medically while doing important work with very sick patients. It requires and allows work with a team that has vitality and in which it is possible to define roles meaningfully, cooperatively, and effectively with relatively less bureaucratic bother than in some settings. It is a revelation to work with some of the nurses and aides who have long-standing experience in home care. At this point in history, it seems as if some of the caring functions that seem less apparent in the hospital may be found in the workers who prefer to be more independent in home care.

Finally, home care can be meaningful and even inspiring. There is no greater reward in medicine, for some, than to assist patients adjust to total disability by becoming able to live in the home they love. In this age of increasing frustration and loss of independence for practitioners, the experience of assisting a patient to a death with dignity and comfort is unforgettable and deeply rewarding. The bonds created with the family through this process are among the most enduring in one's practice career.

## REFERENCES

1. Noble J: Primary Care and the Practice of Medicine. Boston, Little, Brown & Co, 1976

2. Lipkin M, Quill TE, Napodano RJ: The medical interview: A core curriculum for residencies in internal medicine. Ann Intern Med 100:277–284, 1984

3. Bowlky J: Processes of mourning. Int J Psychoanal 42:317–340, 1961

4. Lazare A: Unresolved grief. In Lazare A. Outpatient Psychiatry, pp 498–512, Baltimore, Williams & Wilkins, 1979

5. Lobel B, Hirschfeld RMA: Depression: What we know. (NIMH) USDHHS, PHS, ADAMHA. Washington, DC, Pub. No. (ADM) 85-1318), 1984

6. Beck AT, Resnik HLP, Lettieri DJ: Prediction of suicide. MD, Charles Press, 1974

7. Kaplan HI, Sadock BJ (eds): Comprehensive Textbook of Psychiatry/IV. Baltimore, Williams & Wilkins, 1985

8. Nemiah J: Anxiety states. In Kaplan HI, Sadock BJ (eds): Comprehensive Textbook of Psychiatry/IV, pp 883–894. Baltimore, Williams & Wilkins, 1985

9. Regier DA, Meyers JK, Kramer M et al: The NIMH Epidemiologic Catchment Area Program. Archives of General Psychiatry 41:934–941, 1984

10. Kamerow DB, Pincus HA, Macdonald DI: Alcohol abuse, other drug abuse, and mental disorders in medical practice. JAMA 255:2054–2057, 1986

11. Wells CE: The organic brain syndromes. Psychiatr Clin North Am, August: 319–351, 1972

12. Kaplan HI, Sadock BJ (eds): Comprehensive Textbook of Psychiatry/IV, Chapter 19.2, pp 838–851. Baltimore, Williams & Wilkins, 1985

13. Mumford E et al: The effects of psychological intervention on recovery from surgery and heart attacks: An analysis of the literature. Am J Public Health 72(2):141–151, 1982

14. Beecher HK: Measurement of Subjective Response. New York, Oxford University Press, 1959

15. Shapiro D: Neurotic Styles. New York, Basic Books, 1965

16. Ader R: Psychoneuroimmunology. New York, Academic Press, 1981

17. Ford CV: Somatizing Disorders. New York, Elsevier, 1983

18. Friedland G et al: Lack of transmission of HTLVIII/LAV infection to household contacts of patients with AIDS or AIDS-related complex with oral candidiasis. N Engl J Med, 314(6):344–349, 1986

# 23
# Sociocultural Factors

## ALEX ROSEN

I care as much as to what manner of *man* has a disease, as I care as to what manner of *disease* a man has.—Dr. William Osler

Dr. Osler made the preceding observation at a time in the early 20th century when American medicine was becoming scientific, basing itself on the emerging scientific developments in Europe in the late 19th century. He helped found the Johns Hopkins School of Medicine, which Abraham Flexner, in his historic 1910 report that revolutionized American medical education, hailed as a prototype of the new scientific medicine. Yet, it was the genius of Osler to recognize, as he reflected on a lifetime of clinical practice, that medicine was not only a biologic science, but also a "social" science, since it dealt with people and with behavior, as well as with disease.

A similar observation was made by the 12th century physician and philosopher, Maimonides. In his famous code of ethics, still recited by medical graduates along with the Hippocratic oath, Maimonides advised physicians:

Dear Lord, do not allow me to view my patients merely as vessels of disease.

Although few physicians would quarrel with the philosophy expressed by Osler and Maimonides, they are at times so dominated by "biological reductionism" and high technology that, in actual practice, they often are apt to fail to understand the patient, the total person. This can be seen in the frank, even rueful, observation made by a young medical resident:

Ready for hearts, and lungs, and kidneys, I was instead confronted with a whole person. In the midst of all the familiar precision, of lab values and x-rays, suddenly there were human concerns, grief and heartache, distrust, fear and even anger. So seemingly well turned out as a result of my scientific training, I found myself unexpectedly stumbling; all of us were, with only our own strengths and weaknesses to get us through.

To avoid this "stumbling," the physician with home health-care patients will want to ask himself the same questions that we can conjecture were in Osler's mind as he tried to understand both the disease and the man:

1. Are there family or job stresses that affect the course of the disease and the patient's coping capacity?

2. Is the patient hopeful and cooperative in his own medical care, or dependent, passive, and depressed?

3. Is the patient receptive to professional advice and guidance or are there emotional or cultural hurdles and difficulties?

4. Are there ethnic and religious considerations that affect food, nutrition, and attitudes to disease and self-care?

## THE HISPANIC PATIENT—A CASE ILLUSTRATION

Culturally, "what manner of man" is the Hispanic patient of Puerto Rican background? Particularly, what impact do his cultural characteristics have on his attitude to illness, to seeking health care, to the doctor–patient relationship, and to his health behavior in general? And, most important, how does all this apply to the patient, his care givers, and professionals in home health care?

First, a word of scholarly caution. Although there are a number of identifiable social patterns in Puerto Rican culture (which we will describe below) that have implications for practice with Puerto Rican patients, in individual cases much will depend on the specific patient's experiential, psychosocial, and family history. This means that as in all patient contact, consideration needs to be given to the intervening variables of age, sex, education, job, and individual personality as they affect the impact of these cultural characteristics on a given patient.

The following are specific aspects of Puerto Rican culture that the sensitive professional needs to understand, emotionally as well as intellectually, in order to work effectively with Puerto Rican home care patients and their families. The reader should remember that some of these cultural aspects may be found in any culture. We will first delineate these cultural characteristics and then spell out implications for professional practice.

### Resignation

The Puerto Rican patient, particularly one of recent rural or farm background and low educational status, will often tend to be fatalistic and not struggle energetically against perceived fate. He tends to resign himself to whatever God gave him. He adjusts or adapts to health difficulties rather than struggles to overcome them as his "Anglo" neighbor would do. Fate is something inexorable, and there is nothing to be gained by struggling against it. In rural, agrarian Puerto Rico, the background for so many recent Puerto Rican immigrants to the mainland, the accepted values governing desired behavior include deference to others (especially those in authority), passivity, and submissiveness. As the Puerto Rican immigrant adjusts to mainland values and improves his education and job prospects, this behavior tends to change in the direction of American values of assertiveness and activity.

The challenge to the professional, whether physician, nurse, social worker, therapist, or health aide, will be to individualize patients in the context of their cultural background.

### Confidence and Trust

While achieving rapport and trust is a professional must in all relationships between a professional and a client or patient, it is markedly so in the case of a Puerto Rican patient. Because of his differences in language and educational status, as well as his immigrant status from what is perceived as a poorer, less advantaged home country, the Puerto Rican patient may tend to be cautious in dealing with people in authority. As Ghalt points out

A Puerto Rican client will often not reveal true feelings out of respect for authority. Until "confianza" is established, when two people break down barriers, and see themselves in more familial trusting relationships, much time is wasted...an impersonal institution that requires a person to immediately recount his problems and personal history to a professional is demeaning and alien to the culture of the Puerto Rican.[1]

*Machismo*

The Puerto Rican family is patriarchal, with the father playing a strong role in the family, requiring respect from his wife and children. Much deference and obeisance are given to the father as decision maker and head of the household. However, this status is under strain in the mainland, where women often find employment and begin to challenge the supremacy of the male, who, all too often, because of poor skills, language difficulties, and low educational background, is only sporadically employed in menial positions. There is a negative impact on the male's self-image when opportunities for economic advancement are limited. Such a father will place a good deal of emphasis in the family on the values of "respeto" and "dignidad." When this father becomes a homebound patient, unable to exercise his authority because of disability and unemployment, he will need empathy and sympathetic cultural understanding from both his family and the professionals relating to him in the home health-care setting.

*Religion*

Veneration of Mary, a doctrine of the Catholic Church, is the other side of the coin of the male dominance reflected in machismo. Women are viewed either as pure, sinless, selfless sacrificing mothers or as martyred victims of male egocentrism. These concepts are under the stress and strain of urban, industrialized society, which is so different from the relative simplicity of rural, small-town life in an agrarian society. Only careful interviewing by the professional, carried out with empathy, will reveal the impact of this situation on a particular Hispanic patient and family.

*Attitudes to Color*

In psychological terms, it is vitally important to realize that clarity of cultural identity is a key factor in developing emotional stability and positive self-esteem. A serious threat to these desired characteristics is the differences in attitudes toward skin color in Puerto Rico and on the mainland. In Puerto Rico, the population is descended from a racial mixture of Indians, blacks, and Europeans. They perceive "color" in multiple categories, with a favored shade being "cinnamon." The designation of a person in Puerto Rico in color terms is also influenced by sociocultural factors, in that wealthy, cultured Puerto Ricans are perceived as "whiter" in proportion to their wealth and status. Most important, they do not place the invidious characterization on color status, as is done on the mainland:

When Puerto Ricans arrive on the mainland, they are judged either white or black for the first time, and, if pronounced black, are attributed all of racist stereotypes inflicted on the black people in the U.S.—Enormous problems of identity and disruption are caused in families, particularly when some are considered white or black in the same family.[2]

An example of such personal disruption[3] is that the darker members of immigrating Puerto Rican families often have the most difficulty in adjusting, because of anxiety over conflicting definitions of race and color. Consequently, when Puerto Ricans become clients in social agencies or patients in hospitals or home health-care programs, they often become very sensitive to the color status of the professional. If the professional is white, the Puerto Rican patient may fear that he is viewed stereotypically, if dark-skinned, as "lazy, dirty and incompetent." The patient may fear that the professional does not respect him, that he knows little about him, and that he is unconsciously patronizing. These negative attitudes on the part of the professional are rarely explicitly expressed, but rather conveyed by tone of voice and facial expression. Lower socioeconomic class patients may lack formal education, but they often have remarkable intuitive understanding of those in authority over them.

*Attitude to Achievement*

The distinguished Cornell University sociologist Robin Williams points out in his widely respected book *American Society*[4] that American culture is marked by central stress on personal achievement, especially secular, occupational achievement. The ideal is the self-made man, rising from poverty to become independent, self-reliant, and able to stand on his own two feet. These are the values of an industrialized, urbanized society, fast-moving, energetic, and individualistic.

These values come into conflict with the attitudes of Puerto Ricans coming from a relatively simple agrarian, rural society, where communal interdependence is valued over personal independence; where the emphasis is on "who" a person is rather than "what" he does; where politeness and respect for authority are valued over assertiveness and confrontation. The simpler Puerto Rican culture emphasizes behavior in which children are expected to be submissive and dependent, to have "respeto" for authority and for one's family, and to have regard for one's character and honor.

*Implications for Professional Practice*

1. Differences in socialization norms between Puerto Rican homeland and the mainland represent stress and strain that help explain the behavior of the Puerto Rican in a health-care setting. (It should be emphasized that members of ethnic groups share certain values and cultural characteristics, but they are individuals, affected as well by such intervening variables as age, sex, education, family, and job status.) The professional, whether physician, nurse, social worker, therapist, or home aide, needs to be explicitly aware in terms of cultural knowledge of these socialization differences. This might be termed the cognitive aspect of the professional's responsibility in dealing with culturally different patients and clients.

2. Emotionally, the professional needs to recognize and come to grips with his own attitudes toward cultural differences in patients. These attitudes are often unconscious in nature, and therefore a certain amount of humility, professional introspection, and self-understanding are required for the professional who wants to be truly competent in dealing with rural, racially mixed, and culturally and linguistically different patients. This is not an easy task and requires the same application of intellectual and emotional energy as given to a patient's physical and biochemical problems. Modern medicine increasingly requires humanistic, cultural understanding alongside scientific understanding. They go hand in hand.

3. The professional team will want to make a psychosocial, cultural assessment of the Puerto Rican patient and family, taking into account the variables described above and their implications for a total patient care program in a health-care setting.

4. Behavior has meaning. The great need is to avoid stereotyping and to recognize individualism in the midst of diverse stimuli.

5. In home health care, the active cooperation in health care of the patient and family care partners is of utmost importance to the professional team. Only with cultural sensitivity and empathy on the part of all concerned is this possible to achieve.

## CULTURAL DIFFERENCES AND PATIENTS' BEHAVIOR

### PATIENTS' BEHAVIOR

Modern medical sociology has confirmed Dr. Osler's original sensitive insight in a series of scientific studies. Bloom,[5] in his landmark book, *The Doctor and His Patient,* points out that a patient's behavior cannot be fully understood only on the basis of the patient's physical and biological characteristics. "The past experience of other men in the form of culture enters into almost every event. Each culture constitutes a kind of blueprint for all of life's activities indicating *what must be done, ought to be done, may be done, and must not be done."*

From the perspective of the cultural anthropologist, culture is viewed as a set of guidelines as to how to see the world and how to behave in it. Cecil Helman, an English medical anthropologist[6] concerned with health behavior, sees man as a social animal, organized into groups (family, church, neighborhood) that regulate and perpetuate themselves, and states that it is man's experience as a member of society that shapes his view of the world. It gives him his fundamental values toward basic aspects of life—marriage, children, job, career, leisure activities, and guidelines as to what is wrong and what is right; what is approved in human behavior and what is frowned upon, as we have just observed in the case study of the patient of Puerto Rican background.

### CULTURAL BEHAVIOR

Examples of differential cultural behavior, supportive of Osler's view that both the man and the disease need to be understood, are these brief examples:

> An implicit value assumption in Western society is that man is dominant over the forces of nature, including illness and disease. Thus, there is confidence that scientific medicine in the form of surgery and drugs can modify biological processes, at least to the extent of modern scientific knowledge. On the other hand, in some Eastern philosophies, and among some Hispanics, man is considered helpless before nature and before God. What is ordained will be and God's will be done. These two disparate philosophies have different implications for patient behavior, especially compliance with physician-recommended regimens. This is of vital importance to physicians in home health care where the patient's own active self-care is an essential part of the recovery of the patient.

> Among the very poor and among individuals of low socioeconomic status, even in Western industrialized society, pain and fatigue are often seen as "the way it is supposed to be" and therefore no recourse to a health-care provider is taken.

> In an often-cited study,[7] Koos examined the percentage of respondents in different socio-economic classes, recognizing specific symptoms as needing medical attention. Symptoms such as swelling of ankles, shortness of breath, and weight loss were three times more likely to motivate upper socioeconomic class respondents to go for medical attention than members of lower socioeconomic groups. The intervening variables that seem to affect such care-seeking behavior are the individual's job (its security and flexibility for time off); fear about treatment; ignorance and myths about the health-care system; concerns about cost; relative need for treatment as related to age and role in the family (a blue-collar worker of limited income hesitates to jeopardize family income because of seemingly minor symptoms).

### DISEASE AND ILLNESS

Though obviously related, the terms *disease* and *illness* are not identical and interchangeable. Illness is a wider, if more diffuse, concept than disease. It is the body organ (*e.g.,* the heart) that has the disease; it is the patient who has an illness. There is a need, therefore, to distinguish between disease as conceptualized by physicians and illness as experienced by the patient. The modern physician diagnoses and treats diseases, that is, abnormalities in structure and functioning of body organs and symptoms. It is the patient who suffers an illness, that is, experiences disvalued changes in states of being and in social functioning. Illness is the subjective response of the patient, and of those around him, to his being unwell. In home health care this is of critical importance, for the care partner at home is the key ingredient for a successful program. The physical arrangements at home, though important, are secondary to the social requirement of a truly caring person in the home.

## MEANING OF ILL HEALTH

Ill health includes not only its actual experience by the patient but also the meaning given to the experience by society. For example, a person who has fallen ill might ask himself in self-reproach, "Why has this happened to me?" The illness might be ascribed to life-style behavior, such as lack of exercise, poor nutrition, or deviant sexual practices, as in the case of homosexuals who contract the acquired immunodeficiency syndrome. Some of them wonder whether the illness is punishment for their sexual behavior.

The medical sociologist Dr. Renée Fox, of the University of Pennsylvania Medical Center, states[8] that both the meanings given to an episode of ill health and the patient's affective response to it are profoundly influenced by the patient's social and cultural background as well as by personality traits. In other words, the same disease (*e.g.,* tuberculosis) or symptom (*e.g.,* pain) may be interpreted quite differently by two patients from different cultures. Their unique culture will also affect their subsequent behavior and the sort of treatment they will seek out.

### Two Definitions of Illness

Thus, in the real world of medical care, two definitions of illness are operative, one "clinical," the other "social." The clinical definition of illness can be described according to certain signs and physical and biochemical criteria. The social definition is broader in nature, including the patient's subjective reactions to his status and his resultant behavior. These are products of culture, social variables, and personal history.

Long-term patients, particularly those with chronic illness, are keenly sensitive to these distinctions. One of the difficulties hindering physician–patient communication is the all too prevalent modern physician's preoccupation with the biological–physiological aspects of illness and his relative neglect of psychosocial and cultural factors. Thus, in the initial months after a heart attack, the patient often has symptoms that are both physiological and psychological in origin. Depression may be a result of drug side-effects and reduced heart function. But the etiology may also be the patient's fear of disability and death, or threat to his self-image as a competent, independent person. The modern physician, trained in the high-technology atmosphere of a teaching hospital, often does not give the same rigorous intellectual attention to these two sets of variables, the physical and the psychosocial.

Osler's admonition to look at both the disease and the person who has the disease is therefore particularly valid for the field of home health care. In contrast to the relatively passive, acutely ill hospitalized patient, the individual in home care needs to be active in helping to carry out his medical regimen. Such an individual is a partner in his own self-care, not a passive observer.

### From Dyad to Triad

From Dr. Osler's dyadic formulation of the disease and the man, the addition of a third variable, environment, makes it a triadic formulation: disease, person, and social environment.

This triad is seen in the discharge of the patient from the hospital to *the home.* There is a continuum of care here that must be nurtured if the patient is to make full recovery from the acute illness and its aftermath. Rossman[9] has made a clinical analysis of this continuum into the home, for continuing health-care purposes. For therapeutic purposes, he distinguishes between the comparative environments of the hospital and the home. He holds that there are often unanticipated morbid, iatrogenic consequences, especially for the elderly, on being hospitalized. Confusion and disorientation sometimes result when the elderly patient is thrust into an unfamiliar, even threatening, environment, with many diagnostic procedures (some painful, others unfamiliar and anxiety-producing) and with strange staff members coming and going in an impersonal, often noncommunicating stream. According to Rossman, a depressing consequence of hospitalization, at times, is the *role loss* that may occur. For example, a disabled woman at home can function to some degree as a mother, wife, and caretaker. In the hospital such roles are necessarily given up. Thus, the hospital at times has a blighting effect on supportive, interpersonal relationships, and dilutes long-standing maternal or paternal roles. For the elderly patient, this hospital experience often has an alienating effect. When this is combined with the all too familiar condition among aged patients of weakness, helplessness, and isolation, the consequence of depression is understandable.

## HOSPITAL DISCHARGE

Contrast the typical hospital experience of an elderly patient with what happens (not always, but often, based on factors described below) when the patient is discharged to a supervised home health-care program. The patient's diagnosis and prognosis do not change, but the patient himself changes, especially in his outlook, self-confidence, and sense of psychological security. The patient feels like a "person" again, for now he is part of a supportive, caring family, and of a professional care team. He is in control in his home, in contrast to enforced passivity in the hospital. Surrounded by familiar objects and possessions, he can eat familiar foods at convenience, he can go to the bathroom or kitchen at will, and, to the degree possible, consistent with the nature of disability and chronic disease, he can resume a normal life. A previously anorectic patient in the hospital soon begins eating again in familiar home surroundings. Patients often gain weight, handle pain better, and generally begin to improve their morale.

## ROLE EXPECTATIONS

The behavior involved in role expectation is conceptualized in a significant paper in medical sociology, which has had considerable impact on the thinking of health professionals. The distinguished sociologist, Talcott Parsons, calls attention to the concept that it is not possible to understand illness and patient behavior without an awareness of the "motivational economy" of the social system, and that, correspondingly, the therapeutic process must be treated as part of the same motivational balance. He states

> The fulfillment of role expectations is always one crucial dimension in patient behavior. The sick person is, by definition, in some respect disabled from fulfilling normal social obligations, and the motivation of the sick person in being or staying sick has some reference to this fact. Conversely, since being a normally satisfactory member of social groups is always one aspect of health, mental or physical, the therapeutic process must always have as one dimension the restoration of capacity to play social roles in a normal way.[10]

Thus, one of the clinical values of the home care setting is that it allows, to some degree, the assumption of fairly normal role responsibilities by the patient, and thus enhances the therapeutic process to which Parsons refers.

## THE PATIENT'S SOCIAL CONTRACT

For our purposes in reviewing home health care and the responsibility of the physician, it is important to realize that the definition of illness represents a "social" process. As Helman points out,[6] in most cases a person is defined as "ill" where there is agreement between his perceptions of impaired well-being and the perceptions of those around him, particularly the family. Their cooperation is needed in order for him to adopt the rights and benefits of the "sick role," that is, of the socially acceptable role of the ill person. People who are so defined are able temporarily to avoid their obligations toward the social groups to which they belong, such as family, friends, and work-mates. At the same time, those groups often feel obligated to care for their sick members when they fall ill. As Fox points out,[8] the sick role provides *a semilegitimate channel of withdrawal from adult responsibilities, and a basis of eligibility of care by others*.

This may be termed the psychocultural basis for the "social contract" between the sick patient and the home health-care partners. What needs to be better understood is how different cultural and ethnic groups differ in their acceptance of responsibility to care for the disabled, for dependent parents, and for the aged. Among Italians, for instance, this caring attitude is called "Pietà." It seems a stronger mandate in Italy itself than among acculturated Italians in America.

## CARING PARTNER

The key ingredient to adequate home health care is the attitude of the family, particularly that of the chief care giver, who is often the spouse of the patient, a grown child, or a close relative or friend. This "caring partner" can be taught to give medications and hypodermic injections, dress wounds, and perform other simple but important patient care procedures. This is the physical aspect.

From a psychological point of view, however, the most significant change for the patient on discharge from the hospital and entering a home health-care program is the implicit but potent message (conveyed by the mobilization of resources in the home on the patient's behalf) that the patient is important and is valued and treasured. Elderly and chronically ill patients are particularly vulnerable to feelings of neglect and abandonment. Thus, the reassurance of a comprehensive health-care program, the linch-pin to which is a "caring partner," often performs wonders for the patient's morale.

## THE PATIENT AND THE HOME

The home as a "therapeutic environment" relates to individuals at both ends of the life cycle. Attachment to the home can be seen in the school boy rushing home to the warmth and comfort of family, as well as in the resistance of elderly patients to their institutionalization in a nursing home. Such resistance on the part of the elderly to being separated from their familiar, comforting surrounding is legendary in the home health-care field. They often resist transfer with sometimes seeming irrationality. But validation of this behavior is seen in the confusion and intellectual decompensation and sometimes death that occur in the elderly after their institutionalization.

## THE MEANING OF THE HOME

As Butler has pointed out[11] in commenting on the psychological meaning of the home for the elderly, "the place where one lives is connected with who *one is,* and how one expresses this sense of *self.* Many older people associate home with autonomy and control."

Historically, it is significant to note that a stimulus to the origin of home health care, especially to its growth after World War II, was the negative attitude of veterans to institutionalization, similar in nature to the attitude of the elderly just described. The veterans needing medical care upon discharge from the armed forces preferred to have their treatment at home. They had had their fill with the impersonality of institutional military life. With the availability of automobiles and public transportation, it was feasible for them to become outpatients rather than inpatients. This helped popularize home care as another form of delivery of medical care.

Relevant to our theme of identifying sociocultural factors in home health care is the following experience of wartime England during the bombing raids on English cities. It was found that those children separated from their families when sent to suburban areas where they would be physically safe from aerial bombing paradoxically suffered greater psychological damage than children who remained with their families in the cities vulnerable to bombing. There were detrimental effects on children due to extended maternal deprivation, even though objectively they were in less physical danger. The home, with its attendant strengths of parental and sibling support, even in the midst of aerial bombing, thus was of key importance in the psychological health of children. These two experiences of wartime children and discharged veterans helped the development of home health care in the United States.

## SPECIFIC CULTURAL FACTORS IN HOME HEALTH CARE

The thesis of this chapter is that cultural factors affect the process of health care in a home setting. Following are selected questions relative to cultural factors that should be taken into consideration by the physician developing home health-care programs for his patients.[6]

### FAMILY STRUCTURE

Is there a positive degree of interaction and cohesion in the family? Is there a sense of responsibility to care for the patient, in both physical and psychological terms? Is the patient able to assume the normal role as mother, father, or sibling consistent with the degree of disability? Is there true sharing in the family for assumption of family responsibilities, whether in child-rearing or care of the chronically or terminally ill? Or, is the family fragmented, without the necessary psychological strength and emotional support to care for an ailing family member?

### GENDER ROLES

Is there agreement about who does what in the home, without the stereotyping of so-called woman's work? Is there a mutuality, consistent with the culture of the family, about who works, who stays at home, who prepares the food, and who cares for the children? Is there an effort to involve the patient, as appropriate, in decision-making as to these responsibilities?

### DIET AND NUTRITION

Some ethnic groups have specific food preferences. The physician will need to determine whether these ethnic foods are nutritionally appropriate in light of the patient's specific illness. Holding constant this variable, patients usually tend to fare better eating familiar food. Is there appropriate sensitivity to the clinical implications of culturally influenced food preferences on the part of the physician and other members of the health-care team?

### FOLK MEDICINE

Many ethnic groups often use treatments within the popular or folk sectors. This includes the use of herbal remedies, patent medicine, special diets, and use of lay healers. The patient often does not volunteer such information to the physician for fear he may be misunderstood or ridiculed. Therefore, a mutually trusting relationship between the doctor and the patient is necessary for their mutually respectful discussion as to the relevancy and usefulness of these folk remedies. This should be approached with sympathetic respect, since many of these folk practices have been handed down from generation to generation, and have a strong hold on their practitioners.

## CULTURAL COMPONENTS IN PAIN MANAGEMENT

People respond to pain not only as individuals but also as members of cultural groups. What they share is a common culture and a social heritage, in effect, a guide to social behavior. In a functional interpretation of culture, it is accepted among anthropologists and sociologists that it is a rare human activity that is purely physiologic in nature and not affected by sociocultural considerations. Thus, in childbirth some mothers are stoic and accepting of pain, whereas in other cultural groups, the pain seems magnified. In some groups, for a male to complain of routine pain is considered unmanly.

## CULTURAL DIFFERENTIATION

A most vivid example of cultural differentiation in attitudes toward pain is the experience of the "Hiroshima Maidens." These were Japanese women who were terribly burned in the atomic bombing of Hiroshima and Nagasaki at the end of World War II. Rodney Barker, the author of the book *The Hiroshima Maidens,* comments that there was a distinct difference between American and Japanese attitudes to the pain endured by the women and that this attitude, in turn, affected their coping capacity.

In a letter to *The New York Times* on October 6, 1985, Dr. Barker described these differences:

> For a decade, these women lived as outcasts in a society with few traditions of public or private charity, where *suffering is often seen as a purifying experience* [emphasis added].
>
> Facially disfigured, functionally handicapped, stigmatized by rumors that radiation disease might be contagious or produce genetic defects, they would have lived hard lives in any society. In Japan at that time, their situation was hopeless.
>
> Time spent in America, where it was considered a moral obligation to help others in need, among people whose philosophical and religious outlook enabled the maidens to see themselves as members of the human family, provided them with precisely the therapy they needed to face the future with a broader perspective, with confidence and motivation.[12]

Because of these cultural attitudes to pain, the Hiroshima women markedly improved in their morale, their self-image, and their coping capacity to pain while in the different cultural climate of the United States.

## THE SPOUSE AND PAIN

In pain management in a home health-care program, it is important to note that the spouse of the patient often plays a role that affects the patient's ability to cope with pain.

Dr. Russell Portenoy, of the Pain Service of Montefiore Medical Center, comments

> One of the least recognized and probably most crucial factors in chronic non-malignant pain, is the patient's relationships, not only with a spouse, but with other family members.
>
> Studies have found that 20 to 80 percent of patients with this form of chronic pain, also suffer from depression and that, for some of them, the pain itself is a way of manifesting depression.
>
> For a significant percent of patients, chronic pain has become a way of life. It is the way one lives in the family and interacts with the world at large. The patient and spouse develop a

kind of organic relationship always revolving around the pain. Physicians enlist the help of spouses to break down what they call pain behavior or emotional factors that perpetuate pain.

Though obviously pain has a physiologic reality, the patient's tolerance of pain seems to be strongly affected by the patient's family, by his culture, and by the social environment, particularly by the meaning given by society as to the meaning and nature of the pain and by the emotional support given by the spouse, parents, siblings, and other members of the extended family.

## THE HOSPICE AND PAIN

Another example of cultural sensitivity to patient tolerance of pain is the nature of pain control in some hospice programs. The physician treating the terminally ill patient is faced with the dilemma of either overprescribing and thus possibly creating addiction, or under-prescribing and thus leaving the patient in great pain. Anne Kitterhagen, of the Tacoma, Washington Hospice Program, points out that almost 90% of all hospice patients suffer from cancer.[13] While half of cancer patients have no pain at all, the other half experience moderate to severe distress. Often patients and families feel that pain must accompany terminal illness. Yet upon entering the hospice, they learn otherwise.

Patients get better care in the hospice because it provides better pain control. Pain is often poorly controlled in those patients dying outside of a hospice. Doctors, inexperienced in working with the dying, often needlessly fear that patients will become addicted to drugs. Therefore, doctors may reduce needed drug dosages so pain is never fully relieved or they may withhold drugs until the patient is in deep distress and literally has to beg for relief. Some doctors err on the other side of prescribing. They order dosages that are so high and so frequent that patients are robbed of real life. Patients virtually live out their last precious days in a drugged stupor.

The management of nonmalignant pain is affected by sociocultural factors, as discussed earlier.

## PSYCHOLOGY OF CHRONIC ILLNESS

The chronically ill most often are not able to work or be gainfully employed. In American society, with its strong emphasis on independence and self-support, and on the Puritan ethic, the psychological and emotional consequences of the lack of productive work can be devastating. There is often a resulting lack of self-esteem and self-worth among the chronically ill who find themselves dependent on others. Work represents part of one's identity and status in our society and determines one's standard of living and the kind of friends one has, and it structures one's life. Its absence is often traumatizing, and the patient's self-image as a productive member of society is thus often negatively affected.

The psychology of the chronically ill was summarized by Dr. Stephen Cole,[14] a psychiatrist on the staff of the Veterans Administration Hospital in New York:

Patients with chronic illnesses, such as hypertension, diabetes, arthritis, cerebrovascular and cardiovascular disease, often feel inferior and experience themselves as helpless victims of a disease process out of their control. Demoralized, they become less able to cope with life's problems, and isolate themselves from sources of social support. They then fail to comply with their prescribed regimens of diet, exercise, and medication. This behavior pattern often leads to more severe symptomatology, more frequent flare-ups of the acute phase, and greater utilization of the emergency room, out-patient clinics and hospital beds. For the rest of their lives, many people with chronic illness can only look forward to persistent disability, unemployment, and long periods of hospitalization.

## WHO KNOWS THE PATIENT BEST?

Physician knowledge of the chronically ill patient is often limited, based on brief office visits and hospitalization experiences. Such knowledge is often confined to the disease itself, as if it were independent of the patient. The physician thus usually does not know or seem to care about the resources at home, both in a physical and psychological sense, nor is he sufficiently aware of the patient's coping capacity. He often depends for this information on the nurse or social worker who has been in the home setting to examine and talk with the patient and who tends to be professionally sensitive to the family and to the nurturing components of patient care.

Paradoxically, it is often the least trained home health-care professional, the home health aide, who has the most prolonged and intimate contact with the family and the patient. Therefore, such aides are increasingly being given greater recognition and training in the home care team. They are members of the home health-care team on whom culturally sensitive physicians have learned to depend, both for vital patient information and for facilitation of physician-ordered regimens.

## THE NURTURING–CURING STRAIN

The physician may unconsciously make an invidious distinction between *nurturing,* which he sees as the province of ancillary health-care professionals, and *curing,* which he sees as the province of the physician. Trained in a tertiary, high-technology setting, with emphasis on dramatic, scientific methods of clinical intervention, such a physician may see the chronic patient, especially one with a poor prognosis, as an inappropriate object of his scientific expertise. Dr. Phillip Brickner of St. Vincent's Hospital in New York states the issue as follows:

> Doctors are trained in acute care hospitals, with emphasis on cure. When they face a chronically-ill elderly patient at home there is often a feeling of discouragement; the doctor does not feel the gratification which his hospital experience with the acutely-ill has given him and he is vaguely aware that the chronically ill patient has many psycho-social problems which defy full comprehension and for which his medical education has not prepared him. Doctors often find it difficult to work with such patients, who may have a poor prognosis, and for whose illness scientific medicine has no cure.[15]

Physician attitudes thus become as important a characteristic, for better or worse, of their armamentarium for patient diagnosis and treatment as their body of scientific knowledge.

## PHYSICIAN–PATIENT COMMUNICATION ISSUES

### FACTORS AFFECTING COMMUNICATION

In the last three decades, there has developed, especially as a result of the "Great Society" programs sponsored by Presidents John F. Kennedy and Lyndon B. Johnson, a societal environment characterized by more knowledgeable patients and an active consumer movement. As a further result of improved levels of education and greater media attention to health issues, the patient/consumer has become more assertive and more questioning, even skeptical, of professional behavior. Patient advocates are a phenomenon of this situation.

Many individuals have become more active in maintaining good health, and they tend to carry over such attitudes when they become chronically ill. Therefore, they ask more probing questions, wish to better understand what is going on in their illness, and desire to become a partner in their care, rather than a passive recipient of professional advice. Such patients draw a distinction between a "compliant" patient and a "cooperative" patient. Dr. Louis Pelner describes the distinction as follows:

> A "compliant" patient gives his medical history truthfully and accurately, follows the doctor's orders precisely, answers questions fully, pays his bills on time, realizes that some diseases require a great deal of time to diagnose and treat, and understands that some diseases will even resist medical efforts. "Whatever you say, doctor," characterizes his unquestioning attitude.
>
> A "cooperative" patient, on the other hand, is all of this but with significant differences. He sees himself rather as a partner with his physician in his care, and wants to be privy to his doctor's plans. He answers the doctor's questions, and in turn wants his questions answered. He becomes an interested active participant, not a mere passive recipient. Blind faith is no longer the guiding rod. "I want to know" characterizes his questioning stance to his doctor.[16]

For the chronically ill patient in a home health-care program, this distinction is vital, for such a patient often lives many years with illnesses such as diabetes, cancer, heart disease, and stroke. Typically, he becomes very knowledgeable about the disease. It is his constant companion—and he follows every new advance in the field with assiduous attention. His illness almost becomes a "career" to him. He has many questions to pose to his physician, who sometimes responds tersely, feeling that with his busy office practice he has no time to give a "seminar" to each of his patients. In an educational program developed for diabetic patients that I conducted, it was found that the most frequently expressed complaint among diabetic patients was "my doctor doesn't have time to talk to me."

Such chronically ill patients do not accept the definition of "compliant" as "yielding to a wish, command, or request" as the dictionary defines it. Such phraseology connotes a value system that in some quarters of medicine vests wisdom, authority, and activity in the physician, and, assigns, somewhat stereotypically, ignorance, submission, and inactivity to the patient. This is a most dysfunctional approach to the chronic patient in a home health-care program where the patient needs to be active, not passive, in his care program; knowledgeable, not ignorant; and who desires a mutual give and take in communication, not an imperious one-way channel.


## CONCLUSION

If a grain of sand can be said to represent the world, then the one example of Dr. William Osler can be said to represent our philosophy in patient home health care.

There is need to consider three major factors: the patient's disease, the patient as a total person (of a given culture), and the environment in which care is given. The home care patient is not passive, but active, and a partner with the health-care team in his own treatment. Healing of illness requires more than healing parts of the body; it also requires a strong sincere motivation to communicate with patients in a two-way direction; and the physician needs to gain and earn the patient's trust and confidence if he is to influence the patient's behavior and life-style. The patient is a person, not an object, with rights and a dignity that is not forfeited because he is ill and dependent.

Dr. Stanley Reiser of Harvard Medical School puts it best in his book *Medicine and the Reign of Technology.*[17] He describes a humanist philosophy particularly apropos for the physician relating to home health-care patients.

There is a broadly emerging conviction: that the problems of illness are matched from beliefs, values, and other facets of cultural and mental life. They are best approached through dialogue with the patient and with humanist learning, and these can be as forceful and significant as the biological problems of illness are approached through technology and science.

The healing of illness requires more than healing parts of the body; it also requires intensive efforts to communicate with patients—to gain their trust, and to understand their needs and hopes.

As Dr. William Osler so well put it, there is need to understand both the disease and the man.

# REFERENCES

1. Ghali SB: Culture Sensitivity and the Puerto Rican client. Social Casework 58:459–468, 1977
2. Romero S: Counselling Puerto Rican families. Minority Clients. New York, Family Service Association, 1981
3. Pinderhughes E: Teaching empathy: Ethnicity, race and power at the cross-cultural treatment interface. The American Journal of Social Psychiatry 4(7), 1984
4. Williams R: American Society: A Sociological Interpretation. New York, Alfred Knopf, 1961
5. Bloom S: The Doctor and His Patient. New York, Free Press, 1965
6. Helman C: Culture, Health and Illness. London, Wright-PSG, 1984
7. Koos EL: The Health of Regionville: What the People Thought and Did About It. New York, Columbia University Press, 1954
8. Fox R: Illness. In International Encyclopedia of Social Sciences. New York, Free Press, 1968
9. Rossman I: Clinical Geriatrics, 3rd ed. Philadelphia, JB Lippincott, 1986
10. Parsons T: The social meanings of illness. In Freidson E: Profession of Medicine. New York, Dodd, Mead & Co, 1971
11. Butler R: The aging process. In Rossman I: Clinical Geriatrics, 3rd ed. Philadelphia, JB Lippincott, 1986
12. Barker R: Hiroshima Maidens. New York, Viking, 1985
13. Nassif JZ: The Home Health Care Solution. New York, Harper & Row, 1985
14. Cole S: Remarks to Medical Students in Behavioral Science Course. New York, New York University School of Medicine, 1981
15. Brickner P: Home Health Care for the Aged. New York, Appleton-Century-Crofts, 1978
16. Pelner L: The Ideal Patients. Unpublished manuscript
17. Reiser S: Medicine and Reign of Technology. London, Cambridge, Cambridge University Press, 1978

# 24

# Probate and Legal Issues

MICHAEL D. WITT

The extensive growth in the numbers of patients treated at home has given rise to a need for administrators, health-care providers, and institutions to review their legal relationships with each other, their employees, the health insurance industry, purveyors of durable medical equipment, and, most important, their patients. Federal and state cost-containment efforts have caused a dramatic increase in the scope of services that are being provided at home. The medicolegal issues relating to these services are addressed in this chapter.

## CONCEPTS OF RESPONSIBILITY

While practitioners have considerable autonomy in how, where, and under what circumstances they choose to practice their profession, they are constrained by the profession's canons of ethics, by federal and state laws relating to medical practice, and by various legal doctrines created over time by the judiciary. In general, these doctrines require a practitioner to use care in treating a patient. A patient allows the care to be provided by consenting to a given procedure or treatment. In order to consent to a procedure, a patient must be capable of understanding the risks, benefits, and alternatives to a given procedure. Once care has begun, a practitioner is obliged to continue to treat until the care is completed. The level and type of care that must be provided are measured by comparing the practitioner's actual care level to that of an accepted industry standard of conduct. This standard is established by physicians or other relevant practitioners who testify about the type and quality of care that an average qualified practitioner would provide in a similar medical situation, taking into account advances in the profession. Thus, the practitioner's care is measured against that of an "average" practitioner, similar in training and experience to the practitioner, who is expected to respond in a certain manner. A nurse practitioner, for example, is expected to provide care to the level of care that an average nurse practitioner would provide in a similar situation. The applicable standard of care in a given situation varies with the condition being treated and with the specific medical factors at issue.

The standard of "average" or "reasonable" practice is determined usually by the testimony of qualified expert witnesses. In such a highly regulated, intellectually demanding, and inherently risky area as medicine, it is ironic that physicians do not set standards for testifying in courts of law. Few standards exist for qualifying experts; usually, a medical degree from an accredited medical college and state licensure will suffice. Although a judge will require an expert to have certain minimal qualifications to testify, it is quite irregular for an expert witness to be excluded if the judge believes that he will have something useful to say. A party may ask a court to prevent an expert from testifying, if the credentials of the "expert" are woefully inadequate. The lack of standards often leads to inconsistent results, especially when an expert loses his objectivity and becomes an advocate of the party who retained him. In any event, the expert addresses the facts in a given case and discusses whether, in his or her opinion, the practitioner's care met the "standard" of care in the instant case. A cardiologist will not be held to the same standard of care (and thus not owe the same obligation or duty) to the patient as an orthopedic surgeon. Similarly, the obligation owed to a patient by a licensed practical nurse or a physician's assistant will not be the same as that of a registered nurse. The essence of the obligation is that each practitioner will be held to the level of responsibility and careful practice that is appropriate for his level of training. The professional under review is supposed to attempt only those tasks that are appropriate for his level of training, skill, and expertise. If he attempts to perform treatments or procedures that an average practitioner of similar skill and training would not perform in like circumstances, he enhances his exposure to liability by failing to conform to the expected standard of conduct. If this occurs, the professional is said to have "breached" his obligation or duty to a patient.

A breach of duty occurs only if a duty was owed in the first instance. Simply because a person takes a telephone call from a patient at home, or if other indicia of a provider–patient relationship do not exist, then a duty, and subsequently a breach of a duty, cannot be said to occur.

Once a health-care provider–patient relationship exists, if a patient receives substandard medical care, he can recover only if the breach of the obligation to provide quality care is causally connected to an actual loss or injury. If the breach does not result in an injury to the patient, or if the substandard care is not the proximate cause of an actual injury, then the practitioner is not liable for any loss suffered by a patient.

Most successful claims of professional malpractice seem to arise, in general, because of surprise and dissatisfaction with a result. If a patient receives a frank discussion of the risks and is treated with respect, the practitioner reduces the risk that a patient will bring a lawsuit for any injury that may result from a procedure or treatment. While it is not without exception, a practitioner with a pleasant bedside manner and friendly attitude has a higher likelihood of avoiding a suit than his or her more abrupt colleague. Other common causes of a lawsuit include the failure to refer a patient to an expert on a timely basis, failure to recognize a complication, or a delay in the diagnosis of an illness.

The mere fact that an unfortunate result occurs does not imply or prove that negligence was present. Generally, practitioners are not obligated to warrant a certain result (and should specifically avoid it). If an injury occurs without obvious explanation but normally does not occur without negligence, then the corporate parent or supervising physician may be held liable, whether or not actual negligence on anyone's part can be proven. Examples of such errors include leaving a medical instrument or gauze pad in a wound after a procedure or operating on the incorrect leg. It is not necessary for an injured party to identify the exact breach of an obligation; it is only necessary that an injured party show that the provider–patient relationship existed, and that in the normal course of medical practice instruments or gauze pads are not supposed to be left in the wound.

Once having noted an error, a practitioner should take whatever steps are necessary to minimize the extent of the injury, not only because such care may reduce the damages in a lawsuit, but again, because it constitutes good medical practice.

The supervising practitioner or employer-corporation may be held liable for the negligence of those under their control or employed by the corporation under established principles of agency law. In general, an employer is responsible for any damages that result from the negligence of an employee. A corporation, whether operated on a for-profit or not-for-profit basis, is responsible generally for the acts or omissions of its employees, when its employees are acting in the normal roles and activities of their profession. The corporation must act in a non-negligent fashion in hiring employees and developing proper peer review and quality assurance policies, and assure through its approved policies and procedures that a high level of care is provided by its employees.

Any injury that results from professional malpractice will be reduced to economic terms by an economist. At trial, he or she will attempt to evaluate the cost of an injury through the use of historical and prospective earnings analysis, education, age, life expectancy, job performance, quality of life, and the degree of suffering and pain that has resulted.

## AREAS OF EXPOSURE TO LIABILITY

### CORPORATE

While a corporation cannot, by itself, practice medicine or deliver health-care services, it may still be held liable for the negligent acts of its employees. Also, a corporation is obligated to use diligence in hiring, supervising, training, and retraining individuals. Staffing policy is an area of serious concern in a busy home health-care practice because of the intensive care sometimes provided to individuals at home. If insufficient staffing results in too infrequent visits and an injury results through exacerbation of a condition that could have been more properly treated had proper care been rendered at an earlier time, then the supervising practitioner, the nurse or volunteer providing the care, and the corporate-employer could be held liable for any injury that results. If, for example, a licensed practical nurse could have recognized that a decubitus ulcer was becoming more seriously infected, yet a volunteer, without sufficient training, failed to recognize the gravity of the situation, then the corporation's failure to provide adequate levels of staff support could constitute a breach of the corporation's obligation to provide adequate staffing to treat patients under its care.

The level of supervision required in the home care setting depends on the training and credentials of the person providing the care. If the services of a volunteer are being used, then higher levels of supervision are necessary. If the volunteer is given inadequate instructions or is allowed to perform procedures beyond the scope of his training, then the home health agency may be held liable for any injuries that result from the improper supervision. Further, if more highly trained individuals, such as licensed practical nurses, nurse midwives, or registered nurses, fail to consult with a physician in a case where life-threatening injury may result, then not only may those individuals be held to have breached their obligation to the patient, but the supervising physician and parent corporation could be held liable for any injuries that result as well. The scope of the supervision should be tailored to the training and background of the individual; otherwise, the failure to delineate responsibilities properly, through policy and procedure manuals, may give rise to and enhance exposure to liability.

Ultimately, the corporation or supervising physician will be held liable for any breach of duty that results in injury to the patient. Although many individual practitioners, such as nurse practitioners or nurse midwives, are increasingly treated as separately credentialed practitioners under the law, the legal realities are that physicians or the corporate parents supervising the care of such practitioners have the dubious distinction of being viewed by juries as the responsible parties with the "deep pocket" full of assets. It is therefore incumbent on these supervisors to carefully design and structure relationships with home care givers so as to minimize the risk of suit for improper supervision and control over their employees.

# INDIVIDUAL

Most of the home care givers about whom we are concerned have separate credentialing and licensure requirements that vary from state to state. These practitioners have an individual responsibility to meet these licensing standards. If they do not do so, and a question relating to the quality of their care is raised, it is exceedingly difficult to defend them or the employer that allowed them to practice without a license, without proper credentialing and training, or with a history of suits for malpractice or other questionable practices. Accordingly, careful employment histories and other records should be maintained in case such credentials are brought into question. Frequent and comprehensive continuing education should be required for all practitioners. If certain individuals are noted to have insufficient training or education in a given area, the situation is tenuous at best. If this person's training is supplemented properly and the fact and content of the supplemental courses are carefully documented, then a solid defense to allegations of insufficient training can be raised.

Further, a supervising nurse or physician should review the quality of care rendered by individuals on a routine basis to ensure that the actual situation at a home where treatment is being given is the same as reported by a practitioner. Less-than-professional practitioners could take advantage of a person by not reporting or by delaying the reporting of a mistake or the actual level of ill health of an individual. Such a situation could ruin a home health agency's reputation and referral base, and subject the owners to abject embarrassment. Careful attention to reviewing credentials will minimize the risk of such an occurrence. If an agency has a person of questionable integrity on its staff, especially if it were aware of these questions, it is improperly assuming major risks.

Further, it is critical that medication usage be closely monitored, especially in the elderly. A patient should be carefully observed for evidence of inopportune adverse, allergic reactions. A procedure and checklist for the use of each medication should be developed for the employees' use. Also, if cancer chemotherapeutic agents are administered, exquisite care and preparation must be taken to avoid the risk of extravasation. The practitioners administering such medications should receive sufficient training to monitor the patient properly and to recognize the relevant side-effects. Because these reactions are well known, if a reaction does occur, a practitioner should have thought about and developed a contingency plan to deal with such emergencies. This sort of planning and its documentation are essential to maintaining a home health care group's "legal" health.

Lack of patient compliance with physician orders in the elderly is always a serious issue and should be identified as a significant source of potential injury in the home health-care arena. If noncompliance with prescribed medications is recognized to be the norm in the care of elderly patients, then great care must be taken to circumvent the impact of improper or infrequent medication use on the health of an elderly patient. Once such a problem is recognized, then the practitioner must develop treatment modes that minimize the impact of the problem on the patient's health. Numerous devices are available to assist a practitioner in making sure that a patient takes the proper medication at the proper time. If medication errors and lack of compliance are not recognized, then serious injury (and, thus, serious exposure to a malpractice suit) could result before it is brought to the attention of a knowledgeable practitioner.

The advent of sophisticated technologic aids in treating patients in the home care setting may lead to injury where none was anticipated. Withholding such tools may also lead to such errors. Each practitioner and patient must have clearly drafted protocols to follow when a problem arises.

A frequent error that often leads to increased liability risk is inadequate documentation. If a procedure, event, or observation is not written down, a jury most often will assume that the procedure, event, or observation did not occur. Three or four years may pass before the question of what actually happened is raised. The statute of limitations (namely, the maximum period of time that can elapse before an injured person must bring, or else lose the right to bring, a cause of action against a person) is three years in most jurisdictions. If a practitioner does not document that a certain service was provided, the exact details may be forgotten with the passage of time. The patient, however, will have exquisite recollection of precisely what was said or done. Also, a patient may readily convince a sympathetic jury that a procedure or occurrence did or did not take place. A well-documented physical examination or incident report can forestall this potential source of liability. The best defense in such a situation is to have a thoroughly documented medical record. If such documentation reveals that an injury actually occurred and that proper steps were taken to mitigate the extent of such an injury, then such mitigation and an aura of truthfulness will permeate the courtroom, tending to reduce the award amount.

An error should neither be hidden nor ignored. Instead, it should be addressed in as professional a manner as possible, with appropriate attention given to reducing the patient's anger. Many years of experience suggest that it is the abrupt and terse attention given to a patient who has suffered an injury that results more often in a lawsuit than does an injury expressed and explained in a caring, thoughtful manner.

The frequent checking and monitoring of a given therapy is the most appropriate way to minimize the risk of injury and maximize the benefit of a given approach. If improper or inappropriate communication techniques are used to transmit information, often the patient not only will misunderstand the orders, but also will misinterpret the professional language as lack of attention, care, and support. A close relationship between a patient and a home health care provider will help reduce the risk of a lawsuit.

## CREDENTIALING AND QUALITY OF CARE ISSUES

With the more intensive use of nonphysician practitioners, continuing training and education to ensure quality care must be of constant concern to supervisors. This standard of quality must be assured through an institutionally funded and endorsed training program. Each level of individual must be trained according to the responsibilities of the level, and the services provided by each individual must be consistent with that training. Monitoring of this latter issue is a continuing corporate responsibility. For example, volunteers should be given guidelines as to the scope of their responsibility and the types of issues they are likely to confront, and given specific advice and policies as to how they should react in a given instance. Also, for example, in some jurisdictions a physician's assistant has specific reporting responsibility to a physician. Some of these jurisdictions allow physicians' assistants to prescribe medications in a long-term care setting. If they are improperly trained to monitor and prescribe such medications, or if they are improperly supervised, then both the physician's assistants (PA), individually and the supervising physician may be held liable for any injuries that result. Further, a number of states require a physician to certify, as part of the PA's licensing requirements, that the physician will be financially liable for any injuries that result from care by the PA. Such a heavy burden on physicians may cause them to take care when preparing protocols for the procedures that a PA is able to perform. Again, the most protection that a physician or PA could have is to properly specify and document what procedures he or she is entitled to perform and when and how each was performed, with appropriate monitoring and review of the patient's status.

In some jurisdictions, licensed midwives are allowed to prescribe medications in the course of treating pregnant women. While some states allow these practitioners to be completely autonomous, a number of jurisdictions require a midwife to have close supervision and recourse to an obstetrician. The obstetrical area has given rise to numerous problems for obstetricians and midwives alike. Birth defects in a newborn have the dual disadvantage of most often being unexplainable and often very serious. Out of sympathy for the child and the parent, a jury may blame the injury on anyone caring for the mother, the level of uncertainty and relative lack of knowledge about the birthing process notwithstanding. The costs of caring for a child with a brain injury are enormous. Many obstetricians eschew relationships with midwives because of a perceived enhanced risk of suit even though it is not clear that better care results from hospital deliveries. Certainly, emergency equipment is more available in the hospital.

The goal of a quality assurance and utilization review program (QA) should be to improve the quality of care through the adoption of accepted standards of quality. A necessary corollary is that enforcement of these standards is essential; once established, the court system, through negligence suits, will do so. The QA function could serve as a mechanism to identify areas of weakness such that education and training in that area or other areas could take place, to the benefit of all concerned and to enhance the ability of an agency or a practitioner to defend himself. If an individual attends a continuing education or other class, the fact of attendance should be documented, as well as the substance of the course. If other quality assurance functions are not performed, then the failure to properly supervise and train staff will be raised as evidence of employer deficiencies in case of any suit. Also, failure of proper credentialing may lead to discomfiture by a referring hospital or physician group such that if patient care is not ensured, the economic health of a home health practitioner will soon be endangered.

## INFORMED CONSENT TO TREATMENT

Because of the nature of the home health patient population, many of the individuals are elderly and infirm. Either through the effects of age, disease, or the complexity of medical treatment, a patient may not understand the implications of the treatment being rendered. The patient's voluntary agreement to accept treatment must be elicited. To do so, the patient must be able to agree; inherent in such "agreement" is the ability of a patient to be aware of the nature of his or her disease and the material risks and benefits of the proposed and alternate treatments.

The requirement of "informed consent" has given rise to a new legal theory in many jurisdictions. Practitioners who provide excellent care to a patient may be held liable for an injury because they did not inform the patient about a risk. If a patient is not told about an important or "material" risk, or cannot understand or be made aware of these risks, then the failure to warn a patient about a risk that eventuates is sufficient to maintain a suit on the basis of lack of informed consent alone.

Recent trends appear to suggest that a patient (or the patient's guardian) must be informed of all material risk attendant to the procedure. While the courts have not been precise as to what constitutes a material risk, a general rule of thumb (which is only that) suggests that if the risk of a side-effect of a medication or a procedure exceeds 1%, then the patient should be informed of that risk. If the risk is less than 1%, the judicial decisions do not tend to support the requirement of warning the patient about such side-effects. Medical science, however, is not always as accurate as these judicial decisions imply. Many of the estimates of side-effects are highly speculative and are not the result of scientifically valid studies. In many instances, such reports of an adverse reaction are nothing more than one or more case reports that are cited numerous times in subsequent publications until they become dogma. If a side-effect occurs and the medical literature discusses it, failure to inform a patient of it in advance can give rise to liability. If the incidence of a side-effect is small yet the risk is grave, a physician must use a certain amount of common sense to decide whether to inform a patient of the risk of its occurrence.

One method of reducing this risk of liability is to develop lists of risks of a given procedure or medications with documented risks of greater than 1%. These lists should be developed after careful review of the literature about a given procedure or medication. Before the medication or procedure is prescribed, the risks should be reviewed with a patient, with due regard for thorough documentation in the record. The list of side-effects and the informed consent should be placed in the patient's record and co-signed and dated by the patient, any witness, and the practitioner. If the medications used are known to be dangerous, or have not been used in a given patient before, it may be wise to repeat the session again, giving the patient time to think about the risks. If a family member or other person is present at the time the risks are discussed, that person should be asked to co-sign the medical record attesting to the fact that such side-effects were discussed. Lay language should be used so that the patient understands the nature of the procedure. Also, a checklist should be left with the patient so that he or she can review and assist the practitioner in monitoring for the occurrence of these side-effects. It should be prepared in such a way as to be understandable to the lay person.

The effect of age, dependency, or infirmity and a reduced level of ability to communicate alter the patient's ability to understand the risks of a procedure. Although historically physicians have taken the liberty of substituting their judgment for that of the patient, recent trends in litigation and legislation confirm that the decision maker is the patient, irrespective of his level of mentation. When a patient is mentally unstable or infirm, an alternate decision maker is to be appointed. How this appointment occurs varies from state to state; in most jurisdictions, however, a close friend or relative is appointed as a decision maker for the mentally infirm patient. This can be done in several different ways, the most common of which is the court-appointed guardian. A court-approved guardian makes patient care decisions as the patient would have wished were the patient competent. Most guardians are family members or close friends who are well equipped, by reason of long-term relationships with the ward, to understand the person's personality, wishes, and desires. The tendency is to recognize the patient as the ultimate arbiter of his own destiny. Competent patients are able to determine their destiny, whether it means withholding therapy or life-sustaining treatment devices. Competent patients have this right; they should not lose their right because of their mental weakness, and are entitled to be treated with respect.

If a practitioner is aware that a patient is not competent, it is in the practitioner's best interest to have a guardian be appointed to consent to the proposed therapy. Usually, a petition for temporary and permanent guardianship is filed with the state probate court, along with a psychiatrist's affidavit that the person is no longer competent. A physician's medical certificate stating that the need for continued medical therapy is important must be filed as well. Typically, a court will appoint a guardian *ad litem* (for a specific limited purpose) to meet with the proposed ward and to report his findings to the court. Once appointed, a practitioner must secure the guardian's informed consent to any proposed medical therapy.

In some jurisdictions, a patient can use a "living will" to document the patient's wishes in case he or she becomes incompetent and later requires medical therapy. This document should be prepared as a standard document for all patients to think about when they first come into contact with a home care professional. The patient should review the document, and send it to his or her own attorney to modify it according to the patient's specific situation. If a patient becomes incompetent, the patient will already have expressed desires about treatment and continued care. If the living will is not recognized in a jurisdiction, it still serves the useful purpose of setting forth the patient's intentions when or if he or she becomes incompetent. Provisions relating to irreversible terminal illness, invasive surgical procedures, antipsychotics, appointment of a guardian, life-sustaining medical equipment, including feeding tubes, and any other issue that the patient wants to address relating to his or her medical care, should be included.

Such information could also be placed in a document entitled "durable power of attorney." This document carries less legal weight before a reviewing court because it is executed under less formal circumstances than a living will. It is nonetheless useful to express a patient's wishes in such a document. Each agency should require a patient to execute either a living will or durable power of attorney. Otherwise, except on an emergency basis, the agency cannot treat the patient because he or she cannot consent. If the home care provider does not require a patient to address these issues, not only may an emergency temporary guardianship proceeding be necessary, but a home health agency may have to incur legal fees in having the court appoint a guardian to approve medical treatment. The provider is left in the unenviable position of treating the patient without informed consent or, if therapy is withheld, explaining later in a courtroom why he abandoned the patient. The dilemma may be avoided somewhat through the execution of a valid living will or a durable power of attorney.

The physician used to make these decisions in the best interests of the patient and did so in a kind, gentle, and humane manner. Whether the trend to have treatment decisions made by a guardian is an improvement has not yet been determined. It is clearly cumbersome and costly, and, probably, is no better an alternative.

## MEDICAL RECORDS

The medical record has become critically important as a repository of medical–legal information. It can both assist and injure the treating practitioner. Careful documentation, in most instances, serves to protect the practitioner from the vagaries of human recall and changing perceptions of a patient and the practitioner. The records should include entries relating to social and medical history; a description of life-style; family medical history; a full physical examination, with differential diagnoses, findings, tests, and procedures; a list of prescriptions given and refills, with detailed instructions and treatment rendered to the patient; adverse reactions from recommended treatments; and descriptions of patient compliance, reasons for failure, or refusal of the patient to keep appointments or to follow instructions. Such records should be made in a clear and legible form.

Although the record is created at a patient's home, the practitioner still owes a stringent duty to the patient to maintain the patient record. The medical records should not be available to anyone without the patient's or guardian's express (written) authorization to release the record. The records should be available, generally, only to those medical personnel with a legitimate need to be aware of the patient's medical history. Casual comments to nonprivileged medical personnel or lay persons can constitute a breach of the patient's confidentiality; this breach may result in a compensable injury. Increasing numbers of cases involving nonconsensual disclosure of sensitive medical information, such as psychiatric examinations, results of toxicologic determinations, or other information, have resulted in verdicts against both the person inducing the breach and the person breaching the patient's confidentiality. Family members are not to be apprised of a patient's medical history, prognosis, or diagnosis unless this is authorized by the patient. The patient may intend that the family is not to have access to sensitive medical information. Disclosure to close family members who are not expressly authorized to have access to the patient's confidential medical information is a common error.

The improper release of medical records may expose the home health agency, the practitioner, or other keeper of medical records to liability for breach of the patient's confidentiality. A medical record may be released in response to either a proper judicial order ("court order") or a subpoena issued by an attorney. If a medical records department is served with either a judicial order or a subpoena, several steps should be taken to ensure the patient's confidentiality.

First, the home health agency or other keeper of the record must respond to the court order or subpoena in a responsible and timely manner. Usually, a photocopy, certified to be a true, accurate, and complete copy of the record, is adequate. The person requesting the record can be charged a reasonable fee, payable before receiving the record.

Second, if the record contains very sensitive medical, psychiatric, social service, or other sensitive information, then the person whose medical records have been subpoenaed or requested should be notified immediately, in writing (and in advance of the return date of the subpoena or court order), that his records have been requested by formal court process. This allows the patient to respond by getting an attorney, who may choose to file a motion to quash the subpoena. This may be done on the basis of various common law or statutory privileges, including psychotherapist–patient privilege or social worker–client privilege, or that the records were generated as part of a federally funded alcohol detoxification facility. If the facility or patient does not want to release the information, the proper response is to move to quash the subpoena or ask the court to reconsider the issuance of the court order. A provider cannot simply refuse to produce the records; failure to do so may result in a very angry judicial response, such as a contempt of court citation.

Some state social service agencies have statutory rights and procedures whereby they can gain access to a patient's medical records. In such circumstances, the statutory procedures must be adhered to closely. Without such a statutory procedure, simply because a state social service agency or other state employee requests a medical record does not give them a right to informal (*e.g.,* nonjudicially sanctioned) access to a patient's record. Usually, a subpoena or judicial hearing for review of a social service agency's request is necessary before the record's release can be effected. Failure to do so may very well expose the home health practitioner to a claim for breach of confidentiality.

## COST CONTAINMENT EFFORTS

With the advent of the prospective payment system, a rapidly emerging legal trend, relating to the early release of patients from hospitals, has appeared. On occasion, either through inadvertence or by design, acutely ill patients who are not ready to be discharged are being sent home, either to be treated in the hospital clinic, physician's office, or by practitioners in the patient's home. If this inappropriate discharge results in improper monitoring or treatment, the hospital may be liable for any injuries that result. Further, the home care practitioner might be held to the standard of care that could have been rendered in the hospital. If such acute-care standards of medical practice are applied to the home care setting, it may prove to be quite difficult to refute a presumption that the care would have been better had the patient been treated with the technologic benefits available only at a hospital. While the prospective payment system encourages appropriate, early discharge, great care must be taken to select those patients who are proper candidates for treatment at home and to adopt policies and procedures that ensure the careful monitoring and treatment of these patients.

## HOME BIRTHING

Recent interest in birthing at home has given rise to serious concerns about the quality of care provided by nurse midwives and the level of liability risk attendant to that care. The concern centers on the value of the more highly trained obstetrician at a birth, the use of technologic aids, such as internal and external electronic fetal heart monitoring devices, the availability of emergent cesarean section facilities, and the impact of delay on the health of the fetus in need of emergency care. While many home birth advocates argue the low risk and multiple benefits to the experience, it is, in reality, a high-risk venture. If a child is not healthy at birth, the care provided by a nurse midwife may be scrutinized in a court of law, first, by an obstetrician-expert, who probably disapproves of home-birthing, and second, by a jury who will steadfastly refuse to believe that the quality of care rendered by a midwife in a bedroom is similar to that of a board-certified obstetrician in an acute-care labor and delivery facility. Obstetricians are quick to point out the numerous risks that may eventuate from birthing at home, and such obstetricians would also tend to be more available as expert witnesses against a nurse midwife should an error result, notwithstanding whether the injury could have been prevented in a tertiary-care setting. While the quality of care may not be any better, it is far easier to defend an obstetrician who has used all available medical and technologic resources than any other practitioner who does not have these aids available at a patient's home.

The delay in response time to an obstetric emergency is another serious concern. Again, the nurse midwife will most likely be called on to defend a claim that the delay was responsible for the newborn's injury. Unfortunately, this area of medicine is so unclear that it is sometimes impossible to determine whether an injury resulted from an unfortunate (and unavoidable) occurrence or through the negligence of a health-care practitioner. The risks are enormous, however, as the economic recovery for an injury to a newborn is, on average, very high. In any event, at the present time, more and more pressures will be brought to bear on limiting the availability of home birthing. Many of these risks are avoided through the use of birthing centers that have access to emergency resuscitation equipment and obstetrician care. Because they are less expensive alternatives to a hospital, if the quality of care can be maintained, these birthing centers most likely will be able to circumvent (or limit) the considerable liability impediments that exist in this area.

## ENVIRONMENTAL ISSUES

A major benefit to treating a patient at home is the reduced risk of infection from highly toxic, hospital-indigenous, resistant strains of bacteria. While the patient may still become infected, it is hoped that the risk of serious injury will be markedly reduced. Great care must be taken to train patients in aseptic technique. Frequent monitoring is necessary for signs of infection at the site of catheter or needle insertion. If a patient becomes infected, especially after a surgical procedure, a reviewing court may try to assume that the home care practitioner failed to monitor the risk of infection. If the patient becomes infected in the hospital, at least the patient was followed for signs of infection, with therapy instituted early. This same high standard would probably be required in the home care setting. Any serious delays in treatment that result in injury become areas of exposure to liability.

When potent medications such as antibiotics or anticancer medications are used at home, they must be closely monitored for adverse reactions, using the same parameters for evaluating risks and benefits that would occur in the acute-care hospital setting. Infection control procedures and strict policy guidelines for consultation and referral appear to be necessary to reduce the risk of injury and enhance a practitioner's ability for self-defense in a lawsuit.

If cancer chemotherapeutic agents or other potent medications are used, the practitioner must be certain to comply with Environmental Protection Agency regulations, the "right to know" law, and Occupational Health and Safety Administration directives. Proper attention to disposal of excess or spilled medications may require retaining the services of a firm licensed to dispose of hazardous waste materials.

An area of increasing concern relates to the use of durable medical equipment in the home setting. The decision to use a given equipment supplier should be determined by the supplier's timeliness, attention to quality, and willingness to accept and indemnify the practitioner if an injury is caused by one of its machines. These relationships should be carefully described in well-drafted contracts, primarily because improper usage and insufficient maintenance of equipment are common sources of injury to patients and liability for professionals and equipment suppliers alike. Proper training and familiarity with the equipment and appropriate servicing schedules are essential to reduce the risk of exposure to lawsuit. The equipment vendor should supply maintenance schedules and user's guides. These guides and other descriptive publications are useful to the provider in the event that such equipment malfunctions. Of course, it is important that adherence to the manufacturer's recommendations be thoroughly described and documented.

## CONCLUSION

The home health care provider has enhanced medicolegal risks due to the increasingly complex techniques and procedures being performed at home. Careful monitoring, training, and supervision of these providers are essential to reduce the risks of injury to the patient and lawsuits against a provider. Carefully drafted policies that describe allowed procedures will assist defense counsel in reducing the exposure of the practitioner (and his or her employer) to suit. These policies should be subject to a regular preventive "legal" examination, making certain that the policies comport with appropriate risk management principles, with current law, and with new regulatory and legislative initiatives. Insurance policies, credentialing review procedures, and incident report forms should be reviewed as well.

Documentation of all examinations, conversations, and care rendered, of the nature and extent of informed consent to medical or surgical procedures, and of the administration of and reaction to medications is the best defense against allegations of inappropriate or improper treatment. If an error is discovered, it is better to recognize the error and mitigate the damages through working closely with specialists to reduce the extent of an injury. Often, suits arise because of abrupt and insensitive medical personnel who fail to respond properly to an injury or error and succeed only in angering the patient.

Records should never be altered or misplaced; such actions tend to create a presumption that the practitioner made an error. The credibility of a practitioner in such a circumstance is irrevocably damaged in the eyes of a reviewing jury.

Constant surveillance and attention to quality of care are the best preventive measures to reduce liability in the home care setting. This exciting and innovative area of medicine carries with it great potential for innovation and successful treatment of patients in a less expensive, healthy environment. Spiraling insurance costs and malpractice suits should not impede the progress and growth of this concept. They may do so, however, unless quality patient care is ensured.

# 25
# Financial Issues

MICHAEL R. McGARVEY
RICHARD CONVISER

Medicare and Medicaid were enacted in the United States two decades ago as fee-for-service programs. It is no accident that since that time, the costs of health care in this country have increased several times over. These two governmental programs fueled the dramatic growth in the costs of health care. By 1985, health-care costs in the United States had grown to over 10% of the country's gross national product, or over a billion dollars a day. Hospital care claimed about $420 million of this daily billion; physician services and other personal health care (like pharmaceuticals, home health care, and dentistry), about $190 million each; nursing home care, about $90 million; and other health spending (including biomedical research and medical education), about $110 million.

Early efforts to control rapidly growing costs in the Medicare and Medicaid programs led to the creation of the Professional Standards Review Organizations (PSROs). But by 1980 the rate of inflation in health-care costs had generally become so great that it had galvanized concern among the many large purchasers of health-care benefits: unions, employers, health insurers, and the government. These organizations responded by initiating a variety of cost-containment programs. The strategy of many such programs has been to change the incentive structure under which providers are reimbursed. Specifically, these approaches have sought to create alternatives to the traditional fee-for-service method of reimbursement for health-care services. Many of them show promise. Regardless of their ultimate success, however, these cost-containment efforts will color the way developing modalities of care are perceived. The days of looking at services without considering their costs are gone forever.

The trend toward higher costs has been paralleled by several changes in the health-care delivery system. One of these has been a shift of patients out of acute-care facilities. As cost-containment measures have taken hold, the number of hospitals and hospital beds in this country has declined while the number of alternative-care facilities has grown. Another change has been an increase in the degree to which surviving health-care organizations "vertically integrate" lines of business that were once handled by independent companies. Today's hospitals, for example, may also operate subsidiary businesses, like home health agencies and equipment supply companies, and they may also be involved in preferred provider arrangements with health maintenance organizations (HMOs). Several observers have predicted that within another decade, the majority of health-care services in the United States may be delivered by as few as ten multiply integrated "super-med" firms.

These changes in the health-care delivery system have occurred in the same context as the inflation in health-care costs they have attempted to address: shifting patterns of government reimbursement and regulation. Since 1980 the federal government has been increasingly active in legislating changes aimed at reducing its Medicare and Medicaid expenditures for acute hospital care. As we write, Medicare has adopted a diagnosis related group (DRG) methodology for hospital payment in nearly all states. This prospective payment methodology puts a cap on the reimbursement hospitals receive for all patients with a given diagnosis, with the exception of a small proportion of "outlier" cases. Pediatric and psychiatric inpatient services are exempt from the DRG methodology.

Preliminary studies suggest that the DRG reimbursement system is having the intended effect of shortening hospital lengths of stay. One of its by-products, however, is that patients are being released from hospitals "quicker and sicker"—in the new vernacular of the industry. In consequence, the need for follow-up care in nonacute settings (including the home) is growing. When Topeka Blue Cross adopted a DRG system for all its patients, for example, the number of home health-care agencies in its region tripled within two years.

It is certain that the DRG approach to reimbursement will not be the government's final word on the matter. Experiments are currently underway that enroll Medicare beneficiaries into prospective-payment health maintenance organizations, and further innovations are likely. The government's experimental mood is shared by private payers, which have begun to offer a wide range of alternatives to fee-for-service reimbursement. These include HMOs and preferred provider organizations (PPOs), both of which operate on a capitation (per capita prepayment) basis. Additional cost-containment mechanisms being employed include enhanced analyses of utilization data and benefits design as well as a range of managed care programs. The latter typically require prior approval from payers if health-care services are to reimbursed fully. Also on the horizon is an anticipated glut of physicians in the United States by the end of the century. All these developments point toward an increasingly competitive future health-care environment.

Since the Second World War, many physicians have held that the best medical care can be rendered only in an acute-care facility, where the equipment necessary for technologically advanced diagnosis and treatment is available. Current pressures for cost containment are forcing a reexamination of this assumption, and quality of care information from hospitals to aid in its assessment is now available. The collection of this information (like so many of the other changes we have described) was mandated by the federal government: regulation enacted in 1972 required the review of practices by all institutions and providers participating in Medicare and Medicaid programs.

The end result of all this activity is likely to be a health-care system that is leaner and more cost-effective. Many hope that it will also offer care that is at least equal in quality to the more expensive care offered in the recent past. Whether or not this proves to be true, recent changes in reimbursement methods ensure that the demand for home health care will continue to expand.

## THE CHANGING CONTEXT FOR HOME HEALTH CARE

Prior to 1966, the main call for home health agencies had been for prenatal care, health appraisals for newborn infants, and routine check-ups for well children.[1] As a result of federal legislation in 1966 that approved Medicare funding for home health services, the focus of home care shifted to those with long-term chronic illnesses, and the number of agencies nearly doubled within the next decade. That growth was slowed somewhat in 1974 when a certificate of need (CON) process went into effect for new health-care facilities and services in most states. But more than a dozen states have since removed CON requirements for home health agencies, and additional federal legislation has once again spurred their growth.[1] Between 1969 and 1982, the rate of home health care use by Medicare beneficiaries grew by an average of over 13% annually, and home care expenditures increased by over 22% a year.[2]

By 1980, as noted above, Congress had begun to try to limit the growth of the government's health spending. The implicit assumption it made in limiting spending for treatment in acute-care facilities was that these cutbacks would be compensated for by increases in home health care.[3] To make home health care services more accessible to Medicare beneficiaries, the federal government passed legislation in 1982 relaxing certain qualifications for their use. In particular, a provision was dropped that had limited the number of home health visits to one hundred, as was a requirement for a three-day prior hospitalization and a $60 deductible charge. These changes were intended to foster an expansion of skilled home health care services provided under a physician's order. However, no parallel expansion was mandated for homemaker services. Thus, some policymakers have expressed concern whether home health care will actually substitute for all the services diverted from acute-care facilities, as was assumed.[3]

This question aside, there is no doubt that home care services and expenditures are on an expansion course. A doubling or tripling has been forecast for home health spending in the 1980s, from $6 or $7 billion a year at the decade's start to $17 or $18 billion. Not all of this growth will be in the public sector. In 1974, 46% of all Blue Cross and Blue Shield plans offered their subscribers home health coverage, but by 1983 this percentage had risen to 90%. Among commercial insurers, the change is even more striking: only 5% offered a home health care benefit in 1974, but 81% offered it in 1983.[2] Also contributing to the growth of home care is the aging of our country's population. It has been estimated that of those aged 65 to 74, 10% are in need of home health services, compared with 40% of those over 85 years old.[4] The potential for continued expansion of home health care services among the elderly is great. Between 1967 and 1982, the rate of their use by Medicare patients grew by an average of 13.1% annually, yet during 1982 still only about 4.1% of the Medicare population received home care.[2] Another factor in the growth of home care is increased consumer interest in self-care.[5] Of all settings in which care is administered, the home affords the patient greatest control.[6] Some private health insurers are turning increasingly to home care as a way to shorten hospital stays for mothers of newborn children, thus reducing obstetrical costs.

To what extent home care will help to manage health-care costs remains to be seen. Some preliminary findings suggest that it can achieve considerable savings over acute-care facility costs. Hughes' survey of studies on parenteral antibiotic and nutrition programs in the home, for example, reports daily savings amounting to over 70% of hospital costs.[7] Some analysts caution, however, that such *per diem* comparisons must be made carefully, suggesting that it may be more appropriate to look at "the overall costs of caring for patients with matched diagnoses at home and in the hospital over prolonged periods of time."[8] Cost comparisons of ventilator-dependent patients made on this basis still show that home health care results in five- to tenfold savings over acute-care facilities.[8]

The availability of reimbursement for home care services could, however, actually increase the total costs of health care by encouraging the use of these services by people who would otherwise choose to manage on their own.[8] In addition, what would amount to savings for the health-care *system* might not translate into savings for all the individuals who are insured through it. This depends on whether they are as fully covered for home care as they are for inpatient care.[7] If not, costs might simply be shifted to them.

It seems likely that home health care will prove to be cost-effective for selected types of patients. Equally likely is the prospect that the earlier discharge of patients from acute-care facilities will produce qualitative shifts in the levels of care required in the home. Home care will therefore become more costly, on the average, and some of the global savings expected from the application of DRGs to hospital reimbursement will not materialize.

Scrutiny will then shift from hospitals to home care agencies; there will be calls for a closer examination of home care utilization. Inevitably, too, questions will be raised about its quality. Existing quality-assurance mechanisms will be looked at more closely, and procedures put in place to forestall possible abuses of home care. (The Topeka Blue Cross Plan has taken a proactive approach to this issue by requiring prior approval for patients who receive home care benefits.) Perhaps most important of all, if home care is to become an effective modality of care, physicians will be called upon to learn about its possibilities.

## PHYSICIAN REIMBURSEMENT FOR HOME CARE

The shifts taking place in reimbursement and regulatory patterns, along with increasing competition in the health-care industry, pose threats to the traditional role of physicians. Particularly vulnerable are their independence and the level of remuneration they receive for their services.

Proportionately fewer physicians are involved in private practice than formerly. They are increasingly becoming salaried employees of health-care delivery organizations, such as HMOs, or being enrolled as participants in PPOs. With such institutional arrangements come social controls whose primary goal is often to cut costs—with possible consequences for both physicians' levels of reimbursement and quality of care. By reimbursing physicians on a capitation basis, prepaid plans like HMOs and PPOs theoretically give them an incentive to practice high-quality, lower-cost, preventive medicine. One study has shown that HMO physicians are 50% more likely than others to recommend home health care for patients from their offices.[9] But the financial incentive structure of such plans could still detract from the quality of care simply because physicians' quantitative productivity is so much easier to measure than its quality. For example, PPOs sometimes reimburse physicians partially through bonuses that depend on the extent to which they divert care from acute facilities to less costly alternatives. Although such an incentive structure is not likely to be primary in most physicians' treatment decisions, its qualitative effects still bear watching.

The requirement that home health care take place under a physician's order makes physicians indispensable to its operation, especially since the order typically has to be renewed at set intervals. Unfortunately, however, the increase in physician responsibility resulting from the growth of home care is not likely to be met with a commensurate increase in rewards. This is because most current reimbursement mechanisms remunerate physicians only for direct contact with patients. This criterion is readily accommodated when patients are stationary and grouped together, as they are in acute-care facilities or in nursing homes. It is much more difficult to fulfill this criterion when the primary site for patient care is the home, and when the primary responsibilities for the physician are in the form of paperwork, consulting with the home care staff, and cognitive skills. These services are difficult to reimburse in part because they are so difficult to quantify.

The actual level of physician involvement with home care patients is quite variable. Some physicians take the time to meet with patients and their families to ensure that the latter are well equipped to perform necessary care duties; others are not so generous with their time. The compensation typically offered to both types of physicians for these services is minimal. Medicare does recognize physician consultation with home health agencies as an allowable expense. But this does not necessarily translate directly into physician reimbursement.

As we have noted, a strategy commonly followed today to alter patterns of health-care utilization is to shift the incentive structure under which that care is reimbursed. If home care is to live up to its cost-saving potential, it will be necessary to develop fair reimbursement mechanisms for the physicians who are instrumental in its delivery. One possible route is to follow the lead of HMOs and PPOs, and pay physicians for home care on a capitation basis. This has been done with physicians involved in the federal renal dialysis program. While capitation does not guarantee any particular level of contact between physicians and home care patients, it does give physicians some incentive to monitor the progress of these patients.

Given current reimbursement mechanisms, the shift of patients from acute-care facilities to home care is likely to bring about a decline in physician income. Some physicians have followed the lead of hospitals and have become partial owners of home health care agencies. This move helps to protect their financial interests while assuring them of a greater say in what happens in the home setting. However, it is not without its complications. There is the possibility of conflicts of interest with hospitals, which are typically the primary source of recommendations for home care agencies and may be in the home health-care business themselves. There is also the prospect of conflicts of interest with the physician's role as care giver, although Medicare legislation limits any physician's share of ownership in a home health-care agency to 5%. There is also the likelihood of role conflicts with nurses. Home health care has been their province over the years, and anecdotal evidence suggests that some nurses resent physician attempts to exert more control there. These disadvantages must be weighed against the medical benefits of greater physician involvement in home care.

Such cross-pressures could be relieved by a capitation reimbursement plan for home health physicians. Devising such a plan would present complications of its own, however. The tension often present between cost containment and humanitarian goals would be felt here. Should the home health coverage provided on a capitation basis be all-inclusive for Medicare patients, approximating a nationalized health-care plan? If not, what should be excluded from such coverage? Under what conditions should reimbursement be provided for new medical technology that upgrades definitions of efficiency? These issues suggest that any plan to reimburse physicians for home health care needs to be addressed within the context of broader questions about national health-care priorities.

## CHANGING TECHNOLOGIES AND CHANGING NEEDS IN HOME HEALTH CARE

In recent years, attempts to manage rising health-care costs have had their effects on home care as well. One front on which home care has been vulnerable to cost-cutting has been that of durable medical equipment (DME). Often such equipment has been leased from suppliers for such long periods of time that the cost of leasing it has far exceeded the cost of purchase. The realization of this fact has resulted in new federal regulations requiring the purchase of DME costing under $120.

Nonetheless, the costs of home health care are likely to rise markedly in the next few years. A key factor in this rise is, of course, the earlier transfer of patients from acute-care facilities to the home setting brought on by Medicare's adoption of a DRG hospital payment methodology. This change will increase not only the total number of home care patients, but also the average costs of caring for them. Because such patients will typically need more intense services than those previously using home care, they will require more skilled professional nursing care and more sophisticated technologies. The more complex treatment plans that result will also require a higher level of interaction between physicians and home health care nurses.

It is in part because of technologic developments that home care has become a feasible alternative to acute hospital care for many patients. Some of these developments have been rather straightforward, like movable arms on wheelchairs that allow stroke victims to be helped in and out of bed more readily. But others, through remote monitoring (biotelemetry) and miniaturization, have made high-technology equipment available in the home that was once limited to acute-care facilities. Among the procedures that such equipment has brought into the home are peritoneal dialysis, enteral and parenteral nutrition, respirator and ventilator therapy, and chemotherapy.

While such technologies allow for the care of more seriously ill patients in the home, they also necessitate more stringent requirements for home care. In addition to more advanced training for health-care professionals and added physician responsibility and legal liability, these include stricter environmental precautions and stricter standards for the care, cleaning, and calibration of equipment. These higher levels of training and regulation will add to the costs of some forms of home care, although these costs will presumably still remain lower than those for comparable care in acute-care facilities.

We suggested above that there is a need to rethink methods of reimbursement for physicians involved in home care. There is also a need to reconsider the flat rate at which agencies are currently reimbursed for home health-care visits. This is because the sicker patients who are now referred to home care, in addition to requiring costlier equipment, often require longer and more frequent visits than past home care populations. AIDS patients, for example, may require two to three home visits a day, rather than the one visit required by most other home care patients. To guard against the possible "skimming" of less severe cases by home health-care agencies, and to reimburse agencies fairly for the services they do provide, it would be appropriate to develop severity of illness indicators as a basis for home care reimbursement. Otherwise, caring for severely ill patients can put those home health agencies that accept them at a financial disadvantage.

Severity of illness indicators and new reimbursement methods are not the only innovations necessary in home health care. Others include ways of determining the necessity of services, assuring their quality, and ensuring that those who need home care receive both prompt access to it and timely discharge.

## FURTHER IMPLICATIONS OF THE CHANGING HEALTH-CARE CONTEXT

In the current atmosphere of concern about the rising costs of health care, home health care represents one of several promising alternatives to acute care in traditional settings. When care comes to be spread over a variety of settings, however, it becomes difficult to keep track of all the expenditures that are associated with a single episode of illness. This can defeat the goal of cost management. Further, the quality of care provided in alternative settings is often more difficult to assess than that provided in acute-care settings, where evaluation methods have been refined over a number of years. This can defeat the equally important goal of quality assurance.

For these reasons, several additional pressing needs have to be met in connection with home health care. Foremost among these is the enhancement of methods to assess its quality. Issues to be addressed in this connection include monitoring the length of time from hospital discharge to the initial visit from a home health agency, establishing protocols for infectious diseases, and ensuring the existence of competent and independent utilization review committees. Regulation and licensure requirements from state health agencies could help to achieve these goals. In New York State, home health agencies have been subject to such requirements since the beginning of 1986.

If attempts to manage health-care costs are ultimately to succeed, it will also be necessary to develop ways to manage the financing of episodes of illness across all types of treatment settings. At present, policymakers tend to focus on reducing costs in one type of setting at a time—a strategy that contains some costs but only shifts others. A more comprehensive approach to cost containment would therefore seem to be indicated. This would be facilitated by the development of a full continuum of care, allowing patients to select or be guided to the most appropriate level of care at the right time.

Finally, if quality and cost goals are both to be met, health-care purchasing alternatives should continue to be subjected to scrutiny. The role of physicians in Medicare HMOs and the possibility of social HMOs—meeting a range of patient needs broader than medical care alone—need to be explored more thoroughly. Only through the pursuit of these broader items on a health policy agenda can home care come to be used in the most appropriate ways.

## REFERENCES

1. Cowart M: Policy issues: Financial reimbursement for home care. Family and Community Health 8 (2): 1–10, 1985
2. Coleman JR, Smith DS: DRGs and the growth of home health care. Nursing Economics 2: 391–395, 408, 1984
3. Wood JB, Estes CL: Home health care under the policies of New Federalism. Caring June: 58–61, 1984
4. Johnson KA: Exploring home health care opportunities as a result of the prospective payment system. Caring April: 54–60, 1985
5. Home health care market trends. Caring June: 16–19, 1984
6. Gould EJ: Standardized home health nursing care plans: A quality assurance tool. Quality Review Bulletin 11(11): 334–338, 1985
7. Hughes TF: The economics of home health care. Topics in Hospital Pharmacy Management November: 9–15, 1984
8. Rogatz P: Home health care: Some social and economic considerations. Home Healthcare Nurse 3(1): 38–43, 1985
9. Cassak D: Doctors in home healthcare. Health Industry Today 48(10): 18–25, 1985

# Conclusion: Home Care—The Future

LAWRENCE H. BERNSTEIN
ANTHONY J. GRIECO
MARY K. DETE

The future of home care is assuredly one of greater demand for services of grander scope than have been available in the past. Economic reality is currently stimulating the thrust toward expanded home care. Financial pressure, however, is not the sole reason for embarking on a national commitment to caring for people in their own environment. Home care should not be considered just a segment of the health-care system; it must be viewed as part of a larger societal issue. Keeping patients at home places human and humane values at the highest level.

We believe that most patients can stay at home, with only a few needing placement in an institution, acutely or chronically. Expansion of home services could easily be supported by diverting to the exploration and facilitation of home management of the elderly the resources that would otherwise be needed for nursing home construction. We expect "home care" to become as much a part of our vernacular in the next few years as "nursing home" was during the building boom of a few decades ago. At that time, "nursing home" had a positive connotation. Now, it often is looked upon as a failure of the home system. Institutional care, almost by its very definition, must be somewhat impersonal. Home care, the oldest form of providing for the sick, is by contrast the one modality most capable of identifying and meeting the needs of a specific individual on a truly personal basis. This is not to deny the role of nursing homes; we need a continuum of care, with the nursing home being reserved for but a small subset of patients.

Technologic advances have brought parenteral nutrition, intravenous antibiotics, chemotherapy, respirators, and monitoring into the home. With them have been brought emotional, psychosocial, social, and cultural conflicts, with the burden of these problems falling squarely on the shoulders of the home care team. Thus, the need to relieve the stress of patient and family at home is great. The presence of technology sometimes occurs at the cost of "touching." The physician's role is a pivotal one, particularly as an interface between high technology and the patient.

Throughout this book, one word is used repeatedly: "partnership." The teamwork approach, involving the collaboration of physician, nurse, social worker, technician, pharmacist, nutritionist, aide, family, friends, and the patient, is the key to successful home management. With a large, unstructured team of varying composition and flexible hierarchy, communication among the members requires thought, energy, and planning. Availability of the physician by phone is an essential ingredient. House calls and real involvement in management are the substantive ways in which physicians can effectively participate. But what else should the medical community do to support the goal of expanded care at home?

Home care is in need of clear proof that it is financially and medically valuable. We must develop criteria that are valid for determining success rather than discuss home care in merely subjective terms. We do not want strictly financial criteria—"It costs less money." We need functional criteria—"The patient is more independent." But, in addition, we must determine which groups of patients are most likely to benefit from home care—"Home care is the solution, but what is the problem?" In the long run, we believe that home care will flourish because it is *right*—ethically, financially, medically, socially, and morally. Its time has come again. It works—with technology, but because of people.

# Index

Page numbers followed by *f* and *t* indicate figures and tables, respectively.